GLOBAL COMPARATIVE
ASSESSMENTS
IN THE HEALTH SECTOR
DISEASE BURDEN, EXPENDITURES
AND INTERVENTION PACKAGES

Collected reprints from the
Bulletin of the World Health Organization

edited by

C.J.L. Murray   A.D. Lopez
Harvard University   World Health Organization
Boston, MA, USA   Geneva, Switzerland

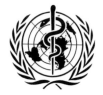

World Health Organization
Geneva
1994

WHO Library Cataloguing in Publication Data

Global comparative assessments in the health sector: disease burden, expenditures and intervention
    packages / edited by C. J. L. Murray & A. D. Lopez.

   1.Health expenditures   2.Cost of illness   3.Disabled
   I.Murray, C. J. L.   II.Lopez, A. D.

ISBN 92 4 156175 0   (NLM Classification: W 74)

The World Health Organization welcomes requests for permission to reproduce or translate its publications, in part or in full. Applications and enquiries should be addressed to the Office of Publications, World Health Organization, Geneva, Switzerland, which will be glad to provide the latest information on any changes made to the text, plans for new editions, and reprints and translations already available.

PRINTED IN BELGIUM
94/10200 – Ceuterick – 10 000

Contents

Foreword:
Comparative health data and analyses

Dean T. Jamison & Jean-Paul Jardel

The World Bank's *World development report 1993: investing in health,* the sixteenth in the World Development Report series, examined the interplay between human health, health policy, and economic development. Underlying the conclusions of *Investing in health* is a series of comparative economic, epidemiological, demographic, and institutional analyses undertaken collaboratively by the World Bank and the World Health Organization. Many of these analyses present original data and interpretations; and most of them are lengthy and somewhat technical. In order to make these analyses more readily available to the policy and scholarly community, we asked the authors to summarize results in a series of relatively brief papers. Eight of these papers have now been published in the *Bulletin of the World Health Organization*—four appeared in June 1994 (Vol. 72, No. 3) and the next group of four appeared in August (issue No. 4). This document reprints those eight papers for wider circulation.

One conclusion of the *World development report* is that a rational evaluation of policies for health improvement requires four basic types of information: a detailed, reliable assessment of demographic conditions and the burden of disease; a complete inventory of available resources for health (both public and private, national and international); an assessment of the institutional and policy environment; and information on the cost-effectiveness of available technologies and strategies for health improvement. It is important in developing national programmes of reform to have this information on a country-specific basis. Comparative data—across countries or across a broad range of interventions—serve both to allow national policy analysts to put their own country's situation into context and, of particular importance, to provide an empirical basis for the search for policy-related determinants of health system performance. Prior to work on the *World development report,* the World Bank prepared an extensive comparative analysis of the cost-effectiveness of interventions for 24 major diseases;[1] yet there was no comparable set of estimates for the global and regional burden of disease resulting from premature mortality and disability to which these interventions might be applied. Nor, indeed, was there much in the way of comparative assessment of resource flows, institutional arrangements or policies for health at the national or international level.[2] The eight papers reproduced in this volume are the results of major analytical efforts undertaken for the *World development report* to address these gaps in comparative data and analyses.[3]

The initial four papers in this compilation describe the methods and main substantive conclusions of the first comprehensive attempt to assess the burden of disease by cause for the world as a whole and for the eight regions into which the analyses undertaken for the *World development report* divided the world. This assessment of the global burden of disease—or GBD— was jointly sponsored by the World Bank and the World Health Organization and brings together the background work of literally scores of contributing specialists; a forthcoming World Bank/WHO book will contain revisions of these estimates along with disease- and risk-factor-specific analyses prepared by the appropriate specialists.

---

[1] See Jamison DT et al., eds. *Disease control priorities in developing countries.* (New York, Oxford University Press for the World Bank, 1993).

[2] WHO publishes an annual comparative compendium, the *World health statistics annual,* that includes cause-of-death statistics. It also publishes an occasional report on the world health situation that provides comparative information on physical inputs, e.g. hospital beds per thousand population; Volume 1 of the eighth such report appeared in 1993. The Organisation for Economic Co-operation and Development provides comparative assessments of health expenditures for its member countries (see, for example, Getzen TE, Pouillier J-P. International health spending forecasts: concepts and evaluation. *Social science and medicine,* 1992, 34: 1057-1068); these have been used for policy analysis of expenditure determinants (see Gerdtham U-G et al. An econometric analysis of health care expenditure: a cross-section study of the OECD countries. *Journal of health economics,* 1992, 11: 63-84). A valuable comparative description of institutions may be found in Roemer MI. *National health systems of the world. Vol. 1: the countries* (New York, Oxford University Press, 1991).

[3] One additional compilation, prepared jointly for the *World development report* and for UNICEF, assesses trends in under-5 mortality rates: see Hill K, Yazbeck A. Trends in child mortality, 1960-1990: estimates for 84 developing countries. Additional background papers for the *World development report* use these (and other) cross-national data sets to assess long-term determinants of the decline in child mortality, the mutual relations between health improvements and economic growth, and the impact of economic adjustment and stabilization programmes on health expenditures.

The initial paper on the GBD, by Murray, describes the methodologies used for quantifying the burden of disease; Murray and Lopez, in another of the papers, provide further discussion of the particular problem of quantifying disability. A third paper provides the first global and regional estimates of numbers of deaths by cause, age and sex; these estimates underlie the summary estimates for total disease burden reported in the fourth paper, which also includes sensitivity analyses and points to directions for further research. In particular that paper points to the importance of completing the initially established agenda of decomposing the GBD not only by disease but also by risk factor and by consequences, e.g. type of disability.

In requesting that an assessment of the GBD be undertaken for the *World development report,* we fully realized that epidemiological and demographic databases for many countries and many diseases were quite weak. One objective of the effort was to make the best possible use of available data by assessing information from a common perspective and by imposing consistency across diseases. (For example, estimates of the number of deaths due to particular diseases published by specialists in those diseases would typically, when added together, exceed total deaths—and often by a substantial margin; hence the need to impose demographically derived consistency constraints.) A second objective was to include the human cost of disability explicitly in the measurement of disease burden by combining estimates of burden from premature mortality with burden from disability. This aspect of the effort also required making the best of often poor and incomplete data. The results are to be interpreted, then, not as definitive assessments but rather as the best available (and only comprehensive) approximations. Naturally the quality of the approximations can be expected to improve with subsequent iterations. [4] The first published GBD estimates—in Appendix B of the *World development*

report—reported the third iteration; the papers in this compilation report on the fourth iteration as well as on the methods used. Specific numbers in these papers will, for this reason, sometimes differ from those in the *World development report*, and subsequent iterations will see further changes.

The fifth and sixth papers present an extensive analysis of global health expenditures; one paper deals with national health expenditures (public and private), and the other deals with international aid to health. The authors estimate that about US$ 1.7 trillion (1.7×10^{12}) was spent on health in 1990 (or 8% of global income); of this total only about 10% (or US$ 170 billion) was spent by the 78% of the world's population living in developing countries. Globally about 60% of expenditure is financed by government (or government mandate), although this percentage is *higher* in the market-oriented economies of the OECD. It is remarkable that such information, which is essential for any reasoned discussion of health finance or health policy, was unavailable prior to the research sponsored for the *World development report 1993.* It is hoped that dissemination of these findings—and of the methods used to estimate expenditures where data have been lacking—will stimulate much needed further research and attention in this area. [5] Clearly, some international mechanism needs to be established that will monitor health expenditures at the national and international level in the future.

The seventh and eighth papers present the methods and preliminary results of analyses based on burden of disease, on health resource availability, and on intervention cost-effectiveness to evaluate alternative allocations of resources. The papers point to reallocation of existing resources that could be expected to improve health conditions substantially in the developing world. In the first of these two papers, Bobadilla, Cowley, Musgrove, and Saxenian describe the methods used to develop the minimum "essential packages" of health services advanced by the *World develop-*

---

[4] Part of the continued improvement to be expected in the accuracy of assessing disease burden will result from ongoing disease-specific analyses; and part will come from country-specific assessments. The first such country assessment—for Mexico in 1991—has just been published (see Lozano R et al. *El peso de la enfermedad en Mexico: un doble reto.* Mexico, Mexican Health Foundation, 1994 (Documentos para el análisis y la convergencia, No. 3). Among other findings, the authors of the Mexican study point to a strikingly high disease burden from injury —50% higher, as a percentage of total burden, than the *World development report* estimates for Latin America as a whole.

[5] The paper that reports on total health expenditure is both pioneering and preliminary; as its authors note, the mandate was to construct the best estimates possible from data sets with important gaps and inaccuracies. A more recent effort by some of the authors to incorporate newly available data from Latin America suggests that the estimates reported here for 1990 need substantial upward revision (see Murray C, Govindaraj R, Chellaraj R. *Health expenditures in Latin America,* forthcoming from the World Bank). Other evidence suggests that health expenditures have rapidly risen in several large Latin American countries in the years since 1990; if these findings also hold for other regions, actual health expenditures in 1994 are likely to be a substantially higher percentage of global income than the 8% reported here for 1990.

ment report and the content of those packages. One of their conclusions is that clinical services can cost-effectively address a substantially larger proportion of the remaining burden of disease than would be addressed by public health interventions. In the second paper of the pair, Murray, Kreuser, and Whang develop and illustratively apply an optimization model that, among other things, allows assessment of the cost-effectiveness of investing in health system components as well as interventions.

This compilation contains the only available comparative assessments of cause of death, disease burden, health expenditures, and international aid for health. In that sense the authors' contributions represent a landmark achievement and provide an invaluable resource for policy analysts and scholars. Yet the very need for the ad hoc assessments that these papers report points to important gaps in the international system for gathering, analysing and distributing policy-relevant comparative data. Without information on how levels and trends in key indicators in their own countries compare with other countries, national reformers will lack benchmarks for judging performance. Likewise students of health systems will lack the empirical basis for forming judgements on which policies work—and which do not. We hope, then, that one follow-on to the analyses reported here will be institutionalization of continued efforts to generate and analyse internationally comparative health data.

Authors

Mr Jamison directed the World Bank team that authored *World development report 1993: investing in health;* he is currently a professor at the University of California, Los Angeles, and Health, Population and Nutrition Adviser (part-time) for the Latin American Region of the World Bank.

Dr Jardel is an Assistant Director-General of the World Health Organization; he chaired the international committee on disease burden assessment that guided preparation of the Global Burden of Disease estimates reported here.

Preface

The eight papers in this volume provide a convenient overview of some of the major research findings to emerge from the World Bank's *World development report 1993: investing in health.* These research papers fall naturally into two broad categories.

The first four papers are concerned with the methods, findings and implications of the global and regional burden of disease assessment prepared for the *World development report.* These papers were originally published in the *Bulletin of the World Health Organization,* Vol. 72, No. 3, 1994. However, two of these papers are reprinted here with much more tabular material (in Annexes) than was possible in the *Bulletin.* Thus, detailed tables giving age-, sex- and cause-specific YLDs (years of life lived with a disability) have been annexed to the paper on "Quantifying disability: data, methods and results". More tables on estimated DALYs have also been annexed to the paper entitled "The global burden of disease in 1990: summary results, sensitivity analysis and future directions". We expect that the addition of these detailed estimates will facilitate global and regional comparative analyses of health status using the DALY indicator.

The second set of four papers is reprinted from the *Bulletin of the World Health Organization,* Vol. 72, No. 4, 1994, without any change.

It should be noted that the grouping of countries in eight regions, as presented here, follows the classification adopted by the World Bank for the 1993 report. "Developed countries" include all those classified as Established Market Economies (EME) or Formerly Socialist Economies of Europe (FSE). All other regional groups are considered as "Developing countries".

A much more detailed account of the methods, assumptions and results for each of the causes assessed in the global burden of disease study is currently being prepared by WHO and the World Bank. In the meantime, we hope that by widely disseminating these summary papers of our methods and findings we will encourage further critical comment on them, and thereby enhance the utility of the burden of disease approach for monitoring health status and for setting health priorities.

C.J.L. Murray
A.D. Lopez

Global burden of disease

Le poids de la morbidité dans le monde

Assessing the health situation in populations has traditionally been carried out on the basis of mortality data, and where available, on the prevalence and/or incidence of disease. A new approach to quantifying the burden of disease has been developed which simultaneously considers both premature death as well as the non-fatal health consequences of disease and injury. The burden of disease approach is based on an incidence perspective and provides an estimate of the number of years of life lost due to premature death (in 1990), and the number of years of life lived with a disability arising from new cases of disease or injury in 1990. These two components constitute the total number of disability-adjusted life years (DALYs) due to disease or injury incurred in 1990. The results of this approach were first utilized in the World development report 1993: investing in health.

The following four articles present, for the first time, details about the methods, assumptions and findings of the global burden of disease methodology. The first article summarizes the principles and properties of the DALY measure. The detailed set of age, sex, cause-specific mortality rates used to estimate the years of life lost from premature death are presented in the second paper. The third article gives details about the estimated years of life lived with a disability, reflecting the likelihood of progressing from disease incidence to disability, the duration of disability, and its severity. The fourth paper provides a summary of the DALYs arising from both components and shows that the results are relatively insensitive to assumptions about parameter values used in the calculation. This article also provides an overview of how the method might be applied to assist countries with their own health situation assessment.

* * *

L'évaluation de l'état de santé des populations s'appuie classiquement sur les données de la mortalité et, lorsqu'elles sont disponibles, sur la prévalence et/ou l'incidence de la maladie. Une nouvelle méthode de mesure quantitative du poids de la morbidité a été mise au point, qui tient compte simultanément du décès prématuré et des conséquences non fatales pour la santé de la maladie et du traumatisme. Cette méthode se place dans la perspective de l'incidence et fournit une estimation du nombre d'années de vie perdues à la suite d'un décès prématuré (en 1990) et du nombre d'années de vie vécues avec une incapacité à la suite des nouveaux cas de maladie ou de traumatisme apparus en 1990. Ces deux éléments entrent dans la composition du nombre total de DALY (disability-adjusted life years: années de vie ajustées sur l'incapacité) dues à une maladie ou à un traumatisme survenus en 1990. Les résultats d'une telle approche ont été utilisés pour la première fois dans le Rapport sur le développement dans le monde 1993: investir dans la santé.

Les quatre articles qui suivent exposent pour la première fois les détails concernant la procédure suivie, les hypothèses, et les résultats de cette méthode de détermination du poids de la morbidité dans le monde. Le premier article résume les principes et les propriétés des DALY. Les taux de mortalité par âge, par sexe et par cause, utilisés pour estimer les années de vie perdues par décès prématuré, sont précisément exposés dans le deuxième article. Le troisième article donne des détails sur le nombre estimé d'années vécues en incapacité, reflétant la probabilité d'évolution depuis la survenue de la maladie jusqu'à l'incapacité, la durée de l'incapacité et sa gravité. Le quatrième article de cette série donne un résumé des DALY imputables à ces deux éléments et montre que les résultats varient relativement peu avec les hypothèses sur les valeurs des paramètres utilisés dans le calcul. Cet article donne également un aperçu de l'utilisation possible de cette méthode pour aider les pays à évaluer l'état de santé de leur population.

Quantifying the burden of disease: the technical basis for disability-adjusted life years

C.J.L. Murray[1]

Detailed assumptions used in constructing a new indicator of the burden of disease, the disability-adjusted life year (DALY), are presented. Four key social choices in any indicator of the burden of disease are carefully reviewed. First, the advantages and disadvantages of various methods of calculating the duration of life lost due to a death at each age are discussed. DALYs use a standard expected-life lost based on model life-table West Level 26. Second, the value of time lived at different ages is captured in DALYs using an exponential function which reflects the dependence of the young and the elderly on adults. Third, the time lived with a disability is made comparable with the time lost due to premature mortality by defining six classes of disability severity. Assigned to each class is a severity weight between 0 and 1. Finally, a three percent discount rate is used in the calculation of DALYs. The formula for calculating DALYs based on these assumptions is provided.

Introduction

This paper provides the technical basis for a new measure of the burden of disease: the disability-adjusted life year (DALY). It is one of four papers in this issue of the *Bulletin of the World Health Organization* on the Global Burden of Disease study (*1–3*); this first one details the conceptual basis for the indicator, the second examines the empirical basis for measuring time lost due to premature mortality by cause, the third describes the time lived with a disability by cause, and the fourth presents summary results and a sensitivity analysis. In this article, the rationale for measuring the burden of disease, the need for a single indicator of burden, some general concepts used in the design of an indicator of the burden of disease, a series of specific value choices, and some computational aspects are analysed in turn.

Why measure the burden of disease?

The intended use of an indicator of the burden of disease is critical to its design. At least four objectives are important.

— to aid in setting health service (both curative and preventive) priorities;

— to aid in setting health research priorities;

— to aid in identifying disadvantaged groups and targeting of health interventions;

— to provide a comparable measure of output for intervention, programme and sector evaluation and planning.

[1] Assistant Professor of International Health Economics, Harvard Center for Population and Development Studies, 9 Bow Street, Cambridge, MA 02138, USA. Requests for reprints should be sent to this address.

Not everyone appreciates the ethical dimension of health status indicators (*4*). Nevertheless, the first two objectives listed for measuring the burden of disease could influence the allocation of resources among individuals, clearly establishing an ethical dimension to the construction of an indicator of the burden of disease.

Single and multiple indicators of disease burden

Since Sullivan's proposal of a composite index of health status incorporating information on morbidity and mortality (*5, 6*), there has been extensive debate on the utility of such single indicators of health status (*7*). For our purposes, this debate on the value of constructing single indicators can be reduced to a basic choice between explicit and implicit valuations. Decision-makers who allocate resources to competing health programmes must choose between the relative importance of different health outcomes such as mortality reduction or disability prevention. Because money is unidimensional, the allocation of resources between programmes defines a set of relative weights for different health outcomes. The only exception to this is in a completely free market for health care where such decisions between competing health programmes are not made by a central authority but by individuals, one health problem at a time. Even in the USA, competitive resource allocation choices are still made for at least subsegments of the population such as Medicaid, Medicare and Veterans Administration beneficiaries. If the process of choosing relative weights of different types of health outcomes is left entirely to the political or bureaucratic process there is a high probability that similar health outcomes may be weighted inconsistently, perhaps

Reprinted from *Bulletin of the World Health Organization*, 1994, **72** (3): 429–445.

3

reflecting the political voices of different constituencies. More importantly, there may be no open discussion or debate on key value choices or differential weightings. The wide variation in the implied value of saving a life in public safety legislation is but one example (8).

Alternatively, we can explicitly choose a set of relative values for different health outcomes and construct a single indicator of health. The black box of the decision-maker's relative values is then opened for public scrutiny and influence. Both this paper and the others in this series on the burden of disease are predicated on the desirability of making implicit values explicit. Development of a single indicator of the burden of disease for use in planning and evaluating the health sector is described below.

Some general concepts

This paper is not intended to present a new paradigm for measuring health, nor to firmly identify one intellectual tradition such as utilitarianism, human rights, or Rawls' theory of justice (9) as the basis for the social preferences incorporated into DALYs. Rather, the majority of the paper is devoted to a discussion of several types of social preferences which must be incorporated into any indicator of health status. In order to derive a usable indicator, a particular stand is also taken on each of the social values described. The philosophical basis for this position will not be argued in detail. For the interested reader, an indicator very similar to DALYs has been developed based on Rawls' device of the "original position". That is a type of thought experiment where a group of individuals, ignorant of each other's social position, age, sex and other characteristics, are asked to choose the values and institutions to govern society. An "original position" could be invoked for a more specific task such as choosing the values to be incorporated in a health indicator.[a, b] Further philosophical treatment is excluded here.

However, four general concepts in the development of DALYs, which have enjoyed wide consensus with the groups involved in the study, are presented. These concepts are not derived from one particular conception of the good and may in fact be based on mutually inconsistent ethical frameworks. Nevertheless, the purpose of this paper is to explain

the technical assumptions underlying DALYs and not to propose a unified ethical framework for all health sector analysis. In our discussion of the details of various social preferences incorporated into the indicator, we make reference to these concepts. The reader who finds these concepts intuitively plausible may feel comfortable with DALYs as a measurement tool.

(1) *To the extent possible, any health outcome that represents a loss of welfare should be included in an indicator of health status*

Any health outcome that affects social welfare should in some way be reflected in the indicator of the burden of disease. In other words, if society would be willing to devote some resources to avert or treat a health outcome, that outcome should be included in the total estimated burden. As will be seen later, this is at odds with one major stream of work on the measurement of disability which ignores all forms of disability below some thresholds of severity and duration. Note that by making reference to the concept of welfare we are not claiming that DALYs are the best measure of the health component of social welfare. Nor that maximizing DALYs gained from health interventions up to some cost per DALY would be consistent with an objective of maximizing social welfare, although this argument has been formally made (10). The link between health maximization, as measured by DALYs or any other measure, and welfare maximization would require another paper to adequately address the complexities of this issue.

(2) *The characteristics of the individual affected by a health outcome that should be considered in calculating the associated burden of disease should be restricted to age and sex*

Every health outcome such as the premature death of a 45-year-old man from a heart attack or permanent disability from blindness due to a road accident in a 19-year-old woman can be characterized by a set of variables. Some of these variables define the specific health outcome itself such as the etiology, type, severity or duration of the disability. Others are individual characteristics such as sex, age, income, educational attainment, religion, ethnicity, occupation, etc. In the most general terms, the task of constructing a burden of disease measure is to take an n-dimensional matrix of information on health outcomes and collapse this into a single number. To transform this complex array of information, what are the variables that should be included or indeed allowed to be considered? Some might argue that all

[a] **Murray CJL.** *Mortality measurement and social justice.* Paper presented at the Annual Conference of the Institute of British Geographers, 5 January 1986, Reading, England.

[b] **Murray CJL.** *The determinants of health improvement in developing countries. Case-studies of St. Lucia, Guyana, Paraguay, Kiribati, Swaziland and Bolivia.* Oxford University D. Phil. thesis, 1988.

the variables may be relevant and none should be excluded *a priori*. At the limit, this is a form of total relativism since every health outcome becomes unique and there is no meaning to an aggregate indicator.

Others might want to include variables that are unacceptable to the authors. The government of South Africa under apartheid implicity put a higher relative weight on health outcomes in whites as compared to blacks. Nearly everyone would agree that attributes such as race, religion or political beliefs have no place in the construction of a health indicator. Some, however, might see a logic of including income or educational status such that the health of the wealthy counted more than the health of the poor. Estimations of the cost of disease (*11, 12*) use methods that value equivalent health outcomes in higher income groups as more costly than the same outcomes in the poor.

The set of variables that can be considered are restricted here to those defining the particular health outcome and individual characteristics that are general to all communities and households, namely age and sex. Daniels (*13*) has argued that differentiation by age should not be viewed as pitting the welfare of one age group against another, but rather as viewing an individual during different phases of the life-cycle. Variables defining subgroups such as income or education, which not all individuals or households can hope to belong to, are expressly excluded from consideration. This is a fundamental value choice founded on our notions of social justice. Some readers, with different values and conceptions of social justice, might conclude that other information should be included in assessing health status.

(3) *Treating like health outcomes as like*

We articulate a principle of treating like health outcomes as like. For example, the premature death of a 40-year-old woman should contribute equally to estimates of the global burden of disease irrespective of whether she lives in the slums of Bogota or a wealthy suburb of Boston. Treating like events equally also ensures comparability of the burden of disease across different communities and in the same community over a period of time. Community-specific characteristics such as local levels of mortality should not change the assumptions incorporated into the indicator design. The value of a person's health status is his or her own and does not depend on his or her neighbour's health status. A concrete example of this will be discussed in the section on the duration of time lost due to premature mortality. The approach presented means that occasionally we will sacrifice consistency with cost-effectiveness

measures but retain comparability of burden across communities and a plausible treatment of equity.

(4) *Time is the unit of measure for the burden of disease*

Many health indicators measure the occurrence of events such as disease incidence or death per unit time and others measure these events per unit population. The units of measure are specific to the entity studied such as infant deaths for the infant mortality rate or measles cases in the measles attack rate. For a composite health indicator, a more general unit of measure is required. The best candidate for a general unit of measure is time itself, denominated in years or days. Using time as the unit of measure also provides a simple and intuitive method to combine the time lived with a disability with the time lost due to premature mortality. Measuring health status using time is not a new idea; the concept of years of life lost from dying young has been in use for nearly 45 years (*14*). The development of time-based measures and the myriad modifications of this approach are explored more fully below.

Incidence versus prevalence perspectives

With time as the chosen unit of measure, the burden of disease could still be an incidence- or prevalence-based indicator. Time lost due to premature mortality is a function of death rates and the duration of life lost due to a death at each age. Because death rates are incidence rates, there is no obvious alternative for mortality to using an incidence approach. There are no calculated measures of the prevalence of the dead. In contrast, for disability both incidence and prevalence measures are in routine use. There are at least two ways of measuring the aggregate time lived with a disability. One method is to take point prevalence measures of disability, adjusting for seasonal variation if present, and estimate the total time lived with the disability as prevalence × one year. The alternative is to measure the incidence of disabilities and the average duration of each disability. Incidence × duration will then provide an estimate of the total time lived with the disability.

If the incidence of disabilities is constant over time and the population age-structure is also constant, then the prevalence and incidence approaches yield exactly the same total amount of time lived with a disability. For nearly all populations the age structure is not constant and for many diseases such as lung cancer, cervical cancer, stomach cancer, HIV infection, and leprosy the incidence is changing over time. For the Global Burden of Disease study, we have chosen to use an incidence perspective for three reasons. First, with the method of calculating time lived with disabilities is more consistent with the method for calculating time lost due to premature mortality. Second, an incidence perspective is more sensitive to current epidemiological trend and will reflect the impact of health interventions more rapidly. The results of the Global Burden of Disease study, presented in Murray et al. (3) have also been calculated using a prevalence approach. These prevalence-based measures of the burden of disease will be published at a later date (15). Third, measuring the incidence or deriving it from prevalence data and information on case-fatality and remission rates imposes a level of internal consistency and discipline that would be missing if the prevalence data were used uncritically.

Specific value choices in designing an indicator of burden

In the following sections, we address in detail the four key social preferences or values that must be incorporated into an indicator of the burden of disease. These are: the duration of time lost due to a death at each age, the value of time lived at different ages, non-fatal health outcomes (converting time lived with a disability to be comparable with time lost due to premature mortality), and time preference.

The duration of time lost due to premature death

Since Dempsey (14) introduced the concept of measuring lost time due to mortality rather than crude or age-standardized death rates, a wide variety of methods for measuring years of life lost have been proposed (16–23). Because the same terms have been used to describe quite different measures of lost time, there is substantial confusion on the precise method used in any particular study.

At least four different methods of estimating the duration of time lost due to premature death are possible. The following terminology is introduced in an attempt to clarify the discussion and comparison of methods: potential years of life lost, period expected years of life lost, cohort expected years of life lost, and standard expected years of life lost. Each measure is defined and its advantages and disadvantages are reviewed. In the earliest literature on measuring years of life lost, there was also considerable debate about the 'zero mortality assumption' (17–19). Using this assumption, calculating the years of life lost due to a particular disease entails recalculating a life-table in the absence of mortality from that cause at any age. Thus the number of years of life lost due to a tuberculosis death at age 40 would be different

from a motor vehicle accident at age 40. Such methods violate the concept of treating like health outcomes identically and are not discussed further.

(1) *Potential years of life lost* are calculated by defining a potential limit to life and calculating the years lost due to each death as the potential limit minus the age at death. The formula for the number of years of potential life lost in a population is in notation:

$$\sum_{x=0}^{x=L} d_x (L-x)$$

where d_x is deaths at age x, and L is the potential limit to life. A wide range of potential limits to life have been in used in practice, ranging from 60 to 85 (16–18, 22–25). The choice of the upper limit is arbitrary and the arguments are made on statistical grounds. Dempsey (14) proposed that the limit to life be selected as life expectancy at birth for a given population. Romeder & McWhinnie (16) have argued that the potential years of life lost should be calculated based only on deaths over age 1 to avoid being too heavily affected by infant mortality. This is a strange argument which has little intuitive appeal. If the indicator is to be used in informing resource allocation decisions, we would not want to ignore infant deaths. Proponents of the potential years of life lost approach, point to its ease of calculation and the egalitarian treatment of all deaths at a given age as equally important in contributing to the estimated total. If the potential limit to life is chosen as close to life expectancy, the results for the younger age groups are not substantially different from those for expected years of life lost (discussed below). The major disadvantage is in the treatment of deaths in the older population. Deaths over the arbitrary potential limit to life, for example 65 as calculated by the Centers for Disease Control (CDC) in the USA, do not contribute to the estimated burden of disease. This runs counter to our first principle because society clearly does care about the health of these groups and expends substantial resources in all countries on their health care. Even in high mortality populations, societies do appear to care about the health of the population over 60 or 70.

(2) An alternative is to calculate the *period expected years of life lost (17–19, 21)*, using the local expectation of life at each age as the estimate of the duration of life lost at each age. Period expected years of life lost has become the standard method of estimating years of life lost in many cost-effectiveness studies

(26, 27). This method is seen as a more 'realistic' estimate of the stream of life gained by averting a death, given competing risks of death in a particular population. More formally,

$$\sum_{x=0}^{x=l} d_x e_x$$

where l is the last age group and e_x is the expectation of life at each age. Because the expectation of life does not drop to zero at an arbitrary age, this method has the advantage of providing a more appealing estimate of the stream of lost life due to deaths in the older age groups. However, application of the period expectation method with locally different values of life expectancy would lead us to conclude that the death of a 40-year-old woman in Kigali contributes less to the global burden of disease than the death of a 40-year-old woman in Paris because the expectation of life at age 40 in Rwanda is lower than in France. Equivalent health outcomes would be a greater burden in richer communities than in poorer communities. As this runs counter to the principle of treating like events as like, this method is not used for estimating disability-adjusted life years.

The claim that period expected years of life lost are a more realistic estimate of the true duration of time lost due to premature mortality rests on three questionable assumptions. First, if a death is averted, that individual will then be exposed to the same mortality risks as the average individual in the population. In other words, the individual whose death is averted would not have a higher risk of subsequent death than the rest of the population. This may not be true for many chronic disabling conditions; likewise, because much mortality is concentrated in the chronically ill, averting a random death from injury may save more years than average expectation. For the population as a whole, the assumption of being exposed to the average mortality risk is reasonable. When evaluating specific interventions in a cost-effectiveness study, care must be taken to evaluate directly this question of interdependent mortality risks.

Second, period life expectancies are calculated based on the assumption that someone alive today will be exposed in the future to currently observed age-specific mortality rates at each age. Twentieth century mortality history demonstrates that this is a completely fallacious assumption, particularly in a population with moderate or high mortality (Fig. 1). Mortality has been declining at a steady pace throughout the last decades so that the life expectan-

Fig. 1. **Period and cohort life expectancy at birth, 1900–1950, USA females.**

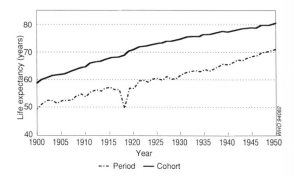

cy of a cohort, the real expectation of life based on the mortality experience of a group over time, is much higher than the period life expectancy based on currently observed rates. Fig. 1 shows how the cohort life expectancy at birth for US females has been 10–15 years higher than period life expectancy from 1900 to 1950.

Third, if we conceive of the burden of disease as the gap between current conditions and some ideal, why would one choose current mortality patterns to define that ideal and the existing gap? Such a standard would also have to be changed each year as life expectancy increases, leading to paradoxical situations where improvements in life expectancy could increase the expected years of life lost due to some large causes.[c]

(3) A third method for estimating the duration of time lost due to premature mortality is defined as *cohort expected years of life lost*:

$$\sum_{x=0}^{x=l} d_x e_x^c$$

where e^c is the estimated cohort life expectancy at each age. Clearly, cohort life expectancies must be estimated since we cannot know today the mortality experience a cohort will experience. However, the estimates based on past patterns of mortality decline are likely to be closer to the truth than period life expectancies. The difference in absolute terms between period and cohort expected years of life lost

---

[c] **Rothenberg R.** *Application of years of life lost to the elderly: demographic influences on a composite statistic.* Presented at 46th Annual Scientific Meeting of the American Geriatrics Society, Boston, MA, 1989.

will be greatest for high mortality populations where substantial absolute mortality decline can be expected in the next decades. Despite the logical advantages of the cohort approach over the period approach, it still suffers from the criticism that it will not treat like events as like because cohort life expectancy will still differ from community to community. While inappropriate for measuring burden of disease, cohort life expectancy is the most attractive method of estimating the benefits of interventions for cost-effectiveness analysis.

(4) The advantages of the cohort expectation approach in the treatment of deaths at older ages and the egalitarian nature of the potential years of life lost methods can be combined. *Standard expected years of life lost* can be defined as:

$$\sum_{x=0}^{x=l} d_x e_x^*$$

where e^* is the expectation of life at each age based on some ideal standard. For DALYs, the standard has been chosen to match the highest national life expectancy observed; Japanese females have already achieved a period life expectancy at birth of close to 82 years. For a specific standard, the expectations are based on model life-table West Level 26 which has a life expectancy at birth for females of 82.5. Using a model life-table makes the standard expectations at each age easily available through publications and software distributed by the United Nations Population Division and eliminates some peculiarities of the Japanese age-specific mortality. Choosing one family of model life-tables over any other makes little or no difference to the results at such a low mortality level. With this indicator, deaths at all ages, even after age 82.5, contribute to the total estimated burden of disease while all deaths at the same age will contribute equally to the total estimated burden of disease.

Should the same standard expectation of life at each age be used for males as well as for females? One could argue on grounds of fostering equity that a male death at age 40 should count as the same duration of life lost as a female death at age 40. There appears, however, to be a biological difference in survival potential between males and females (28, 29). The average sex differences in life expectancy at birth in low mortality populations is 7.2 years (30). Not all this difference is biological; a large share is due to injury deaths among young males and higher levels of risk factors such as smoking. If we examine

high-income groups in low-mortality populations, the gap in life expectancy between males and females narrows considerably. Fig. 2 shows the differences in life expectancy by income groups in Canada (31). Where males are not exposed to high risks due to occupation, smoking, alcohol or injuries, the residual gap in life expectancy is narrowing dramatically. Projecting this forward, the ultimate gap in life expectancy at birth between the sexes is likely to approach 2 or 3 years. Independent estimates of the biological differences in survival potential have generated similar estimates (33). For the burden of disease study, we have chosen to use a life expectancy at birth of 80 for males and 82.5 for females from model life-table West.

In summary, the duration of time lost due to premature mortality can be measured by at least four different methods. Fig. 3 shows a comparison for a hypothetical population where period life expectancy at birth is 55. Four terms have been introduced to try and clarify the different methods of calculation, although this terminology is not yet in general usage. For the calculation of DALYs, we have chosen to use the standard expected years of life lost method with slight differences in the standard for males and females. To illustrate, the first two columns of Table 1 provide an abridged listing of the standard male and female expectancies used.

Social value of the time lived at different ages

In all societies social roles vary with age. The young, and often the elderly, depend on the rest of society for physical, emotional and financial support. Given different roles and changing levels of dependency with age, it may be appropriate to consider valuing the time lived at a particular age unequally. Higher

Fig. 2. **Differences in life expectancy at birth for males and females, by income quintile, in urban Canada, 1986.**

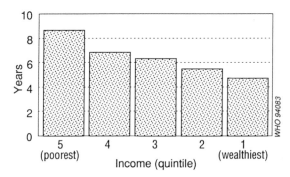

Fig. 3. **Duration of time lost due to premature mortality at each age.**

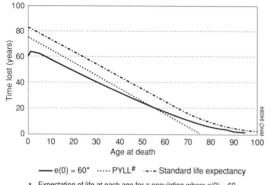

- e(0) = 60* ····· PYLL# ·-·- Standard life expectancy

* Expectation of life at each age for a population where e(0) = 60

\# Potential years of life lost

Table 1: **Standard life expectancy and DALYs lost due to premature death at each age**[a]

Age	Life expectancy		Death DALYs	
(years)	Females	Males	Females	Males
0	82.50	80.00	32.45	32.34
1	81.84	79.36	33.37	33.26
5	77.95	75.38	35.85	35.72
10	72.99	70.40	36.86	36.71
15	68.02	65.41	36.23	36.06
20	63.08	60.44	34.52	34.31
25	58.17	55.47	32.12	31.87
30	53.27	50.51	29.31	29.02
35	48.38	45.56	26.31	25.97
40	43.53	40.64	23.26	22.85
45	38.72	35.77	20.24	19.76
50	33.99	30.99	17.33	16.77
55	29.37	26.32	14.57	13.92
60	24.83	21.81	11.97	11.24
65	20.44	17.50	9.55	8.76
70	16.20	13.58	7.33	6.55
75	12.28	10.17	5.35	4.68
80	8.90	7.45	3.68	3.20

[a] Life expectancy is calculated for the age at the beginning of the interval.

weights for a year of time at a particular age does not mean that the time lived at that age is *per se* more important to the individual, but that because of social roles the social value of that time may be greater. Fig. 4 illustrates graphically two contrasting approaches to the value of the time lived at different ages: uniform value or unequal age weights with more importance given to time in the middle age group.

Unequal weights can be justified within two different conceptual frameworks. First, the theory of human capital views individuals as a type of machine with costs of maintenance and expected output. The value of time at each age for this human production machine should be proportionate to productivity. Several of the original proponents of measuring the years of life lost proposed measures of working years of life lost (17–19). Piot & Sundaresan calculated the years of healthy living in the productive age groups as a health sector outcome measure.[d] Several World Bank authors (33, 34) have used productivity weights in the calculation of years of life gained in cost-effectiveness studies. Barnum (34), in particular, suggests using average wage rates by age as the weighting factors. The logical extension of the human capital approach would be to weight time by other human attributes that correlate with productivity such as income, education, geographical location or even, in some economies, ethnicity. The obvious inequity is why no-one explicitly calls for this extension, even though it would only be

logically consistent. Because of this apparent inconsistency in the application of the human capital concept and because the human capital approach inadequately reflects human welfare, productivity weights are not used in the development of disability-adjusted life years.

Alternatively, we can view unequal age-weights as an attempt to capture different social roles at different ages. As all individuals can aspire to belong to each age group in his or her lifetime, Daniels argues that it is not unjust to discriminate by age (13). The concept of dependency and social role is broader than formal sector wage productivity and is not linked to total income levels. Unequal age-weights also has broad intuitive appeal. There has been little formal empirical work on measuring individual preferences for age-weights in the community; however, informal polling of tuberculosis programme managers by the author in an annual training course has revealed that everyone polled believes that the time lived in the middle age groups should be weighted as more important than the extremes. Not surprisingly there was no consensus on the precise weights to be used, only on the general functional form.

Having chosen to use unequal age-weights to capture different social roles through the life-cycle, how should specific weights be selected? With little empirical work on preferences for age-weights based on differing social roles as opposed to productivity, the only option was to use a modified Delphi method

---

[d] **Piot M, Sundaresan TK.** *A linear programme decision model for tuberculosis control. Progress report on the first test-runs.* Unpublished WHO document No. WHO/TB/Techn. Information/ 67.55, 1967.

Fig. 4. **Age-weight function.**

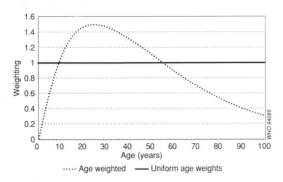

..... Age weighted   —— Uniform age weights

with a group of public health experts. One must also choose between establishing a set of discrete weights for each age or define a continuous mathematical function for the weights at each age. Discrete age-weights allow for great flexibility in the pattern chosen but require time-consuming iterative computations in their application.

For reasons of convenience, it is preferable to define a continuous age-weighting function. Functions of the form:

$$Cxe^{-\beta x}$$

where β is a constant having the general form shown in Fig. 4. This conforms to the basic age-weighting pattern desired. Only a narrow range of β provides reasonable age patterns, approximately between 0.03 and 0.05. Based on informal polling of the advisory board for this study, we chose a β of 0.04. As discussed by Murray et al. (3), the results are largely insensitive to the specific β chosen but are sensitive in certain qualitative ways to the difference between equal and unequal age-weights.

The constant C in the equation is chosen so that the introduction of unequal age-weights does not change the global estimated burden of disease from the total that would be estimated with uniform age-weights. Its value thus depends on the age and sex pattern of results of the global burden of disease in real populations detailed in Murray et al. (3). In another article on the global burden of disease published in this issue of the *Bulletin*, C equals 0.16243. If the age-weighting function were changed, for example by altering β, the constant would necessarily change as well.

Non-fatal health outcomes

Measuring non-fatal health outcomes in terms commensurate with time lost due to premature mortality

has been the subject of extensive research for three decades (35). Disease-specific measures such as attack rates date from the nineteenth century, but more general measures of non-fatal health outcomes became a major issue in the 1960s. A series of authors formulated models for composite indicators of mortality and morbidity (5, 6, 36–39).[e] While each indicator had notable differences, they all defined a series of health states ranging from health to death, a series of weights reflecting the severity of these states and in some cases probabilities of movement from one state to another over time. Since these pioneering studies, intellectual efforts have evolved on three largely independent lines. Remarkably, for reasons of disciplinary focus, geographical and institutional locus, and types of health systems, the different strands of work on measuring non-fatal health outcomes have proceeded in relative isolation (40). The result is substantially different vocabulary, methods, and objectives and not surprisingly confusion. To provide the context for the disability-adjusted life year approach, the three domains of work will be briefly outlined.

Joint measures of non-fatal health outcomes and premature mortality were obviously of use in cost-effectiveness analyses of health projects (41–43). Consequently one line of development has been pursued by health economists interested in using the measures at the level of the individual or beneficiaries of a specific intervention. The now familiar term, the quality-adjusted life year (QALY), has become a standard tool in health programme evaluation in industrialized countries (43–45). In the work on QALYs, the focus has been on developing sophisticated methods for measuring individual preferences for time spent in different health states. For example, Nord (46) reviews five approaches developed to elicit utility weights for health states. Boyle & Torrance (47) have discussed a comprehensive system of health states, but this has yet to be applied. For most cost-effectiveness studies, health states have been defined *ad hoc* for a particular intervention such as coronary artery bypass grafting (48). The dimensions of physical, mental or social function within each state has received little attention in the QALY literature.

The second school of work has been the burgeoning field of health status indicators pursued largely in North America (see 49–51 for proceedings of three general conferences). Rather than the emphasis on choosing utility weights as in the estimation of QALYs field, the major thrust has been

---

[e] See footnote d on page 9.

defining the precise dimensions of health status and practical survey instruments for measurement. Beginning initially with a narrow vision of disease, the measures have progressively incorporated variables related to physical function, mental function, and more recently social function (52). The term health-related quality of life has been used for this broader vision. The indicators themselves are weighted aggregates of a multitude of variables measuring specific functions or dimensions of physical, mental and social function. Research on new survey instruments has explored the differences between self-reported, proxy reported, independently observed, and objective functional tests. Reliability, various forms of validity (although rarely criterion validity), and feasibility of application are the basis for choice between indicators. The weights used in collapsing measurements of multiple variables into a single indicator have not been as much a topic for concern as in the QALY literature; frequently they are chosen on arbitrary grounds such as equal weighting.

The third cluster of work on measuring non-fatal health outcomes also dates from the early 1970s. A World Health Organization initiative in collaboration with the WHO Centre for the Classification of Diseases in Paris, and various nongovernmental organizations led to the publication of a draft classification of impairments, disabilities and handicaps in 1975[f] and the *International classification of impairments, disabilities and handicaps* (ICIDH) in 1980 (53). The conceptual framework that emerged from this process is substantially different from the QALY or health status index approaches. In the manual of the ICIDH, a linear progression from disease to pathology to manifestation to impairment to disability to handicap is proposed. Impairment is defined at the level of the organ system, disability is the impact on the performance of the individual, and handicap is the overall consequences, which depend on the social environment. For example, a loss of a finger or an eye is an impairment. The consequent disability may be the loss of fine motor function or sight. Depending on the need in particular environments, the loss of function could lead to a handicap or disadvantage. The loss of fine motor function may be a greater handicap, in this terminology, for a concert violinist than for a bank-teller. Note the major difference between this approach which sees handicap as a completely different axis from disability and the health status field which adds social function

as one more in a long list of variables incorporated in a measure of health-related quality of life.

Both the World Health Organization and the United Nations Statistical Division have adopted the ICIDH. Currently, other countries are adopting the ICIDH as the basis for measuring disability and handicap. Le Réseau d'Espérance de Vie en Santé (REVES) is an independent network of academics and government agencies that are concerned with quantifying healthy life (54). In line with the ICIDH, REVES has proposed three indicators: impairment-free life expectancy, disability-free life expectancy, and handicap-free life expectancy (55). Reflecting the concerns of some associations of people with disabilities and handicaps, some members of REVES are actively opposed to the use of weights for different health states in calculating composite health indicators. *De facto*, in any of the health expectancies, weights of 0 and 1 are used somewhat arbitrarily. These health expectancies, such as disability-free life expectancy, weight all the time spent with a moderate or severe disability as equal to the time lost due to premature mortality, a weight of one. Mild disability is given a weight of zero. The threshold below which disability is weighted with zero is not clearly defined in this literature. Often a threshold is justified by pointing out that nearly everyone has some mild impairment, disability or handicap so that if milder outcomes were included, health expectancies would approach zero in all environments. If weights between zero and one were chosen as in DALYs, this would not occur.

Given the diverse approaches to measuring non-fatal health outcomes, many possible strategies could have been used for measuring the burden of disease. Prior to the Global Burden of Disease study, the only effort to evaluate the burden of disease due to disability and premature mortality by cause for an entire population was the Ghana Health Assessment Project (25). While that study was path-breaking, it did not publish the methods or rationale used for defining, measuring and weighting disability. Learning from past experience, we chose to deal more directly with disability measurement issues and to develop a practical approach that could be applied to over 100 diseases and their sequelae. Four key issues had to be addressed: defining disability classes, separating duration and severity, mapping diseases through to disabling sequelae, and choosing weights for different classes.

In the terminology of the *International classification of impairments, disabilities, and handicaps*, we have chosen to measure disability, not handicap. Handicap or disadvantage is an attractive concept because it focuses on the impact, given a particular social context of the individual. In some cases, simi-

---

[f] **Wood PHN.** *Classification of impairments and handicaps.* Unpublished WHO document No. WHO/ICD9/REV.CONF/75.15, 1975.

lar disabilities may lead to a greater handicap for an already disadvantaged person than for the more fortunate. In many cases, however, allocating resources to avert handicap, as opposed to disability, could exacerbate inequalities. The manual of the ICIDH itself gives the following example: "Subnormality of intelligence is an impairment, but it may not lead to appreciable activity restriction; factors other than the impairment may determine the handicap because the disadvantage may be minimal if the individual lives in a remote rural community, whereas it could be severe in the child of university graduates living in a large city, of whom more might be expected." (53, p. 31).

Pursuing handicap could and probably would lead us to invest in avoiding mental retardation in the rich and well-educated but not in the poor. On even the most minimal principles of equity, this is unacceptable. The principle of treating like events as like requires using disability instead of handicap.

Having decided to measure disability, the challenge is to develop a way of capturing the multiple dimensions of human function in a simple scheme. Six disability classes have been defined between perfect health and death. Each class represents a greater loss of welfare or increased severity than the class before. Disabilities in the same class may restrict different abilities or functional capacities but their impact on the individual is considered to be similar. Table 2 provides a definition of each of the six classes. Limited ability has been arbitrarily defined as a 50% or more decrease in ability.

The classes are also defined operationally. A class is defined by the set of disabling sequelae included in that class. For those who work with individuals with a disability, looking at the set of disabling sequelae included in that class may make it much clearer what a Class 3 disability is. Operational validation forces us to ask: are the disabling sequelae in each class approximately similar and does each class represent a group os sequelae more severe than

the class before? As explained below, the final distribution of disabling sequelae by class was subject to the review of an independent group of experts.

The separation in the development of the disability-adjusted life year of duration of disability and severity must be emphasized. Severity of a disability could be a function of duration. A similar loss of function is argued to be worse per unit time if it is expected to be permanent than temporary. Man can endure suffering if the prospect of relief is near. In DALYs, severity or class weights are not a function of the time spent in each class but only of the class itself. This allows comparisons between the time lived with short- and long-term disabilities with the time lost due to premature mortality. A numerical example illustrates: 100 people each losing 0.1 of a DALY is a burden equal to 1 person losing 10 DALYs. We should note that experience in Oregon, with the application of cost-effectiveness to health resource allocation decisions, demonstrated that many individuals are against the separation of severity and duration (56). Through a series of town meetings, priorities for intervention based solely on cost-effectiveness criteria were modified. Analysis of these modifications demonstrated a concern for a larger quantum of benefits accruing to individuals as compared to the same number of QALYs accruing to more individuals (57). This concern would be captured better through a series of dispersion weights that adjusted for DALYs by the size of the health gain affecting the individual because part of this effect relates to the duration of time lost due to mortality rather than just the severity of the disability. Because experience is limited only to Oregon, we have not introduced dispersion weights into the analysis and have maintained the separation of disability duration and severity.

A major obstacle between public health studies on particular diseases and work on disability has been the absence of a probability map from disease

Table 2: **Definitions of disability weighting**

	Description	Weight
Class 1	Limited ability to perform at least one activity in one of the following areas: recreation, education, procreation or occupation.	0.096
Class 2	Limited ability to perform most activities in one of the following areas: recreation, education, procreation or occupation.	0.220
Class 3	Limited ability to perform activities in two or more of the following areas: recreation, education, procreation or occupation	0.400
Class 4	Limited ability to perform most activities in all of the following areas: recreation, education, procreation or occupation	0.600
Class 5	Needs assistance with instrumental activities of daily living such as meal preparation, shopping or housework.	0.810
Class 6	Needs assistance with activities of daily living such as eating, personal hygiene or toilet use.	0.920

through to impairments and disabilities. On paper arrows may be drawn from disease all the way to handicap, but even those who work on disability can rarely provide concrete information on the probability that someone with a particular disease will go on to suffer disabilities of differing severity. For the Global Burden of Disease study, such a mapping from disease through impairment to disability was developed. The details of the map and specific problems encountered are discussed in Murray & Lopez (2).

To compare the time lived in six disability classes with the time lost due to premature mortality, a weight for each class is required. At least five types of methods have been proposed to elicit preferences for health states from individuals (45, 46): rating scales, magnitude estimation, standard gamble, time trade-off, and person trade-off. In brief,

(a) rating scales ask individuals to place different states on a scale from 0 to 100;

(b) magnitude estimation asks direct questions about the relative value of the time spent in one state compared to another;

(c) standard gambles ask individuals to choose between the certainty of living in a health state versus a chance of getting well at a probability p and dying at probability $1-p$;

(d) time trade-offs elicit how much time an individual would exchange living in one state versus being healthy, such as 0.4 years of healthy life versus 1 year in a particular health state; and

(e) in person trade-offs, individuals are asked to choose between curing a certain number of individuals in one disability class versus another number in a different class.

Time trade-off questions differ from the other methods because they confound questions of the utility of time spent in disability classes and the time preference rate discussed below. The last three methods all try to elicit the point at which the individual is indifferent between the two choices being offered. When the individual is indifferent the two outcomes are then equivalent and a weight is derived. Specific weights depend not only on the type of question used but on the group of respondents. Health care providers, patients, families of patients, and the general public may give different results to a specific question (46). The specific weights may depend on the question and respondent type but the ordinal ranking of health states is often less sensitive to the specific formulation.

Weights for the six classes have been chosen by a group of independent experts who had not been involved in the estimation of the incidence, duration or mortality of any disease, convened at the Centers for Disease Control. They chose weights based on both the word definitions and the set of disabling sequelae in each class. De facto, they used a magnitude estimation method to choose a number between 0 and 1 for each of the six classes. Their votes were averaged to generate the final class weights provided in Table 2. How much do the specific weights matter? For classes 3 through 6, even if the weight is changed up or down by 0.1 it will have only a minor effect on the estimated burden of disease by cause. For Classes 1 and 2, however, the incidence times duration of disability is much higher and a change of weight from 0.05 to 0.1, for example, could have a significant effect on the results. Future work at the country level and at the global and regional level will benefit from a broader exercise to elicit weights for the six disability classes.

Time preference

At the simplest level, time preference is the economic concept that individuals prefer benefits now rather than in the future. The value of goods or services today is greater than in one or ten years. If offered the choice between 100 dollars from a completely reliable source today or 100 dollars in 1 year, most will prefer their money today. If offered 110 in one year versus 100 today, some may choose the 110 dollars. The bank interest rate on a savings account is the rate at which individuals are willing to forego consumption today for consumption in the future. The market rate of interest is the aggregate rate at which individuals in society as a whole discount future consumption. It is standard practice in economic appraisal of projects to use the discount rate to discount benefits in the future (58). The process of discounting future benefits converts them into present-value terms which can then be compared with project costs also discounted if they are spread over more than one year to determine cost-effectiveness.

However, despite the uniform use of discounting in cost-benefit and cost-effectiveness analysis, there is no consensus on the conceptual justification for discounting or on the appropriate discount rate (59, 60). Simplifying, there are two approaches to choosing the discount rate. One can use the social opportunity cost of capital as captured by the market rate of return on investment. Distortions of the market caused by corporate taxation and other interventions can complicate determining the social opportunity cost of capital. In practice, discount rates based on the social opportunity cost of capital are high (between 8% and 15%). The World Bank and the U.S. Congressional Budget Office have used a 10% discount rate for many years in project appraisal (61). Studies of long-term return on investments, however, suggest a lower discount rate of 1–3%. The alternative concept is that society, like individuals, has a social time preference which should be used for discounting future benefits to society. This rate is thought to be lower than the market rate of interest (closer to 1–3%) (59).

Discounting years of health life or their equivalent has been used since Piot & Sundaresan in 1967 in many cost-effectiveness analyses.[g] However, as health policy researchers have become more familiar with time preference, discounting health benefits has become highly controversial (62–75). While a detailed discussion of arguments for and against discounting is beyond the scope of this paper, a brief review of some arguments for social time preference may put discounting in a sharper perspective.

• First, individuals may have a pure time preference for no clear reason except myopia. Myopia is not a persuasive basis for social time preference. There is no reason to value welfare *per se* today more than welfare *per se* of the same individuals. Nor is there a reason for society to value the welfare *per se* of those alive today more than the welfare *per se* of those who are yet to be born.

• Second, if consumption is expected to grow in the future and there is decreasing marginal utility of consumption, then a marginal unit of consumption in the future will lead to less utility in the future and should be discounted. This logic for a positive discount rate may be reversed for health benefits. Disability-adjusted life years represent a measure of time gained or lost in the future. Time gives the potential to consume and derive utility; it is not equivalent to a fixed number of units of consumption. In fact, in the face of growing consumption a future DALY may yield more utility than a current DALY.

• Third, there is uncertainty correlating with time so that future outcomes need to be discounted to reflect the finite but non-zero risk that society will not exist at that time. Or in a less extreme form, it may be reasonable to expect an individual to incorporate his or her future risk of death each year into individual time preference, on average about 1% per year. For society, the equivalent risk of extinction will be much lower. Defining a plausible risk of social extinction is difficult, but attempts have been made to use certain probability distributions for estimates of uncertainty correlating with time.

• Fourth, Keeler & Cretin (75) have formalized a commonly appreciated problem known as the time paradox. If one argues that health benefits should not

be discounted or should be discounted at a rate lower than monetary costs, one will always choose to put off investing in a health project until the future. Benefits will be the same in present-value terms because they are not discounted. But the costs in present-value terms will be lower if the project is deferred to the future. Costs are lower because the budget could be invested and yield a positive return. A thousand dollars today will turn into $1100 or $1050 in a year. Only when costs and benefits are discounted at the same rate do we become indifferent to the time when a project is implemented. The time paradox depends on three critical assumptions: (a) the opportunity for health intervention will be the same in the future with similar costs and benefits, (b) it is politically feasible for society to receive more resources for health in the future in exchange for putting off current expenditure, and (c) the rate of return in other sectors or in financial markets is higher than in the health sector. If any of these do not hold, the time paradox is no longer relevant.

• Fifth, if health benefits are not discounted, then we may conclude that 100% of resources should be invested in any disease eradication plans with finite costs as this will eliminate infinite streams of DALYs which will outweigh all other health investments that do not result in eradication.

Recognizing that the debate on discounting health benefits will not be resolved in the near future, we have chosen a low positive rate of 3 percent for the calculation of DALYs. This is consistent with the long-term yield on investments. There is also a precedent in the World Bank Disease Control Priorities Study (27) that used a 3 percent rate. It avoids the difficulty of the time paradox and of overvaluing eradication programmes when no discount rate is used. Murray et al. (3) provide the sensitivity of the Global Burden of Disease results to varying the discount rate between zero and ten percent.

Introducing discounting into the computation of DALYs raises a number of technical questions. It complicates the choice between incidence and prevalence perspectives. With discounting, even with constant incidence rates, the number of DALYs computed using an incidence perspective for disability will be lower than using a prevalence perspective, because the stream of disability into the future will be discounted so that the last years in the stream will count much less than the first. Second, years of life lost due to premature mortality and years lived with a disability must be compared carefully. If we calculated the time lost from premature mortality which will occur in the future from current disease incidence, we get a different result than if we calculate the time lost due to premature mortality occurring

---

[g] See footnote *d* on page 9.

this year. Even if death rates were constant over time, discounting would introduce a difference. The only practical solution, however, is to assess the time lived with a disability by using current incidence and the time lost due to premature mortality by using current death rates.

Third, we can calculate the discounted stream of lost life due to premature mortality at age a by discounting the number of years as estimated from the standard.

$$\frac{1}{r} - \frac{e^{-rL}}{r}$$

where r is the discount rate and L is the standard expectation of life at age a. An expectation of life is the average number of years expected, but expected deaths will be distributed over many ages. Because discounting is a nonlinear function, the average of a discounted distribution is not equal to the discounted value of the average of a distribution. A more precise estimate of the discounted life expectation would take into account the distribution of the ages of death. Discounting the survivorship function, however, yields results that are only marginally different. The discounted duration of time lost due to premature death at each age, calculated using the survivorship function method, for females ranges from 0.8% to 2.3% (from 1% to 3% for males) less than the direct method. Because of the minor differences and the tremendous advantages of defining a single formula for calculating DALYs, the direct method for discounting has been chosen.

DALY formula

In summary, the disability-adjusted life year is an indicator of the time lived with a disability and the time lost due to premature mortality. The duration of time lost due to premature mortality is calculated using standard expected years of life lost where model life-table West with an expectation of life at birth of 82.5 for females and 80 for males has been used. Time lived at different ages has been valued using an exponential function of the form $Cxe^{-\beta x}$. Streams of time have been discounted at 3%. A continuous discounting function of the form $e^{-r(x-a)}$

has been used where r is the discount rate and a is the age of onset.[h] Disability is divided into six classes, with each class having a severity weight between 0 and 1. Time lived in each class is multiplied by the disability weight to make it comparable with the years lost due to premature mortality.

A general formula for the number of DALYs lost by one individual can be developed:

$$\int_{x=a}^{x=a+L} DCxe^{-\beta x}e^{-r(x-a)}dx$$

The solution of the definite integral from the age of onset a to $a+L$ where L is the duration of disability or time lost due to premature mortality gives us the DALY formula for an individual:

$$-\left[\frac{DCe^{-\beta a}}{(\beta+r)^2}\ [e^{-(\beta+r)(L)}\ (1+(\beta+r)(L+a))-(1+(\beta+r)a)]\right]$$

where D is the disability weight (or 1 for premature mortality), r is the discount rate, C is the age-weighting correction constant, β is the parameter from the age-weighting function, a is the age of onset, and L is the duration of disability or time lost due to premature mortality. This formula can be conveniently written in a spreadsheet cell to facilitate calculation of DALYs. In the specific form used for calculating DALYs, r equals 0.03, β equals 0.04, and C equals 0.16243. The general form of the DALY formula facilitates the sensitivity testing presented in Murray et al. (3). Fig. 5 presents the number of DALYs lost due to a death at each age for a male and a female. This pattern is the aggregate results of the duration of time lost due to premature mortality, age-weighting and discounting but the figure does not reflect any disability.

---

[h] Note that in a continuous discount function r is not precisely the same as r in the discrete form. The formula for the discrete form is simply $1/(1+r)^t$. If the discount rate in the discrete formula is r, then the equivalent result is achieved with a continuous discount rate of $ln\ (1+r)$.

Fig. 5. **DALYs lost due to death at each age.**

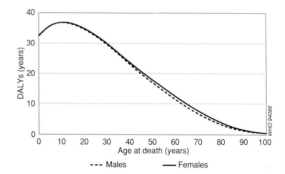

--- Males   —— Females

Conclusion

Disability-adjusted life years as an indicator is consistent with a long line of work on composite indicators of non-fatal health outcomes and premature mortality. While DALYs must be viewed as only one more step in a long development process, there are several aspects about them that are worth noting when comparing DALYs by cause, age, sex, and region with other indicators.

• The particular set of value choices — the duration of life lost, the value of life lived at different ages, comparison of the time lived with a disability with the time lost due to mortality, and the time preference — all differ from past indicators. They have been selected in such a way that the indicator is comparable across a wide range of environments. We also believe that value choices reflect a broad consensus among those practising international public health. However, as the sensitivity analysis shows (3), many of the conclusions of the Global Burden of Disease study are unaffected by changes in those parameters.

• Apart from the specific value choices, the major difference between DALYs and more widely available measures such as potential years of life lost is, of course, the inclusion of the time lived with a disability. As demonstrated elsewhere (3), 34% of the global burden of disease is due to disability; some causes such as neuropsychiatric diseases appear as major problems using DALYs but not using potential years of life lost.

• Estimates of the burden of disease denominated in DALYs can easily be used in conjunction with the literature on cost-effectiveness of health interventions. For example, the largest compendium of international health interventions has reported results in terms of cost per DALY (27). This facilitates using estimates of the burden of disease in determining health resource allocations.

• The more original aspect of DALYs is not their design but the successful application of the indicator to measure the burden of disease for over 100 diseases in eight regions for five age groups among males and females. While details such as the distribution of disabling sequelae by class are bound to be changed in the future as more information is obtained, it is already established as a feasible alternative for assessing the burden of disability and premature mortality.

Acknowledgements

This work would not have been possible without the tremendous efforts of Caroline Cook. Extensive comments from P. Musgrove, M. Reich and A. Lopez were very helpful. J.-L. Bobadilla, D. Jamison, J. Zeitlin, W. Whang, J. Kim, S. Anand, J. Koplan, K. Hill, J.-M. Robine, R. Wilkins and R. Rannan-Eliya provided constructive comments and suggestions for improvement.

Résumé

Mesure quantitative du poids de la morbidité: base de calcul des années de vie ajustées sur l'incapacité

La prise de décision concernant la ventilation des ressources pour la santé exige la connaissance d'un indicateur du poids de la morbidité. Il faut en outre disposer d'un indicateur unique car, en fin de compte, c'est l'ensemble des événements de santé qui sont rapportés aux dépenses de santé. Pour élaborer un indicateur du poids de la morbidité, quatre principes généraux ont été utilisés et articulés. Tout d'abord, dans la mesure du possible, tout événement qui représente une perte de santé doit être inclus dans un indicateur de l'état de santé. Deuxièmement, les caractéristiques du sujet qui présente l'événement de santé dont on tiendra compte dans le calcul du poids de la morbidité correspondant, seront limitées à l'âge et au sexe. Troisièmement, des événements identiques seront considérés de manière identique, à savoir que le décès d'une femme de 40 ans au Burundi est censé avoir la même valeur dans le poids de la morbidité mondiale que le décès d'une femme de 40 ans à Boston (Etats-Unis d'Amérique). Quatrièmement, le temps est utilisé comme unité de mesure commune du poids dû au décès prématuré et à l'incapacité. Les années de vie ajustées sur l'incapacité (DALY: *Disability Adjusted Life Years*) sont calculées en faisant intervenir la notion d'incidence et de durée et non celle de prévalence.

Quatre choix sociaux, ou préférences, doivent être inclus dans tout indicateur du poids de la morbidité. On envisage tout d'abord les années perdues par suite d'un décès prématuré. Depuis l'introduction de ce concept en 1947, quatre méthodes sont utilisées: les années potentielles de vie perdues, les années de vie perdues attendues pour la période, les années de vie perdues attendues pour la cohorte, et les années de vie perdues attendues standardisées. De manière à traiter comme il convient les décès dans la population de 60 ans et plus, et à traiter de manière égale tous les décès au même âge dans toutes les populations, nous avons utilisé la méthode des années de vie perdues attendues standardisées.

C'est la table de mortalité modèle Ouest, avec une espérance de vie à la naissance de 82,5 ans pour les femmes et de 80 ans pour les hommes qui a été choisie comme norme pour les femmes.

Le deuxième choix social examiné est la valeur du temps vécu aux différents âges. Toutes les durées pourraient être considérées comme égales. Cependant, on peut tenir compte du fait que les jeunes et les personnes âgées sont dépendants des adultes d'âge intermédiaire. Les différences de rôle social ont été explicitement introduites dans le calcul des DALY en utilisant une fonction exponentielle de forme xe^{-bx} pour pondérer l'âge. S'appuyant sur le consensus du groupe consultatif réuni pour l'étude, une forme spécifique a été choisie pour b.

Troisièmement, le nombre d'années passées avec une incapacité de gravité plus ou moins grande doit être comparé au nombre d'années perdues par décès prématuré. Les publications sont nombreuses sur la mesure des événements de santé non fatals et peuvent être regroupées arbitrairement en trois catégories: celles qui s'apparentent à l'économie de la santé traditionnelle et s'attachent plus particulièrement aux QALY (*Quality Adjustments of Life Years*: années de vie sauvées ajustées sur la qualité), celles qui s'intéressent à la qualité de vie liée à la santé et celles qui utilisent la CIH (*Classification internationale des handicaps: déficiences, incapacités et désavantages*). Pour pouvoir mesurer comparativement les années vécues avec une incapacité et la mortalité, six classes d'incapacité ont été définies, de l'état de santé parfait au décès. Une définition descriptive est formulée pour chacune des classes. Ce qui est encore plus important est que chacune est en outre définie opérationnellement par un ensemble de séquelles incapacitantes consécutives à la maladie ou au traumatisme inclus dans chaque classe. Le coefficient de pondération va de 0 à 1, et a été choisi pour chacune des classes par un groupe d'experts indépendant n'ayant pas connaissance des détails de l'étude.

Quatrièmement, il est tenu compte de la notion économique d'actualisation de préférence temporelle. Qu'il s'agisse des individus ou de la société, tous tendent à préférer des avantages immédiats à des avantages différés. Il est tenu compte de cette préférence temporelle dans le calcul, en appliquant un taux d'actualisation aux avantages différés. L'utilisation d'une préférence temporelle positive dans l'analyse d'une suite de bénéfices pour la santé comme les années de vie sauvées est très contestée. Nous conformant à plusieurs précédents bien établis, nous avons utilisé un taux d'actualisation de 3%. La formule de calcul des DALY est ensuite indiquée, accompagnée de certaines réflexions sur les avantages et les inconvénients de cet indicateur comparé aux autres indicateurs de l'état de santé.

References

1. **Murray CJL, Lopez AD.** Global and regional cause-of-death patterns in 1990. *Bulletin of the World Health Organization*, 1994, **72**: 447–480.
2. **Murray CJL, Lopez AD.** Quantifying disability: data, methods and results. *Bulletin of the World Health Organization*, 1994, **72**: 481–494.
3. **Murray CJL, Lopez AD, Jamison DT.** The global burden of disease in 1990: summary results, sensitivity analysis and future directions. *Bulletin of the World Health Organization*, 1994, **72**: 495–509.
4. **Power M.** Linear Index Mortality as a measure of health status (Letter). *International journal of epidemiology*, 1989, **18**: 282.
5. **Sullivan DF.** *Conceptual problems in developing an index of health.* US Public Health Service Publication Series No. 1000. Vital and Health Statistics Series 2. No. 17. Bethesda, MD, National Center for Health Statistics, 1966.
6. **Sullivan DF.** A single index of mortality and morbidity. *Health reports*, 1971, **86**: 347–354.
7. **Holland WW, Ipsen J, Kostrzewski J.** *Measurement of levels of health.* Copenhagen, WHO Regional Office for Europe, 1979.
8. **Jones-Lee MW.** *The value of life: an economic analysis.* London, Martin Robertson, 1976.
9. **Rawls J.** *A theory of justice.* Cambridge, Harvard University Press, 1971.
10. **Garber AM, Phelphs CE.** *Economic foundations of cost-effectiveness analysis.* Cambridge, MA, 1992 (National Bureau of Economic Research Working Paper 4164).
11. **Max W, Rice DP, MacKenzie EJ.** The lifetime cost of injury. *Inquiry*, 1990, **27**(4): 332–343.
12. **Rice DP, Kelman S, Miller LS.** Estimates of economic costs of alcohol and drug abuse and mental illness 1985 and 1988. *Public health reports*, 1991, **106**(3): 280–292.
13. **Daniels N.** *Just health care.* New York, Cambridge University Press, 1985.
14. **Dempsey M.** Decline in tuberculosis. The death rate fails to tell the entire story. *American review of tuberculosis*, 1947, **56**: 157–164.
15. **Murray CJL, Lopez AD.** *The global burden of disease and injury.* Geneva, World Health Organization (in preparation).
16. **Romeder JM, McWhinnie JR.** Potential years of life lost between ages 1 and 70: an indicator of premature mortality for health planning. *International journal of epidemiology*, 1977, **6**: 143–151.
17. **Greville TNE.** Decline in tuberculosis: the death rate fails to tell the entire story. *American review of tuberculosis*, 1948, **57**: 417–419 (comments on M. Dempsey's articles).

18. **Haenszel W.** A standardized rate for mortality defined in units of lost years of life. *American journal of public health*, 1950, **40**: 17–26.

19. **Dickinson FG, Welker EL.** What is the leading cause of death? Two new measures. *Bulletin of the Bureau of Medical Economics of the American Medical Association*, 1948, **64**: 1–25.

20. **Robinson HL.** Mortality trends and public health in Canada. *Canadian journal of public health*, 1948, **39**(2): 60–70.

21. **Kohn R.** An objective mortality indicator. *Canadian journal of public health*, 1951, **42**: 375–379.

22. **Murray CJL.** The infant mortality rate, life expectancy at birth and a linear index of mortality as measures of general health status. *International journal of epidemiology*, 1987, **16**(4): 101–107.

23. **Feachem R et al.** *The health of adults in the developing world*. Oxford, Oxford University Press (for the World Bank), 1992.

24. **Anonymous.** Leads from the MMWR. Years of potential life lost before age 65 — United States, 1987. *Journal of the American Medical Association*, 1989, **261**: 823–827.

25. **Ghana Health Assessment Project Team.** A quantitative method of assessing the health impact of different diseases in less developed countries. *International journal of epidemiology*, 1981, **10**: 73–80.

26. **Drummond MF, Stoddard GL, Torrance GW.** *Methods for the economic evaluation of health care programmes*. Oxford, Oxford Medical Publications, 1987.

27. **Jamison DH et al.,** eds. *Disease control priorities in developing countries*. Oxford, Oxford University Press (for the World Bank), 1993.

28. **Ruzicka LT, Lopez AD,** eds. *Sex differentials in mortality: trends, determinants and consequences*. Canberra, Australian National University, 1983.

29. **Heligman L.** Patterns of sex differentials in mortality in less developed countries. In: Ruzicka LT, Lopez AD, eds. *Sex differentials in mortality: trends, determinants and consequences*. Canberra, Australian National University, 1983: 7–32.

30. **United Nations.** *World population prospects, 1992 assessment*. New York, United Nations, 1992.

31. **Wilkens R, Adams O, Brancker A.** Changes in mortality by income in urban Canada from 1971 to 1986. *Health reports*, 1989, **1**(2): 137–174.

32. **Pressat R.** Surmortalité biologique et surmortalité sociale. *Revue française de sociologie*, 1973, **14**: 103–110.

33. **Prost A, Prescott N.** Cost-effectiveness of blindness prevention by the Onchocerciasis Control Programme in Upper Volta, *Bulletin of the World Health Organization*, 1984, **62**: 795–802.

34. **Barnum H.** Evaluating healthy days of life gained from health projects. *Social science and medicine*, 1987, **24**: 833–841.

35. **Clearing House on Health Indexes.** *Bibliography on health indexes*. Hyattsville, MD, National Centre for Health Statistics, 1993, issue #3.

36. **Chiang CL.** *An index of health: mathematical models*. (Public Health Services Publications 1000 Series 2. No. 5). Washington, DC, National Centre for Health Statistics, 1965.

37. **Fanshel S, Bush JW.** A health-status index and its application to health services outcomes. *Operations research*, 1970, **18**: 1021–1066.

38. **Patrick DL, Bush JW, Chen MM.** Methods for measuring levels of well-being for a health-status index. *Health services research*, 1973, **8**: 228–245.

39. **Berg RL.** Weighted life expectancy as a health status index. *Health services research*, 1973, **8**: 153–156.

40. **Koplan JP.** Health promotion, quality of life, and QALYS: a useful interaction. In: *Challenges for public health statistics in the 1990s. Proceedings of the 1989 Public Health Conference on Records and Statistics*. Bethesda, Department of Health and Human Services, 1989: 294–298 (Publication No. PHS 90–1213).

41. **Torrance G, Thomas WH, Sackett DL.** A utility maximization model for evaluation of health care programmes. *Health services research*, 1972, **7**: 118–133.

42. **Weinstein M, Stason WB.** *Hypertension: a policy perspective*. Cambridge, Harvard University Press, 1976.

43. **Zeckhauser R, Shephard D.** Where now for saving lives? *Law and contemporary problems*, 1976, **40**(b): 5–45.

44. **Kaplan RM, Bush JW, Berry CC.** Health status: types of validity and the index of well-being. *Health services research*, 1976, **11**: 478–507.

45. **Torrance GW.** Measurement of health state utilities for economic appraisal: a review. *Journal of health economics*, 1986, **5**: 1–30.

46. **Nord E.** Methods for quality adjustment of life years. *Social science and medicine*, 1992, **34**: 559–569.

47. **Boyle MH, Torrance GW.** Developing multiattribute health indexes. *Medical care*, 1984, **22**: 1045–1057.

48. **Williams AH.** Economics of coronary artery bypass grafting. *British medical journal*, 1985, **291**: 326–329.

49. **Lohr KN, Ware JE Jr**, eds. Proceedings of the advances in health assessment conference. *Journal of chronic disease*, 1987, **40**(suppl 1): 1S–191S.

50. **Lohr KN,** ed. Advances in health status assessment: conference proceedings. *Medical care*, 1989, **27**(suppl): S1–S294.

51. **Lohr KN.** Advances in health status assessment: fostering the application of health status measures in clinical settings. Proceedings of a conference. *Medical care*, 1992, **30**(5) supplement: MS1–MS293.

52. **Greenfield S, Nelson EC.** Recent developments and future issues in the use of health status assessment measures in clinical settings. *Medical care*, 1992, **30**(5) supplement: MS23–MS41.

53. *International classification of impairment, disability and handicap*. Geneva, World Health Organization, 1980.

54. **Réseau Espérance de Vie en Santé.** *Statistical world yearbook. Retrospective 1993 issue*. Montpellier, INSERM, 1993.

55. **Robine JM, Mathers CD, Bucquet D.** Distinguishing health expectancies and health-adjusted life expectancies from quality-adjusted life years. *American journal of public health*, 1993, **83**: 797–798.

56. **Oregon Health Services Commission.** *Prioritization of health services: A report to the Governor and*

Legislature. Portland, State of Oregon, 1991.
57. **Hadorn DC.** Setting health care priorities in Oregon: cost-effectiveness meets the Rule of Rescue. *Journal of the American Medical Association*, 1991, **265**: 2218–2225.
58. **Dasgupta P, Marglin S, Sen A.** *Guidelines for project evaluation*. New York, United Nations, 1972.
59. **Lind R.** *Discounting for time and risk in energy policy*. Baltimore, Johns Hopkins University Press, 1982.
60. **Little I, Mirrlees J.** *Project appraisal and planning for developing countries*. London, Heinemann, 1974.
61. **Hartman RW.** One thousand points of light seeking a number: A case study of CBO's search for a discount rate policy. *Journal of environmental economics and management*, 1990, **18**: S3–S7.
62. **Martens LLM, van Doorslaer EKA.** Dealing with discounting. *International journal of technology assessment in health care*, 1990, **6**: 139–145.
63. **Fuchs V.** *The health economy*. Cambridge, Harvard University Press, 1986.
64. **Fuchs V, Zeckhauser R.** Valuing health — a priceless commodity? *American economic review*, 1987, **77**: 263–268.
65. **Hammit J.** Discounting health increments. *Journal of health economics*, 1993, **12**: 117–120.
66. **Krahn M, Gafna A.** Discounting in the economic evaluation of health care interventions. *Medical care*, 1993, **31**: 403–418.
67. **Olsen J.** On what basis should health be discounted. *Journal of health economics*, 1993, **12**: 39–53.
68. **Viscusi WK, Moore M.** Rates of time preference and valuations of the durations of life. *Journal of public economics*, 1989, **38**: 297–317.
69. **Johannesson M.** On the discounting of gained life-years in cost-effectiveness analysis. *International journal of technology assessment in health care*, 1992, **8**: 359–364.
70. **Anonymous.** Discounting health care: only a matter of timing? *Lancet*, 1992, **340**: 148–149.
71. **Parsonage M, Neuberger H.** Discounting and health benefits. *Health economics*, 1992, **1**: 71–76.
72. **Cairns J.** Discounting and health benefits: another perspective. *Health economics*, 1992, **1**: 76–79.
73. **Messing SD.** Discounting health: the issue of subsistence and care in an underdeveloped country. *Social science and medicine*, 1973, **7**: 911–916.
74. **Ganiats TG.** On sale: future health care. The paradox of discounting. *Western journal of medicine*, 1992, **156**: 550–553.
75. **Keeler E, Cretin S.** Discounting of life-saving and other nonmonetary effects. *Management science*, 1983, **29**: 300–306.

Global and regional cause-of-death patterns in 1990

C.J.L. Murray[1] & A.D. Lopez[2]

Demographic estimation techniques suggest that worldwide about 50 million deaths occur each year, of which about 39 million are in the developing countries. In countries with adequate registration of vital statistics, the age at death and the cause can be reliably determined. Only about 30–35% of all deaths are captured by vital registration (excluding sample registration schemes); for the remainder, cause-of-death estimation procedures are required. Indirect methods which model the cause-of-death structure as a function of the level of mortality can provide reasonable estimates for broad cause-of-death groups. Such methods are generally unreliable for more specific causes. In this case, estimates can be constructed from community-level mortality surveillance systems or from epidemiological evidence on specific diseases. Some check on the plausibility of the estimates is possible in view of the hierarchical structure of cause-of-death lists and the well-known age-specific patterns of diseases and injuries.

The results of applying these methods to estimate the causes of death for over 120 diseases or injuries, by age, sex and region, are described. The estimates have been derived in order to calculate the years of life lost due to premature death, one of the two components of overall disability-adjusted life years (DALYs) calculated for the 1993 World development report. Previous attempts at cause-of-death estimation have been limited to a few diseases only, with little age-specific detail. The estimates reported in detail here should serve as a useful reference for further public health research to support the determination of health sector priorities.

Introduction

Reliable information on global and regional deaths by cause are an essential input to planning, managing and evaluating the performance of the health sector in developing countries. The numbers of deaths by cause influence the manner in which resources are allocated to different service programmes and research activities. An accurate assessment of current death rates by cause in different regions also forms the baseline against which new health programmes must be evaluated. Without a reasonable baseline, we shall not, in 5 or 10 years from now, be able to assess what has worked and what has failed. In addition, reliable information on deaths by cause is an essential input to the assessment of the cost-effectiveness of new technologies for disease control and health promotion. The epidemiological transition, where the cause-of-death structure shifts profoundly from infectious to chronic diseases, is under way in most middle-income countries and among the richer communities in low-income countries (1, 2). Estimating the cause-of-death pattern for 1990 will also provide a quantification of the extent to which this pattern has changed in different regions and for the developing world as a whole.

While data on deaths by cause are required for objective planning and evaluation of the health sector, the available datasets are wholly inadequate. A decade ago, claims concerning child and adult mortality by disease-specific programmes at the World Health Organization and by individual disease experts exceeded the total deaths in each age group by two- to threefold. Through the efforts of the World Bank and WHO, more consistent estimates of mortality, by cause, under age 5 have been developed although these still remain uncertain. Moreover, no plausible or consistent estimates for death over age 5 exist despite their increasing importance in the context of the epidemiological transition. The purpose of the present analysis is to redress these gaps in critical information. We present summary results from the Global Burden of Disease study, which involved over 100 disease experts (see Acknowledgements) and was a basic input into the World Bank's *1993 World development report: Investing in health (3).*

[1] Assistant Professor of International Health Economics, Harvard Center for Population and Development Studies, 9 Bow Street, Cambridge MA 02138, USA. Requests for reprints should be sent to this author.

[2] Scientist, Tobacco or Health Programme, World Health Organization, Geneva, Switzerland.

Reprinted from *Bulletin of the World Health Organization*, 1994, **72** (3): 447–480.

21

Attempts to estimate global mortality by cause are not new. The basic problem is that reliable vital registration data, with the cause of death coded by a physician, are available for only a small number of mostly developed countries (4). Estimates of mortality by cause need to be based on other approaches for virtually all of the populations of sub-Saharan Africa, most of Asia, the Middle East and North Africa. Indirect techniques to do this were first developed by Preston to model the relationship between total mortality and cause-specific mortality for broad groups of causes, based on an analysis of historical vital registration data for the developed and a few developing countries (5). In particular, cause-specific mortality was postulated to be a *linear* function of total mortality. Preston's work has formed the basis of nearly all subsequent approaches to estimating causes of death in regions without vital registration. Several others have refined the approach by estimating equations for specific age groups, incorporating more recent data or examining more detailed lists (6–9).[a]

It is axiomatic that models only capture the relationship between cause-specific mortality and total mortality present in the countries with data. As few developing countries (particularly those with higher mortality) have good vital registration data, these model estimates are largely based on the experience of developed countries with a low mortality. Even the historical data for moderate levels of mortality in developed countries included in Preston's analysis tend to underestimate the mortality from communicable diseases. The relevance of models built on historical data is also affected by problems of diagnostic quality, revisions to the International Classification of Diseases, and basic differences in disease epidemiology in different regions. Furthermore, changes in cause-specific mortality with respect to total mortality are difficult to interpret in view of the parallel decline in the proportion of deaths coded to senility and ill-defined conditions. Our premise is that model estimates of cause-specific mortality are reasonable for large groups of causes. Model-based estimates for detailed causes, however, are probably not valid.

Recent studies have employed alternative procedures for estimating specific causes of death based on a review of data from disease-specific surveillance systems and the epidemiological literature (10, 11). Estimates of mortality from a particular cause such as malaria can be built up from epidemiological data on incidence, remission, and case-fatality rates. The major limitation of the epidemiological approach to cause-of-death estimation is the lack of data for many diseases in many regions. There is also a tendency for the epidemiological approach to yield higher estimates than vital registration or model-based estimates, possibly because disease-specific analyses tend to be more inclusive than exclusive.

The estimates presented in this report use a combination of data sources and approaches, exploiting vital registration data where available, using models of the epidemiological transition to estimate broad causes, and supplementing these with a distillation of disease-specific data sources. Not only have estimates been derived for very many more causes than previous attempts at global estimation, but they have also been presented for specific age groups. In considering several competing and exhaustive causes simultaneously, we have also been constrained by independent estimates of total mortality by age. This is clearly not relevant for disease-specific estimates carried out in isolation and is a major reason why the estimates reported here for several diseases are lower than previously claimed.

Methods

Cause-of-death estimates for the developing and developed world depend first on estimates of the total mortality by age and sex. These deaths can then be attributed to particular causes. The analysis in this study is based on the following eight geographical regions as given in the *World development report 1993* (3): the Established Market Economies (EME), the Former Socialist Economies of Europe (FSE), Latin America and the Caribbean (LAC), China (CHN), India (IND), Other Asia and Islands (OAI), Middle Eastern Crescent (which includes North Africa, the Middle East, Pakistan and the Central Asian Republics of the Former Soviet Union) (MEC), and Sub-Saharan Africa (SSA). The demographic estimates of mortality by age and sex have been developed by the World Bank. The database for estimating child mortality is unquestionably much better developed than that for adult mortality (12). Indeed, there is considerable controversy among demographers over the levels of adult mortality in some developing regions without good vital registration systems, where mortality was estimated indirectly from census and survey data. For example, the United Nations Population Division and the World Bank estimates of adult mortality by age and sex can differ by as much as 50%, but in general the differences are smaller.

---

[a] **Bulatao RA, Stephens PW.** *Estimates and projections of mortality by cause: a global overview, 1970–2015.* Unpublished manuscript prepared for the World Bank, 1991.

The cause-of-death groupings and detailed causes examined were initially developed by Murray et al. (9). Their system was extensively modified for the Global Burden of Disease study, preserving however the division of mortality into three large groups: communicable, maternal and perinatal (I); noncommunicable (II); and injuries (III). These are then further subdivided into several more specific causes. A list of causes selected for the study is given in the Annex. Clearly, this list, by being selective, has omitted some causes which, with further analysis, may justifiably be included in the future.

Our approach to attributing death to one single cause is based on the principles of the international classification of diseases: each death is coded to the underlying cause that initiated the sequence of events leading to death. For example, a patient with lung cancer who dies from respiratory failure from a post-obstructive pneumonia is coded to lung cancer. In the case of young children, where several causes may contribute significantly to death, the underlying cause has been selected as the primary cause of death, based on expert opinion about the nature of disease interactions at these ages. One disease can also be a risk factor for another. A patient with cirrhosis who dies from an oesophageal variceal bleed will be coded to cirrhosis despite the fact that his or her cirrhosis may have been caused by hepatitis B infection at an early age. Finally, deaths attributed to senility and ill-defined causes have been proportionately allocated either (if under age 5) to the communicable, maternal and perinatal causes, or (if older) to noncommunicable causes.

Our estimates of mortality by cause have been constructed from three types of estimates. First, for regions or parts of regions with good vital registration data, we have used deaths coded by the vital registration system according to the ninth revision of the International Classification of Diseases. This includes all deaths in the Established Market Economies and Former Socialist Economies, 61% of deaths in Latin America and the Caribbean, 23% of those in the Middle Eastern Crescent, and 11% of those in Other Asia and Islands (Table 1). As China does not have a complete vital registration system, a random sample of the population was monitored through the Disease Surveillance Points (DSP) system (13), in which teams (including a physician) review hospital records or interview the family to determine the cause for each death. However, not all deaths in the surveillance sites are captured by the DSP system. Underreporting is estimated at 10.8% in urban areas and 15.3% in rural areas. According to other methods for assessing completeness such as the Brass "growth-balance" method (14), the World Bank has estimated that underregistration of deaths in China is closer to 30%. Hence for China, an adjustment for underreporting was first made using the World Bank-estimated underreporting ratio, and then distributed across urban and rural areas on the basis of the information from the DSP system. For India, the Survey of Causes of Death (rural) provides useful information on lay-reported causes of death. This system collects information via a "verbal autopsy" on about one-half of 1% of all rural deaths in India, based on about 1300 primary health care centres

Table 1: **Methods for estimating causes of death and percentage of deaths registered, by region**

Region[a]	Percentage of deaths registered	Sample registration[b]	Non-registered deaths		
			Groups I, II and III	Detailed causes[c]	Adjustment algorithm[d]
EME	99				
FSE	99				
CHN		DSP		EPI	
LAC	61		Models	EPI/m	X
OAI	11		Models	EPI/m	X
MEC	23		Models	EPI/m	X
IND		SCD (R)	SCD (R)	EPI	
SSA			Models	EPI/m	X

[a] EME, Established Market Economies; FSE, Former Socialist Economies of Europe; CHN, China; LAC, Latin America and the Caribbean; OAI, Other Asia and Islands; MEC, Middle Eastern Crescent; IND, India; SSA, Sub-Saharan Africa.
[b] DSP = Disease Surveillance Points system in China. SCD (R) = Survey of Causes of Death (rural) in India.
[c] EPI = epidemiological estimates. EPI/m = epidemiological estimates and model estimates.
[d] X indicates that an adjustment algorithm was used.

spread throughout the country. This dataset has been used to establish the size of Groups I, II and III and for some finer information on injuries (Table 1).

The second main source is model-derived estimates of cause-of-death patterns based on total age-specific mortality. Building on the original work of Preston, we examined the relationship between Groups I, II and III mortality and total mortality for each age group. Data for the latest available year and a year from the 1950s from all countries, assessed as having complete and reliable vital registration, were included to expand the number of countries with moderate or high mortality in the sample. The relationship between Groups I and II and total mortality is non-linear; at higher mortality rates, Group I begins to increase faster. As a result, linear regression equations will tend to underestimate Group I mortality, particularly at higher mortality levels. To address this bias, natural log regression equations were used; the predicted mortality for Groups I, II and III from the equations was then adjusted to equal the total mortality. With a few exceptions, the coefficients for total mortality and the intercept were statistically significant (<0.05). Group III (injuries) had non-significant intercepts at ages 0–4, 15–29, 60–69 and 70+ years. It is important to emphasize, however, that because many of the slopes and intercepts in the age group 70+ were not significant, we have less confidence in predicting even the highest level disaggregration of mortality into the causes for this age group.

The third source of estimates is built up from studies by disease experts on the regional epidemiology of specific diseases. Specialists in diseases or injuries contributed their assessment of incidence, prevalence, remission and case-fatality rates based on review of existing data for each disease. These estimates were carefully evaluated for internal consistency utilizing a competing-risks computer model. Any internal inconsistencies were reviewed with disease experts and revised. The age pattern of predicted mortality by cause was also carefully reviewed for plausibility.

Estimates for Groups I, II and III totals, by age and sex, for the EME and FSE regions were based on vital registration data. For MEC, OAI and LAC regions, vital registration data for the subcomponent of the respective region with good registration were combined with model estimates for the residual parts. In China, the adjusted data from the Disease Surveillance Points system were applied to the total urban and rural population. In India, the Survey of Causes of Death (rural) system was used (15). For Sub-Saharan Africa, the Groups I, II and III totals were based solely on model estimates. All those regions or subregions with model estimates were subject to revision as discussed below.

The following approach was used for the detailed causes. For EME and FSE regions, only minor adjustments were made to the vital registration data for deaths due to HIV infection. For LAC, vital registration data were used for the subregion with good registrations and this age-sex-specific distribution of causes (within Groups I, II, and III) was then used in the other parts of that region. For example, the percent of Group II mortality due to lung cancer within any age-sex group would be taken to be approximately similar in the areas with and without registration. Adjustments in both subregions were made for some Group I causes, (e.g., vaccine-preventable diseases) based on specific epidemiological data. For China, the age-specific proportions suggested by the DSP system were adopted with minor adjustments. For the majority of OAI, MEC, India, and Sub-Saharan Africa, most of the estimates were based on the epidemiological approach. Alternative methods were developed for clusters of causes including cancers, neuropsychiatric disorders, cardiovascular diseases, chronic respiratory diseases, and injuries as outlined below.

Total cancer deaths for OAI, MEC, IND, and SSA regions by age groups were based on the models. These were then distributed by site as follows. Firstly, the distribution of deaths by site was obtained by multiplying the incidence recorded at IARC (International Agency for Research on Cancer) regional cancer registries and the case-fatality rates recorded in cancer registries with the best follow-up by IARC (16). This distribution of deaths was then applied to the total number of cancer deaths suggested by the models to yield the estimated deaths by site.

For these same four regions, the total deaths by age and sex for neuropsychiatric causes were based on the models, whereas the estimates for detailed causes were based on the average percent distribution of mortality within each age-sex group recorded by vital registration systems in the other four regions (i.e., EME, FSE, LAC and CHN). A similar approach was taken for estimating asthma and chronic obstructive pulmonary disease (COPD) from total chronic respiratory mortality, based on vital registration data disaggregrated into the ICD 3- and 4-digit codes for about 20 countries. A large number of deaths in China coded to cor pulmonale were transferred to COPD, based on discussions with those familiar with the cause-of-death coding applied in the DSP system.

Estimates of total cardiovascular mortality for OAI, MEC, IND, and SSA regions were based on the models. Four detailed causes, or groups of causes, were identified: rheumatic heart disease, ischaemic heart disease, cerebrovascular disease, and a new category entitled "inflammatory heart disease" (pericarditis, endocarditis, myocarditis and cardiomyopathies). Small autopsy series, clinical case studies and limited survey data suggest that this last category is an important cause of death in high mortality populations. For each of these four causes, local studies have been used to qualitatively score the relative risk of each cause in each region. Using actual data from EME, FSE, LAC and CHN, these qualitative scores have been converted into percent distributions by cause for each age and sex group. (This is an obviously crude approach given the importance of cardiovascular causes of death, but it does provide preliminary estimates of the possible mortality due to cardiopathologies in high-mortality populations).

Because the pattern of injury mortality by detailed cause is highly variable across regions and within regions, no satisfactory method is available to predict local injury patterns; in China, for example, suicides and drownings predominate. We have therefore used the average percent distribution of injuries by age and sex for EME, FSE, LAC and CHN to estimate the pattern of detailed injuries for the other four regions, supplemented by the available epidemiological information on injury patterns.

Initial estimates of Group I mortality (communicable, maternal or perinatal), based on the epidemiological approach (i.e., summation of estimates by experts in specific diseases), considerably exceeded the total Group I mortality by 200–300% for men in some age groups in MEC, OAI, IND, and SSA. In these regions, therefore, the reduction in cause-specific Group I numbers to equal Group I deaths produces particularly important differences between the present and previous estimates. As all epidemiological estimates were subject to the same critical review, they were all considered equally plausible. Hence, an algorithm was developed to proportionately reduce all Group I causes equally.

Essentially, the algorithm was as follows: if the overestimation was less than 10%, then all causes were equally reduced to sum to the total available Group I mortality for that age-sex group. Otherwise an alternative Group I total was defined for each age-sex group using the constant (intercept) in the regression equation, plus 1 standard deviation (Fig. 1).

Adjustments were then also made so that Groups I, II and III summed to the total mortality. This new equation defined the Group I upper bound. Where Group I was overestimated by more than 10%, each cause was automatically reduced by 10%. If the resulting estimate was outside of the Group I upper bound, the upper-bound estimate of Group I was used instead and the detailed causes were proportionately reduced to equal the new Group I total. If the

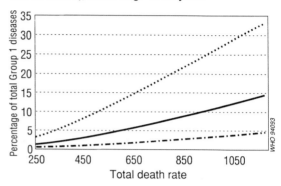

Fig. 1. **Predicted Group I versus total standardized death rates, plus and minus 1 standard error (top and bottom curves), females age 45–59 years.**

resulting estimate, after a 10% reduction, was smaller than the Group I upper bound, then the estimates were used without further modification. Fig. 1 illustrates how the width of the confidence band increases dramatically with rising overall mortality, based on the estimates for women aged 45–59 years.

Results

Fig. 2 illustrates the profound differences in cause-of-death structure between developed and developing regions due to differences both in population age structure and, more importantly, in the age-specific mortality rates for different groups of diseases. Group I (communicable, maternal or perinatal causes) accounts for 40% of the deaths in developing regions but only 5% of deaths in developed regions. Group III (injuries) causes roughly the same proportion (8–9%) of deaths in both regions but are twice as common among males than females.

For the developing regions as a whole, one in every two deaths now occurs from noncommunicable diseases. Indeed, the ratio of deaths from Group II to Group I causes, which is a rough indicator of the epidemiological transition, is about 5 in China, and 2 in Latin America, compared with about 17 in developed regions and unity elsewhere in the developing world, except for Sub-Saharan Africa where Group I causes are still 2–3 times more common than Group II. The relative importance of injuries (Group III) in the cause-of-death structure is least in the industrialized countries and India (6–6.5% of all deaths), rising to just under 10% in Eastern Europe and Latin America, and to almost 12% in China.

Detailed mortality estimates for 120 causes by age and sex, separately for developed and developing regions, are given in the Annex; to facilitate the

Fig. 2. **Probabilities of dying from three groups of causes for males and females, by age group and region, 1990.**
(EME, Established Market Economies; FSE, Former Socialist Economies; CHN, China; LAC, Latin America and Caribbean; OAI, Other Asia and Islands; MEC, Middle Eastern Crescent; IND, India; SSA, Sub-Saharan Africa).

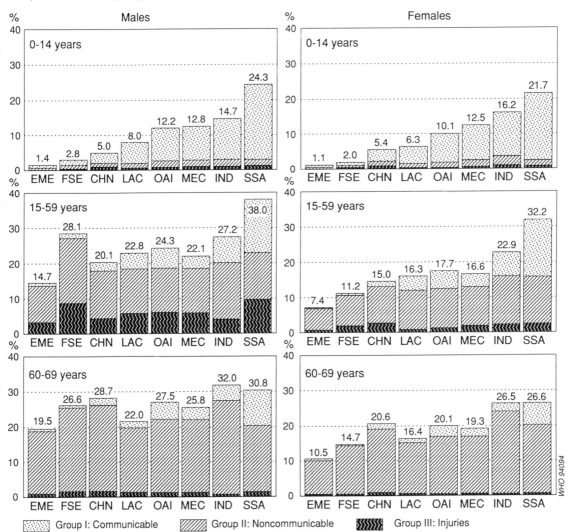

computation of rates, this tabulation also gives the estimated populations at risk in 1990, by age and sex, for the two broad regions.

It is important to note, however, that there is substantial epidemiological diversity among both developed and developing countries. Some populations in Latin America and East Asia have patterns of mortality similar to those in industrialized countries and very different from those in other developing regions. Death rates are considerably higher in Eastern Europe than in other developed countries.

These differences are clear from Fig. 2 which shows the risks of dying for three age groups (0–14, 15–59, and 60–69 years) from the three broad groups of causes in each region.

On average, a newborn child in the Established Market Economies has only a 1% chance of dying before reaching adulthood (age 15 years), which is markedly lower than the 20–25% risk in Sub-Saharan Africa. Almost all of this excess mortality arises from Group I causes. The risk of childhood death is also comparatively low in China, with the probability of dying being roughly similar for boys and girls. The only other region with a relatively small difference in survival chances between males and females is MEC; otherwise, male death rates are considerably higher than those for females and are due almost entirely to the higher death rates from Group I causes.

During adulthood (15–59 years) the risk of death in all regions is largely determined by the noncommunicable diseases, although Group I causes still contribute significantly in Sub-Saharan Africa and, to a lesser extent, in India. The risk of death from injuries is a major public health problem among males in all regions, but is particularly high (one-third of the overall risk) in FSE. Interestingly, the risk of death in adulthood (15–59 years) from noncommunicable diseases is higher for both men and women in all developing regions compared with the Established Market Economies, something which is not widely appreciated but is consistent with the pattern observed in the industrialized countries earlier this century. The excess is less marked for males, however, owing to the impact of tobacco (17). Smoking-related mortality is one of the principal factors underlying the comparatively high risk of death (18.5%) from noncommunicable diseases among adult males in Eastern Europe, typically accounting for about 40% of male deaths at these ages. At older ages (60 to 69 years), mortality is dominated by the noncommunicable diseases, although even at these ages a substantial risk of death from communicable diseases in Sub-Saharan Africa remains. At these ages, the comparative advantage in survival prob-ability enjoyed by the EME countries is considerably less (the excess compared with SSA and IND being 1.5–2), which reflects the progressive convergence of mortality risks with advancing age.

Developed regions (11 million deaths)

Comparatively few deaths in developed countries are now due to communicable, maternal or perinatal causes (see Table 2). Of half a million such deaths, a quarter of a million involve respiratory infections in middle age or particularly old age, and should perhaps be considered together with the noncommunicable respiratory deaths. The remainder include perinatal conditions (90 000 deaths, virtually all occurring in the first few weeks of life), and HIV infection (40 000 deaths in 1990, but with substantial increases expected).

Where communicable diseases are rare, the large majority of the deaths are due to noncommunicable diseases: cardiovascular diseases alone cause 5.3 million deaths a year (half of them from ischaemic heart disease and a quarter from stroke), malignant neoplasms caused 2.4 million deaths (0.5 million from lung cancer, plus 0.25 million from other tobacco-related cancers, such as mouth, pharynx, oesophagus, pancreas and bladder), and the most important remaining category is respiratory disease, which causes 0.5 million deaths (chiefly from chronic obstructive pulmonary disease). The importance of diabetes is underestimated in these Tables, because it can also cause death indirectly, by increasing the incidence of heart disease and stroke.

Table 2: **Distribution of deaths from three groups of causes, by region, 1990**

Region[a]	I. Communicable, maternal and perinatal causes		II. Noncommunicable causes		III. Injuries		Total
	No. of deaths (× 1000) attributed to:						
EME	439	(6.2)[b]	6 238	(87.6)	445	(6.2)	7 121
FSE	136	(3.6)	3 264	(86.8)	362	(9.6)	3 762
CHN	1 343	(15.1)	6 519	(73.4)	1 023	(11.5)	8 885
LAC	966	(32.3)	1 733	(57.9)	293	(9.8)	2 992
OAI	2 306	(41.8)	2 736	(49.6)	477	(8.6)	5 519
MEC	2 026	(46.2)	1 966	(44.8)	392	(8.9)	4 384
IND	4 060	(43.3)	4 700	(50.2)	611	(6.5)	9 371
SSA	5 415	(68.2)	1 898	(23.9)	624	(7.9)	7 937
World	16 690	(33.4)	29 055	(58.1)	4 227	(8.5)	49 971

[a] EME, Established Market Economies; FSE, Former Socialist Economies; CHN, China; LAC, Latin America and the Caribbean; OAI, Other Asia and Islands; MEC, Middle Eastern Crescent; IND, India; SSA, Sub-Saharan Africa.
[b] Figures in parentheses are percentages.

Developing regions (39 million deaths)

Age 0–14 years (15 million deaths). At present, about 13 million children aged 0–4 years die each year in the developing regions, the three chief causes being conditions arising in the perinatal period, diarrhoea, and acute respiratory infections. Other leading causes include measles, malaria, tetanus and pertussis. There are about another 2.2 million deaths each year at ages 5–14 in the developing regions, of which 1.3 million involve communicable diseases (primarily the same ones that dominate the under-5 pattern, but with the notable addition of 150 000 deaths from tuberculosis). Injuries (most notably from drowning or motor vehicles) are a major cause of death throughout childhood, accounting for almost one million deaths a year.

Age 15–59 years (10 million deaths). One in 5 male deaths and, significantly, one in 3 female deaths, among adults are due to Group I conditions. Tuberculosis is a leading killer of young adults, claiming over 1.2 million lives each year, as are maternal causes, acute respiratory infections, HIV infection, malaria, diarrhoeal diseases, and syphilis. Significantly, the noncommunicable diseases dominate the cause of death structure, accounting for half of all deaths in this age group. The principal causes of premature adult mortality are similar for the developing and developed regions. In addition, several sites of cancer are major causes of adult death in developing countries, most notably liver cancer, oesophageal cancer and oropharyngeal cancer, with the mortality in each case being higher for males than females. Lung cancer is already a major cause of adult male mortality in developing countries. Pericarditis, endocarditis, myocarditis and cardiomyopathies, as well as rheumatic heart disease, are significant causes of death among adults.

Among the injuries, in addition to motor-vehicle accidents and drownings, occupational injuries claim the lives of about 86 000 male workers and some 27 000 female workers at ages 15–59 years. There is also a very substantial mortality among adults due to suicide (480 000 deaths, 45% of whom were women) and war (about 160 000 males and 70 000 females).

Comparative mortality is perhaps better assessed by examining the *risks* of death. The probability of adult death from selected causes, as well as broad groups of causes, is shown in Table 3. What is most striking about this Table is the comparatively poor survival chances of adult males in Eastern Europe. Almost 3 in 10 males reaching age 15 can expect to die before age 60, twice the level in the industrialized countries and higher than anywhere else in the world, except Sub-Saharan Africa. Much of this excess is attributable to higher mortality from inju-

ries, heart disease, stroke and lung cancer. The risk of female mortality varies from 7% in the industrialized countries to 31% in Sub-Saharan Africa. Among African men, the risk of death from tuberculosis is currently four times that from AIDS.

Age 60+ (14 million deaths). Only about 10% of deaths in old age are due to Group I causes, primarily tuberculosis and acute respiratory infections; the vast majority of deaths at older ages, as in developed countries, are from noncommunicable diseases. The leading causes of death are chronic diseases similar to those identified at earlier ages of adulthood; details of the numbers of deaths estimated in 1990 can be ascertained from the Annex.

Discussion

The estimates presented here agree reasonably well with those previously reported for specific diseases or groups of diseases. They do not agree exactly, however, and we believe it is important to emphasize why. More than 100 diseases and injuries have been analysed, substantially more than the one to five conditions which have generally been estimated in specific disease reviews. This fact alone will tend to lead to lower mortality estimates simply on the basis of competing causes. Unlike many previous discussions of specific causes of death, we have been constrained to make the cause-specific deaths by age and sex sum to the total mortality for each age and sex group. Awareness of competing causes of child mortality has naturally led over the past five years to estimates that are more consistent with each other. The same cannot be said of estimates of the adult causes of death which have not been compared with each other in a consistent fashion.

The approach followed in this analysis is to try to exploit all existing data sources, based on a prudent assessment of their completeness, reliability and relevance. Public health research has led to a very substantial amount of data from community surveys, registration systems and the like which can provide important insights into cause-of-death patterns. Vital registration, or sample vital registration, or surveillance systems (where complete registration is not feasible) will always be the method of choice to provide continuous mortality data, provided that the cause of death is reliably certified. The goal of adequate registration of vital events is still beyond the means of many developing countries; in the meantime, much can be learned from other sources including hospital-based data, partial registration, and community studies that inform public health priorities.

Neither the accuracy, nor the inaccuracy of the estimation procedures employed in this study should

Table 3: Probability of dying (in %) between ages 15 and 60 years for males (M) and females (F) from selected causes, by region, 1990[a]

	Established Market Economies		Formerly Socialist Economies of Europe		China		Latin America and the Caribbean		Other Asia and Islands		Middle Eastern Crescent		India		Sub-Saharan Africa	
	M	F	M	F	M	F	M	F	M	F	M	F	M	F	M	F
All causes	14.67	7.35	28.09	11.24	20.11	14.97	22.82	16.35	24.28	17.71	22.09	16.64	27.21	22.88	38.04	32.16
Group I	*0.88*	*0.26*	*0.98*	*0.35*	*2.15*	*1.64*	*4.28*	*4.02*	*5.48*	*5.07*	*3.50*	*3.71*	*7.10*	*6.77*	*14.97*	*16.28*
Tuberculosis	—[b]	—	0.54	—	1.45	0.98	2.02	1.15	4.18	2.31	2.75	1.64	4.37	2.33	7.98	5.10
HIV infection	0.57	0.10	—	—	—	—	0.67	0.13	—	—	—	—	—	—	2.04	2.30
Diarrhoeal diseases	—	—	—	—	—	—	0.16	0.28	0.25	0.28	0.26	0.32	0.45	0.44	0.29	0.34
Malaria	—	—	—	—	—	—	0.11	0.12	0.38	0.42	—	—	0.14	0.14	0.97	1.14
Respiratory infections	0.19	0.10	0.33	0.11	0.11	—	0.50	0.62	0.45	0.49	0.27	0.33	0.79	0.80	0.71	0.84
Maternal conditions	—	—	—	—	—	0.31	—	0.68	—	1.30	—	1.11	—	2.03	—	3.64
Group II	*10.38*	*6.04*	*18.50*	*9.09*	*13.91*	*10.50*	*12.81*	*11.18*	*12.93*	*11.41*	*12.84*	*11.10*	*16.37*	*13.73*	*13.32*	*13.47*
Stomach cancer	0.33	0.18	0.95	0.43	1.06	0.58	0.35	0.18	0.39	0.22	0.36	0.23	0.37	0.21	0.30	0.31
Colorectal cancer	0.37	0.28	0.39	0.35	0.25	0.23	0.16	0.17	0.12	0.14	0.11	0.11	0.12	—	—	—
Liver cancer	0.16	—	—	—	1.81	0.59	—	—	0.66	0.20	0.15	0.10	0.14	—	0.79	0.35
Lung cancer	1.14	0.40	2.14	0.25	0.65	0.34	0.35	0.10	0.59	0.20	0.72	0.17	0.38	—	0.24	0.10
Diabetes mellitus	0.20	0.14	0.15	0.15	0.14	0.17	0.54	0.72	0.37	0.57	0.60	0.83	0.49	0.65	0.13	0.24
Rheumatic heart disease	—	—	0.30	0.33	0.39	0.64	—	0.14	0.11	0.32	0.15	0.39	0.35	0.86	0.33	0.94
Ischaemic heart disease	2.19	0.56	5.34	1.33	0.87	0.45	2.04	1.06	2.68	1.33	1.95	0.82	2.61	1.09	0.81	0.40
Cerebrovascular disease	0.63	0.42	1.93	1.29	2.06	1.75	1.52	1.46	0.96	1.23	1.41	1.50	1.08	1.32	1.73	2.16
Inflammatory cardiac diseases	0.22	0.08	0.29	0.11	0.20	0.17	1.09	0.77	0.75	0.58	1.03	0.69	2.31	1.48	2.21	1.60
Chronic obstructive lung disease	0.18	0.10	0.52	0.15	1.22	0.98	0.31	0.23	0.23	0.24	0.30	0.25	0.36	0.36	0.26	0.33
Asthma	—	—	0.12	—	—	—	0.10	0.12	—	0.12	—	0.12	0.11	0.18	—	0.16
Cirrhosis of the liver	0.71	0.26	0.45	0.16	1.00	0.47	1.38	0.43	1.17	0.50	0.70	0.36	1.42	0.58	1.30	0.64
Group III	*3.41*	*1.04*	*8.60*	*1.80*	*4.06*	*2.82*	*5.73*	*1.15*	*5.86*	*1.23*	*5.74*	*1.84*	*3.75*	*2.38*	*9.75*	*2.41*
Road traffic accidents	1.19	0.39	2.25	0.45	0.85	0.32	1.60	0.37	1.61	0.29	1.14	0.26	1.05	0.22	2.06	0.27
Suicide	1.00	0.35	1.89	0.42	1.27	1.65	0.37	0.12	1.21	0.35	0.88	0.32	0.58	0.50	1.52	0.34
Homicide and violence	0.34	0.10	0.75	0.23	0.23	0.10	1.47	0.13	0.66	0.10	0.46	—	0.20	—	0.87	0.10
War	—	—	—	—	—	—	0.22	—	—	—	1.61	0.73	—	—	2.47	1.23

[a] Probabilities have been estimated using the formula $1-e^{(-({}_{15}M_{15}+{}_{15}M_{30}+{}_{15}M_{45}))}$ where $_xM_y$ is the death rate from y to age y + x. Cause-specific risks are adjusted to sum to total mortality risk.

[b] Dash (—) equals less than 0.1 percent.

be exaggerated. Vital registration is likely to provide a good and, in many cases, a very good basis for determining the causes of death. Nevertheless, even these returns are often faulty, suffering from poor medical certification practices, diagnostic biases, sociocultural influences and so on. In the absence of vital registration, well-focused, well-maintained disease surveillance systems in defined populations can be expected to yield good epidemiological data on the causes of death. Their utility, as for vital registration, depend clearly on good coverage of events, reliable certification, and internationally comparable diagnostic procedures. Lay-reporting systems are likely to be only of use for determining broad cause-of-death categories, but even these "real" data may be preferable to indirect estimates from models of the mortality transition. Such models, as used in this study, are predicated on the average experience of the more developed countries at earlier stages of epidemiological transition and thus inherently assume the same cause-level relationships for contemporary developing countries. This is clearly highly contentious and we have therefore tried to adjust the model-based estimates, wherever possible, using direct epidemiological evidence. In some cases (such as for cancer), we have preferred to use the indirect estimates of mortality, suggested by the models, rather than estimates based on cancer incidence because the level of underreporting by registries in some areas (e.g., India) seemed to us to be sufficiently high to invalidate this approach.

Communicable, maternal and perinatal causes remain an important unfinished agenda in the developing world, much more so in Sub-Saharan Africa, India, the Middle-Eastern Crescent, and Other Asia and Islands. Some causes of mortality are now well recognized but still remain major public health challenges including acute respiratory infections, diarrhoeal diseases, measles, tetanus, HIV infection, malaria, and maternal causes. Other Group I causes such as syphilis, meningitis, and especially tuberculosis are underappreciated as causes of mortality. Models of the epidemiological transition imply a steady decline in communicable, maternal and perinatal mortality through time. It would be foolhardy, however, to take such a complacent attitude towards Group I mortality in light of their continued high levels in many parts of the world and increasing trends for some diseases, e.g., HIV infection and possibly malaria.

While recognizing the need for continued vigilance over communicable, maternal and perinatal mortality, it is important to realize that globally the noncommunicable diseases have already emerged as the leading causes of death in developing regions. Even in poor countries, the epidemiological transi-

tion is under way with profound implications on the demand for health care to address the burden of chronic diseases. Moreover, with a number of cost-effective interventions targeted to communicable disease mortality in children, it is reasonable to expect the proportion of mortality due to noncommunicable diseases to increase. At present, the *risk* of death from noncommunicable diseases during adulthood (15–60 years) is considerably higher in the developing world than in the Established Market Economies, suggesting that the future, in effect, has already arrived.

This article does not provide information on the time trend in noncommunicable diseases. The historical, statistical returns for developed countries and data for those developing countries with long series of vital registration data suggest that age-specific rates of noncommunicable diseases have declined throughout most of this century. Specific trends in noncommunicable diseases as well as the overall trend are hard to predict, as most of our causal models do not explain the sustained decline observed over the past century. While this decline is likely to continue, behavioural change in many developing regions may slow or alter this trend. Something like 50–60% of adult males in developing countries are regular smokers, and on current trends an epidemic of smoking-related mortality is inevitable (18). As a consequence, increases in lung cancer, other cancers causally related to smoking, chronic lung diseases, and cardiovascular diseases may be expected.

The estimates reported here are the result of applying several different approaches, analysing numerous data sources (some of which were not previously available), and making a large number of decisions about the relative validity of one estimate versus another. We hope that by publishing these estimates, despite their imprecision, we will encourage not only the further development of methods and data sources to improve on them, but also provide a reference to guide policy in assessing the major public health issues contributing to the disease burden at the end of this twentieth century. We have emphasized the importance of developing a baseline estimate of the cause-of-death pattern in all age groups in developing and developed regions for the purposes of planning, managing and evaluating health sector investments. Equally important for a comprehensive assessment of population health status are non-fatal health outcomes, which have not been addressed here. Mortality data, despite their limitations, are more widely available than comparable information for morbidity or disability; hence the estimation of cause-of-death patterns, despite the substantial uncertainty involved, is more reliably informed by empirical data. Nevertheless, there is clearly an urgent need for comprehensive and comparable data on non-fatal health outcomes. The broader issue of measuring both mortality and disability is addressed by the Global Burden of Disease study which provides a new integrative framework for assessing and monitoring the health of populations (*19–21*).

Acknowledgements

We should like to acknowledge the financial and/or technical support of the Edna McConnel Clark Foundation, the Rockefeller Foundation, the World Bank, and the World Health Organization. We would particularly like to thank Richard Peto for his comments on earlier drafts of this article and Caroline Cook for her tireless efforts. The following individuals generously contributed time and technical advice to this undertaking: C. Abou-Zahr, M. Adams, M. Adrian, P. Arthur, R. Ashley, A. Ashworth-Hill, K. Bailey, D. Barmes, L. Barnes, R. Beaglehole, M. Belsey, R. Berkelman, S. Berkley, S. Berman, P. Blake, B. Bloom, M. Blossner, J.L. Bobadilla, L. Brabin, U. Brinkman, J. Broomberg, C. Broome, R. Bumgarner, D. Bundy, A. Burton, J. Campbell, P. Carlevaro, P. Cattand, J. Cattani, M. Chamie, L.C. Chen, C-M. Chen, E. Cooper, P. Cowley, D. Daumerie, P. Desjeux, H. Emblad, R. Etzel, J. Ferlay, P. Fine, J. Fomey, J.C. Funck, A. Galazka, M. Garcia, M. Garenne, S. Gillespie, T. Godal, A. Goerdt, J. Gorstein, S. Gove, R. Govindaraj, M. Grant, R. Guidotti, W. Gulbinat, I. Gyarfas, F. Hamers, H.R. Hapsara, J. Harris, L. Heise, L. Heligman, P. Heller, J. Hempel, K. Hill, A. Hill, C.J. Hong, H. Jamai, D. Jamison, J.P. Jardel, E. Jimenez, F. Kaferstein, A. Kalache, M. Kane, P. Kenya, N. Khaltaev, D. Kilpatrick, H. King, B. Kirkwood, A. Kochi, J. Kumaresan, M.H. Leclerq, N. Lee, L. Lloyd, J. Lob-Levyt, L. Lopez Bravo, D. Mabey, A. Mann, P. Mahapatra, I. Martin, G. Mayberly, P. McKeigue, A. Measham, G. Medley, M. Menchaca, M. Mercier, T. Mertens, E. Michael, M. Michaud, A. Moncayo, R. Morrow, Y. Motarjemi, K. Mott, S. Nadeen, D. Negrel, W. Newbrender, M. Noel, G. Oakley, M. Orzeszyna, M. Parkin, D. Peterson, A. Pio, P. Pisani, A. Preker, J. Pronczuk, E. Pupulin, X. Qiao, G. Quinke, C. Ramachandran, R. Rannan-Eliya, H. Remme, J.M. Robine, C.J. Romer, M. Rosenberg, R. Rothenberg, P. Sandiford, N. Sartorius, A. Schapira, E. Sherwin, A. Silman, G. Smith, P. Smith, B. Smutharaks, J. Stjernsward, R. Stoneburner, T. Studwick, M. Subramanian, D. Symmons, M. Thuriaux, B. Thylefors, I. Timaeus, A. Tomkins, C. Torel, J. Tulloch, P. Vaughn, S. Vidwans, F. Vinicor, V. Waldman, G. Walker, D. Weil, J. Wenger, W. Whang, E. Wheeler, R. Wilkins, G. Yang, R. Yip, Z. Yusef, and A. Zwi. However, the views expressed in the article are entirely those of the authors.

Résumé

Répartition mondiale et régionale des causes de décès en 1990

Depuis longtemps, les renseignements sur les causes de décès sont la base statistique utilisée pour faciliter la détermination des priorités de santé et surveiller l'efficacité des interventions. Les données fiables sur les causes de décès sont toutefois loin d'être largement disponibles. Le présent article donne pour la première fois des estimations mondiales et régionales complètes des causes de décès pour les huit régions du monde définies par la Banque mondiale dans son *Rapport sur le développement dans le monde* de 1993, séparément pour les hommes et pour les femmes et pour plus de 100 causes de décès. Ces estimations ont été établies pour les classes d'âge suivantes: 0–4, 5–14, 15–44, 45–59, 60–69 et 70 ans et plus. Les tentatives antérieures pour donner des estimations mondiales et régionales des causes de décès se sont limitées à une seule cause de décès, tout au plus à quelques-unes, et à une tranche d'âge particulière (en général, le nourrisson et le jeune enfant), ou bien ont donné des estimations pour des catégories de causes de décès très larges, d'une utilité douteuse pour définir le besoin en stratégies d'intervention de santé ciblées.

Plusieurs sources de données ont été utilisées pour procéder aux estimations. L'enregistrement des statistiques de vie, soit pour la population entière d'un pays (lorsque ces données existent), soit pour un échantillon de sites d'enregistrement, a été utilisé lorsqu'il était disponible, en ajustant sur la sous-déclaration et les erreurs de déclaration de la cause initiale de décès. Pour les populations pour lesquelles ces données n'existaient pas, on a mis au point des modèles de relation niveau-cause de décès, d'après ce que l'on sait dans les pays où les données sur les causes de décès sont fiables depuis une quarantaine d'années. Ces modèles ont fourni une estimation préliminaire de la structure des causes de décès, qui a par la suite été révisée en s'appuyant sur des études au niveau de la communauté et les statistiques hospitalières. Les modèles (établis en prenant ± un écart type de la constante de régression) ont également produit un algorithme statistique servant à déterminer les limites de plausibilité des estimations.

D'après ces méthodes, les maladies non transmissibles, et principalement les maladies cardio-vasculaires, les cancers et les pneumopathies chroniques, sont les premières causes de décès dans le monde et sont maintenant devenues des causes majeures de décès dans les pays en développement. Ainsi, en 1990, d'après nos estimations, 14,3 millions de personnes sont décédées de maladies cardio-vasculaires (5,1 millions de cardiopathie ischémique, 4,6 millions d'accident cérébro-vasculaire) et 6,1 millions des suites d'un cancer (dont près d'un million d'un cancer du poumon). Si la *proportion* de décès par maladie chronique majeure est plus faible dans les pays en développement que dans les régions développées, les *risques* de décès sont supérieurs pour de nombreuses causes, en particulier chez les hommes. Il apparaît donc qu'il est urgent d'intervenir contre les maladies non transmissibles, et en particulier contre les habitudes nuisibles pour la santé sous-jacentes à leur étiologie, et ce quel que soit le niveau de développement sanitaire des pays, mais plus encore dans les pays en développement, qui comme la Chine ont fait des progrès considérables dans la lutte contre les maladies infectieuses.

Il reste toutefois que la liste est encore longue des mesures à prendre pour diminuer considérablement la mortalité prématurée par les maladies infectieuses majeures; en effet, dans leur ensemble, ces maladies tuent environ 16,7 millions de personnes chaque année qui, à un demi-million près, vivent toutes dans des pays en développement. Les premières causes de décès en 1990 par cette catégorie de maladie sont notamment les infections respiratoires aiguës (4,3 millions de décès), les maladies diarrhéiques (2,9 millions), les causes périnatales (2,5 millions), la tuberculose (2,0 millions), la rougeole et le paludisme (près d'1 million de décès pour chacune de ces maladies). Les traumatismes (intentionnels ou autres) sont des causes très importantes de décès à tous les niveaux de développement sanitaire, le nombre résultant de décès étant estimé à 4,3 millions en 1990, dont 850 000 par accident de la route, 800 000 par suicide, 380 000 par noyade et 300 000 par homicide et faits de guerre.

Ces estimations devraient être périodiquement remises à jour au fur et à mesure que des données plus récentes et plus fiables seront disponibles. Elles devraient fournir en attendant une base d'information utile permettant de fixer des priorités sanitaires dans le monde.

References

1. **Omran AR.** The epidemiological transition: a theory of the epidemiology of population change. *Milbank Memorial Fund quarterly*, 1971, **49**: 509–538.
2. **Frenk J et al.** Elements for a theory of the health transition. *Health transition review*, 1991, **1**: 21–38.
3. **The World Bank.** *World development report 1993. Investing in health*. New York, Oxford University Press, 1993.
4. **Ruzicka LT, Lopez AD.** The use of cause-of-death statistics for health situation assessment: national and international experiences. *World health statistic quarterly*, 1990, **43**: 249–259.
5. **Preston SH.** *Mortality patterns in national populations*. New York, Academic Press, 1976.
6. **Hull TH et al.** A framework for estimating causes of death in Indonesia. *Majalah demografi Indonesia*, 1981, **15**: 77–125.
7. **Lopez AD, Hull TH.** A note on estimating the cause of death structure in high mortality populations. *Population bulletin of the United Nations*, 1983, **14**: 66–70.
8. **Hakulinen T et al.** Global and regional mortality patterns by cause of death in 1980. *International journal of epidemiology*, 1986, **15**: 226–233.
9. **Murray CJL, Yang G, Qiao X.** Adult mortality: levels, patterns and causes. In: Feachem, RGS et al., *The health of adults in the developing world*. Oxford, Oxford University Press (for the World Bank) 1993: 23–111.
10. **Lopez AD.** Causes of death in the industrialized and developing countries: estimates for 1985–1990. In: Jamison, DT et al., eds. *Disease control priorities in developing countries*. Oxford, Oxford University Press (for the World Bank), 1993: 35–50.
11. **Pisani P, Parkin DM, Ferlay J.** Estimates of the worldwide mortality from eighteen major cancers in 1985: implications for prevention and projections of future burden. *International journal of cancer*, 1993, **55**: 891–903.
12. **United Nations.** *Child mortality since the 1960s: a database for developing countries*. New York, United Nations, 1992.
13. **Department of Hygiene and Immunization, Ministry of Public Health and Chinese Academy of Preventive Medicine.** 1990 annual report on disease surveillance in China. *Diseases surveillance report 1*. Beijing, Hua Xia Publishing House, 1992.
14. **Brass W.** *Methods for estimating fertility and mortality from limited and defective data*. Chapel Hill, NC, Carolina Population Centre, Laboratories for Population Studies, 1975.
15. **Registrar-General, Government of India.** Survey of causes of death (rural). *Annual report 1988*. New Delhi, Government of India, 1990.
16. **Parkin DM, Pisani P, Ferlay J.** Estimates of the worldwide incidence of eighteen major cancers in 1985. *International journal of cancer*, 1993, **54**: 594–606.
17. **Peto R et al.** Mortality from tobacco in developed countries: indirect estimates from national vital statistics. *Lancet*, 1992, **339**: 1268–1278.
18. **Peto R, Lopez AD.** Worldwide mortality from current smoking pattern. In: Durston B, Jamrozik K., eds. *Tobacco and health 1990: the global war*. Proceedings of the Seventh World Conference on Tobacco or Health. Perth, Health Department of Western Australia, 1990: 66–68.
19. **Murray CJL.** Quantifying the burden of disease: the technical basis for disability-adjusted life years. *Bulletin of the World Health Organization*, 1994, **72**: 429–445.
20. **Murray CJL, Lopez AD.** Quantifying disability: data, methods and results. *Bulletin of the World Health Organization*, 1994, **72**: 481–494.
21. **Murray CJL, Lopez AD, Jamison DT.** The global burden of disease in 1990: summary results, sensitivity analysis and future directions. *Bulletin of the World Health Organization*, 1994, **72**: 495–509.

Annex

Estimated deaths (in thousands) by age, sex and cause, 1990: Developed Regions

No. of deaths (in thousands)

Cause of Death (ICD 9)	Both sexes	Males								Females							
		0-4	5-14	15-29	30-44	45-59	60-69	70+	All ages	0-4	5-14	15-29	30-44	45-59	60-69	70+	All ages
Population (in millions)	1,144.0	40.1	80.7	130.0	130.4	93.1	48.4	33.1	555.8	38.2	77.1	125.0	129.2	97.8	60.7	60.3	588.2
All Causes	10,883.1	123.1	28.7	190.6	357.5	886.9	1,181.8	2,782.1	5,550.6	90.5	17.1	61.8	143.0	422.9	767.1	3,830.2	5,332.5
I. Communicable, maternal & perinatal	574.7	73.3	1.5	9.9	32.1	30.9	29.3	138.7	315.8	52.0	1.3	4.8	8.3	9.2	16.0	167.1	258.9
A. Infectious & parasitic	153.0	8.6	–	8.1	27.4	20.0	12.2	23.5	100.4	6.5	–	2.2	4.7	4.8	6.6	27.2	52.7
A1. Tuberculosis	37.5	–	–	1.0	5.4	8.9	6.0	7.6	29.0	–	–	–	–	1.3	1.8	4.4	8.5
A2. Syphilis	1.1	–	–	–	–	–	–	–	–	–	–	–	–	–	–	–	–
A3. HIV	42.8	1.1	–	5.6	18.4	8.7	–	1.2	35.6	1.1	–	1.5	3.3	–	–	–	7.2
A4. Diarrhoeal diseases	6.9	2.1	–	–	–	–	–	–	3.4	1.8	–	–	–	–	–	1.4	3.5
a. Acute watery	6.6	2.0	–	–	–	–	–	–	3.2	1.7	–	–	–	–	–	1.3	3.4
b. Persistent	–	–	–	–	–	–	–	–	–	–	–	–	–	–	–	–	–
c. Dysentery	–	–	–	–	–	–	–	–	–	–	–	–	–	–	–	–	–
A5. Pertussis	–	–	–	–	–	–	–	–	–	–	–	–	–	–	–	–	–
A6. Measles	–	–	–	–	–	–	–	–	–	–	–	–	–	–	–	–	–
A7. Tetanus	–	–	–	–	–	–	–	–	–	–	–	–	–	–	–	–	–
A8. Meningitis	10.1	2.6	–	–	–	–	–	–	5.8	1.8	–	–	–	–	–	–	4.3
A9. Malaria	–	–	–	–	–	–	–	–	–	–	–	–	–	–	–	–	–
A10. Trypanosomiasis	–	–	–	–	–	–	–	–	–	–	–	–	–	–	–	–	–
A11. Chagas disease	–	–	–	–	–	–	–	–	–	–	–	–	–	–	–	–	–
A12. Schistosomiasis	–	–	–	–	–	–	–	–	–	–	–	–	–	–	–	–	–
A13. Leishmaniasis	–	–	–	–	–	–	–	–	–	–	–	–	–	–	–	–	–
A14. Onchocerciasis	–	–	–	–	–	–	–	–	–	–	–	–	–	–	–	–	–
B. Respiratory infections	330.0	12.4	–	1.8	4.7	11.0	17.1	115.3	163.1	9.3	–	1.2	2.1	4.3	9.4	139.9	166.9
C. Maternal causes	3.0	–	–	–	–	–	–	–	–	–	–	1.5	1.5	–	–	–	3.0
C1. Haemorrhage	–	–	–	–	–	–	–	–	–	–	–	–	–	–	–	–	–
C2. Sepsis	–	–	–	–	–	–	–	–	–	–	–	–	–	–	–	–	–
C3. Eclampsia	–	–	–	–	–	–	–	–	–	–	–	–	–	–	–	–	–
C4. Hypertension	–	–	–	–	–	–	–	–	–	–	–	–	–	–	–	–	–
C5. Obstructed labour	–	–	–	–	–	–	–	–	–	–	–	–	–	–	–	–	–
C6. Abortion	1.1	–	–	–	–	–	–	–	–	–	–	–	–	–	–	–	1.1
D. Perinatal causes	88.7	52.3	–	–	–	–	–	–	52.4	36.2	–	–	–	–	–	–	36.3
III. Injuries	806.6	12.5	16.3	139.1	149.8	122.0	55.9	75.8	571.4	8.4	7.3	30.7	33.4	36.1	27.6	91.9	235.2
A. Unintentional	557.7	11.8	14.8	95.3	93.4	79.1	37.1	55.4	386.8	7.7	6.5	20.5	18.8	21.3	18.0	78.2	170.9
A1. Road traffic accidents	218.8	2.3	6.2	60.2	39.4	26.9	13.0	14.4	162.3	1.5	3.4	14.6	9.4	8.7	9.0	12.0	56.5
A2. Poisoning	55.8	–	–	5.4	15.2	14.1	3.9	1.9	41.9	–	–	1.5	3.0	3.9	2.0	2.5	13.9
A3. Falls	96.7	–	–	3.3	6.0	7.8	5.8	21.2	45.2	–	–	–	–	1.8	3.1	44.5	51.4
A4. Fires	17.9	1.1	1.4	1.4	2.3	2.3	1.3	2.1	11.0	–	–	–	–	–	–	2.7	6.9
A5. Drowning	35.6	2.0	3.4	7.2	7.4	4.9	2.0	1.8	28.7	–	–	–	1.4	1.2	–	1.8	6.9
A6. Occupational	21.9	–	–	2.9	8.8	6.7	–	–	18.8	–	1.0	–	1.4	–	–	–	3.1
B. Intentional	248.9	–	1.5	43.8	56.4	43.0	18.8	20.4	184.6	–	–	10.2	14.6	14.8	9.6	13.7	64.3
B1. Self-inflicted	189.5	–	–	27.7	40.2	35.8	16.7	19.1	140.4	–	–	6.4	9.9	12.1	8.4	12.1	49.1
B2. Homicide and violence	59.3	–	–	16.1	16.1	7.1	2.1	1.3	44.1	–	–	3.8	4.6	2.7	1.3	1.6	15.2
B3. War	–	–	–	–	–	–	–	–	–	–	–	–	–	–	–	–	–

A dash (–) indicates less than 1000 deaths.

Estimated deaths (in thousands) by age, sex and cause, 1990: Developed Regions

No. of deaths (in thousands)

Cause of Death (ICD 9)	Both sexes	Males								Females							
		0-4	5-14	15-29	30-44	45-59	60-69	70+	All ages	0-4	5-14	15-29	30-44	45-59	60-69	70+	All ages
II. Noncommunicable	9,501.8	37.3	10.9	41.6	175.5	733.9	1,096.6	2,567.6	4,663.4	30.1	8.5	26.3	101.3	377.6	723.4	3,571.2	4,838.4
A. Malignant neoplasms	2,430.8	2.3	4.3	12.3	50.2	279.7	401.8	603.4	1,353.9	1.8	3.1	9.2	51.9	181.2	263.7	565.9	1,076.8
A1. Mouth and oropharynx	50.5	-	-	-	2.8	14.9	11.8	9.6	39.3	-	-	-	-	2.1	2.7	5.8	11.2
A2. Oesophagus	57.7	-	-	-	1.3	12.3	14.5	15.2	43.3	-	-	-	-	1.7	3.2	9.2	14.3
A3. Stomach	244.0	-	-	-	5.6	32.0	42.3	63.0	143.4	-	-	-	4.2	13.7	22.4	59.8	100.6
A4. Colorectal	280.4	-	-	-	4.0	22.5	37.9	71.2	136.1	-	-	-	3.6	17.7	31.6	91.2	144.3
A5. Liver	43.9	-	-	-	-	7.7	11.1	10.5	30.5	-	-	-	-	1.7	3.9	7.5	13.4
A6. Pancreas	96.3	-	-	-	1.5	9.1	14.8	23.5	49.1	-	-	-	-	5.0	10.9	30.4	47.2
A7. Lung	526.4	-	-	-	9.8	93.8	140.2	157.8	402.1	-	-	-	3.4	21.2	38.7	60.8	124.4
A8. Breast	174.9									-	-	-	15.5	45.8	43.7	69.3	174.9
A9. Cervix	31.5									-	-	-	4.6	7.7	8.0	10.7	31.5
A10. Ovary	55.7									-	-	-	2.7	12.6	16.2	23.7	55.7
A11. Prostate	107.7	-	-	-	-	4.3	19.6	83.6	107.7								
A12. Bladder	70.8	-	-	-	-	6.9	13.4	29.6	50.9	-	-	-	-	1.8	4.1	13.7	20.0
A13. Lymphoma	96.2	-	2.2	2.2	4.2	9.8	12.9	21.2	51.0	-	-	1.2	2.2	5.9	10.4	25.0	45.1
A14. Leukemia	76.7	1.7	-	2.9	3.3	6.5	9.3	17.4	41.8	-	1.2	1.7	2.6	4.9	6.8	17.2	34.9
B. Diabetes mellitus	176.5	-	-	-	3.2	9.7	16.5	38.5	68.7	-	-	-	1.8	7.7	20.9	76.6	107.8
C. Nutritional/endocrine	73.6	1.4	-	1.2	1.6	3.7	5.8	17.4	31.7	1.2	-	1.3	1.3	3.3	5.1	29.0	41.9
C1. Protein-energy malnutrition	6.3	-	-	-	-	-	-	1.8	2.3	-	-	-	-	-	-	3.6	4.0
C2. Anaemia	16.7	-	-	-	-	-	-	4.5	7.1	-	-	-	-	-	-	7.2	9.7
D. Neuro-psychiatric	232.1	2.3	1.8	7.2	12.6	17.8	16.3	55.3	113.3	1.9	1.4	3.3	5.4	8.8	11.7	86.5	118.8
D1. Psychoses	15.7	-	-	-	-	1.1	1.0	3.8	6.8	-	-	-	-	-	-	7.4	8.9
D2. Epilepsy	12.7	-	-	1.5	2.3	1.8	-	-	7.8	-	-	-	1.0	-	-	1.0	4.9
D3. Alcohol dependence	21.8	-	-	-	4.1	7.6	3.7	1.8	17.6	-	-	-	-	1.7	-	-	4.2
D4. Alzheimer & other dementias	94.8	-	-	-	-	2.4	5.2	26.6	36.0	-	-	-	-	1.7	4.8	50.9	58.7
D5. Parkinson disease	30.2	-	-	-	-	-	1.6	13.6	15.5	-	-	-	-	-	1.1	13.4	14.7
D6. Multiple sclerosis	8.4	-	-	-	-	1.2	-	-	3.4	-	-	-	1.1	1.7	1.2	-	5.0
E. Cardiovascular diseases	5,328.0	2.2	1.0	11.1	74.4	318.8	510.3	1,483.0	2,400.7	1.9	-	5.3	24.0	125.9	333.9	2,435.6	2,927.3
E1. Rheumatic diseases	45.7	-	-	-	2.4	5.6	4.0	3.9	16.6	-	-	-	1.8	7.5	8.0	11.4	29.1
E2. Ischaemic heart disease	2,678.0	-	-	2.4	38.7	190.7	298.8	752.7	1,283.4	-	-	-	6.0	49.9	163.3	1,174.9	1,394.6
E3. Cerebrovascular diseases	1,447.9	-	-	2.3	12.8	61.1	109.5	379.0	565.4	-	-	1.5	7.6	40.6	100.8	731.5	882.5
E4. Inflammatory cardiac diseases	135.7	-	-	1.8	5.3	11.4	14.3	37.2	70.7	-	-	-	1.8	4.4	7.8	49.6	64.9
F. Respiratory	508.7	1.0	-	2.0	5.0	30.5	67.1	202.6	308.7	-	-	1.4	2.8	12.7	31.4	150.6	199.9
F1. Chronic obstructive lung disease	358.3	-	-	-	1.1	18.9	50.7	157.0	228.0	-	-	-	-	7.5	22.9	99.1	130.2
F2. Asthma	34.1	-	-	-	1.3	3.3	3.6	7.3	16.6	-	-	-	1.1	2.3	3.2	10.2	17.6
G. Digestive	427.2	1.7	-	2.7	21.5	58.3	56.8	91.1	232.5	1.1	-	1.5	7.8	23.7	34.7	125.5	194.7
G1. Peptic ulcer disease	46.3	-	-	-	1.6	5.0	5.9	13.6	26.3	-	-	-	-	1.2	2.7	15.7	20.0
G2. Cirrhosis	146.3	-	-	-	12.1	33.8	28.1	22.6	97.4	-	-	-	4.2	11.9	13.5	18.8	48.8
H. Genito-urinary	168.9	-	-	1.3	3.5	8.7	13.8	55.9	83.7	-	-	-	2.5	7.2	12.3	61.7	85.1
H1. Nephritis/nephrosis	99.8	-	-	-	2.6	5.9	8.3	30.9	49.2	-	-	-	1.5	4.1	7.2	36.8	50.6
I. Musculo-skeletal	37.2	-	-	-	-	1.3	2.0	6.0	10.4	-	-	-	1.2	2.7	4.1	17.9	26.7
J. Congenital	60.8	25.3	1.6	2.0	1.3	1.1	-	1.0	33.1	20.7	1.4	1.4	1.2	1.1	-	1.3	27.7

A dash (-) indicates less than 1000 deaths.

Estimated deaths (in thousands) by age, sex and cause, 1990: Developing Regions

No. of deaths (in thousands)

Cause of Death (ICD 9)	Both sexes	Males 0-4	5-14	15-29	30-44	45-59	60-69	70+	All ages	Females 0-4	5-14	15-29	30-44	45-59	60-69	70+	All ages
Population (in millions)	4,123.4	281.2	470.5	605.9	383.7	219.3	88.4	48.9	2,097.9	271.1	448.4	577.7	366.8	213.3	90.2	58.0	2,025.5
All Causes	39,088.0	6,485.0	1,160.0	1,400.0	1,564.0	2,615.0	2,963.0	4,670.0	20,857.0	5,958.0	1,060.0	1,221.0	1,188.0	1,841.0	2,211.0	4,752.0	18,231.0
I. Communicable, maternal & perinatal	16,115.0	5,538.6	632.7	413.5	385.4	510.0	386.9	472.3	8,339.4	5,038.1	648.4	643.3	490.0	294.3	246.4	415.1	7,775.6
A. Infectious & parasitic	9,301.1	2,814.0	512.7	373.3	358.5	471.2	239.8	223.0	4,992.5	2,650.6	512.4	359.2	293.7	248.3	115.4	129.0	4,308.6
A1. Tuberculosis	1,978.0	34.3	66.8	165.7	217.3	369.1	193.9	173.7	1,220.8	37.3	84.6	160.6	152.4	164.4	79.2	78.7	757.2
A2. Syphilis	192.3	40.5	-	35.9	19.7	5.1	-	-	102.6	36.7	-	28.0	19.5	4.5	1.2	-	89.7
A3. HIV	248.0	29.1	4.7	53.8	29.1	8.9	2.8	1.4	129.9	26.7	4.9	48.0	31.1	5.5	1.2	-	118.2
A4. Diarrhoeal diseases	2,865.8	1,262.8	102.7	27.4	19.6	14.5	9.5	17.4	1,453.9	1,211.4	107.8	27.8	21.8	15.5	6.8	20.7	1,411.8
a. Acute watery	1,546.7	634.7	78.0	21.8	15.8	11.2	7.6	14.0	783.1	609.1	81.7	22.0	17.6	11.9	5.3	16.0	763.6
b. Persistent	871.3	439.2	4.9	-	-	-	-	-	444.1	421.1	5.2	-	-	-	-	-	427.2
c. Dysentery	447.8	188.9	19.8	5.6	3.8	3.4	1.9	3.4	226.8	181.1	20.9	5.8	4.2	3.6	1.4	4.0	221.0
A5. Pertussis	321.1	145.8	21.9	-	-	-	-	-	167.7	131.4	22.0	-	-	-	-	-	153.4
A6. Measles	1,006.2	441.8	69.2	-	-	-	-	-	511.1	420.7	73.9	-	-	-	-	-	495.0
A7. Tetanus	504.6	231.6	13.9	2.9	2.2	3.8	2.3	1.7	258.4	218.6	14.1	2.9	2.4	4.2	2.1	1.9	246.2
A8. Meningitis	231.7	70.5	30.0	8.8	4.2	4.9	3.0	1.5	143.1	50.1	17.8	10.1	4.8	2.4	2.2	1.3	88.6
A9. Malaria	926.3	331.5	75.7	32.5	19.1	10.2	3.6	1.9	474.5	300.5	77.0	33.2	23.7	11.3	3.9	2.3	451.9
A10. Trypanosomiasis	55.1	1.5	10.2	7.1	3.6	4.8	-	-	28.2	2.7	9.1	6.8	4.4	3.2	-	-	26.8
A11. Chagas disease	23.1	-	-	-	2.7	3.4	2.3	2.2	11.5	-	1.1	3.2	3.2	3.6	1.9	1.8	11.6
A12. Schistosomiasis	37.6	-	4.7	4.6	9.1	2.5	1.8	-	23.8	-	2.0	2.5	1.6	6.6	-	-	13.8
A13. Leishmaniasis	53.7	4.1	13.0	7.0	4.6	1.2	-	-	30.2	3.1	11.4	4.6	3.1	1.1	-	-	23.5
A14. Onchocerciasis	29.8	-	-	2.7	1.4	6.1	4.8	2.4	17.4	-	-	1.9	1.2	4.6	3.1	1.7	12.4
B. Respiratory infections	3,984.4	1,371.2	119.9	40.2	26.9	38.9	147.1	249.3	1,993.5	1,339.1	123.6	42.0	30.1	38.9	131.1	286.1	1,990.9
C. Maternal causes	427.7										12.4	242.1	166.1	7.1			427.7
C1. Haemorrhage	129.5										3.6	73.7	49.7	2.4			129.5
C2. Sepsis	79.1										2.5	44.2	31.3	1.2			79.1
C3. Eclampsia	44.5										1.3	25.4	17.1	-			44.5
C4. Hypertension	31.4										-	17.4	12.6	-			31.4
C5. Obstructed labour	40.4										1.2	22.6	16.0	-			40.4
C6. Abortion	60.2										1.8	34.6	22.9	-			60.2
D. Perinatal causes	2,401.8	1,353.3							1,353.4	1,048.4							1,048.5
III. Injuries	3,420.1	253.9	256.9	716.8	508.1	267.2	124.6	136.0	2,263.6	233.4	149.9	292.4	165.9	113.7	69.2	132.0	1,156.5
A. Unintentional	2,236.7	216.8	222.7	415.1	299.6	183.6	81.3	94.9	1,514.0	192.2	127.0	129.8	77.5	64.8	40.7	90.7	722.7
A1. Road traffic accidents	637.0	27.7	55.0	167.0	123.6	63.7	26.2	21.6	484.7	22.2	35.4	33.4	21.1	18.8	10.0	11.3	152.2
A2. Poisoning	131.8	12.6	5.3	17.2	21.8	17.8	5.8	6.8	87.3	6.5	5.2	11.8	8.1	3.9	3.5	5.4	44.5
A3. Falls	168.2	10.3	7.9	19.2	15.4	15.9	10.5	18.5	97.7	11.9	4.4	2.6	2.5	6.6	8.5	34.0	70.4
A4. Fires	82.5	17.9	5.5	6.0	5.3	3.6	1.9	6.6	46.7	12.4	7.8	3.9	2.1	1.9	2.0	5.7	35.7
A5. Drowning	348.5	58.6	66.2	57.3	22.3	12.5	5.5	7.7	230.1	47.8	30.1	17.2	6.9	5.5	3.6	7.2	118.3
A6. Occupational	115.3	-	-	23.7	42.3	20.3	1.4	-	87.8	-	-	7.3	13.2	6.4	-	-	27.5
B. Intentional	1,183.4	37.2	34.2	301.7	208.5	83.6	43.3	41.0	749.6	41.2	22.9	162.7	88.4	48.9	28.6	41.3	433.9
B1. Self-inflicted	628.6	-	11.2	121.5	98.4	57.1	34.3	36.6	359.2	-	8.1	112.1	54.5	36.3	22.6	35.9	269.4
B2. Homicide and violence	233.1	10.6	6.9	83.8	53.5	18.6	5.5	2.7	181.6	14.6	4.3	11.3	10.3	4.8	2.7	3.5	51.5
B3. War	321.8	26.5	16.1	96.4	56.6	7.8	3.5	1.7	208.8	26.6	10.5	39.3	23.6	7.8	3.2	1.9	113.0

A dash (-) indicates less than 1000 deaths.

Estimated deaths (in thousands) by age, sex and cause, 1990: Developing Regions

No. of deaths (in thousands)

Cause of Death (ICD 9)	Both sexes	Males 0-4	5-14	15-29	30-44	45-59	60-69	70+	All ages	Females 0-4	5-14	15-29	30-44	45-59	60-69	70+	All ages
II. Noncommunicable	19,552.8	692.5	270.4	269.7	670.5	1,837.8	2,451.4	4,061.7	10,254.0	686.5	261.7	285.2	532.1	1,433.0	1,895.3	4,204.9	9,298.8
A. Malignant neoplasms	3,697.9	16.2	51.0	56.4	145.6	547.0	672.5	678.0	2,166.7	26.9	13.4	47.9	161.7	420.0	402.0	459.3	1,531.3
A1. Mouth and oropharynx	315.2	—	1.0	4.5	12.0	31.0	80.4	82.1	211.4	—	—	2.6	8.4	16.7	37.1	38.2	103.8
A2. Oesophagus	331.8	—	—	1.7	8.5	56.4	76.8	76.6	220.3	—	—	1.3	3.6	25.8	40.9	39.9	111.5
A3. Stomach	522.1	—	—	3.4	14.0	88.7	117.4	113.4	337.3	—	—	3.5	14.0	42.4	56.1	68.6	184.8
A4. Colorectal	215.0	—	—	3.8	7.8	20.3	39.2	44.6	116.0	—	—	2.0	7.7	17.9	32.8	38.2	99.0
A5. Liver	419.5	—	1.7	7.3	45.3	106.7	77.7	60.2	299.3	—	2.2	2.2	13.6	33.9	32.7	36.8	120.2
A6. Pancreas	72.5	—	—	—	1.7	10.4	14.7	16.3	44.0	—	—	—	1.1	6.1	9.6	11.3	28.5
A7. Lung	440.5	—	—	3.9	7.8	81.3	117.2	117.7	329.0	—	—	1.2	4.2	26.6	34.5	44.8	111.4
A8. Breast	157.6	—	—	—	—	—	—	—	—	—	—	5.7	26.2	56.9	32.0	36.7	157.6
A9. Cervix	183.4	—	—	—	—	—	—	—	—	—	—	6.1	24.3	72.6	39.0	41.1	183.4
A10. Ovary	50.7	—	—	—	—	—	—	—	—	—	—	3.0	9.9	15.2	10.2	11.4	50.7
A11. Prostate	104.8	—	—	—	—	9.0	44.2	51.0	104.8	—	—	—	—	—	—	—	—
A12. Bladder	79.6	—	—	—	1.5	10.8	22.6	25.7	61.4	—	—	—	1.0	3.5	6.2	7.2	18.3
A13. Lymphoma	121.3	2.9	11.5	5.1	6.6	11.5	19.8	19.6	77.1	—	—	1.8	5.5	7.9	11.9	13.6	44.2
A14. Leukemia	142.7	6.3	17.5	7.7	10.4	8.2	16.1	12.4	78.6	5.4	5.6	8.6	—	8.8	9.2	10.7	64.1
B. Diabetes mellitus	483.1	—	—	5.4	13.2	47.8	76.0	56.0	198.4	—	—	8.3	8.7	66.6	113.9	86.3	284.7
C. Nutritional/endocrine	577.7	118.5	10.7	27.3	24.2	18.4	34.9	32.2	266.2	126.5	27.6	24.6	20.1	30.2	27.7	54.8	311.5
C1. Protein-energy malnutrition	206.6	65.8	5.9	2.1	2.3	4.3	2.7	10.4	91.8	82.0	5.6	2.1	1.3	1.6	5.0	17.2	114.8
C2. Anaemia	146.6	19.9	6.0	5.4	2.5	5.7	5.0	8.2	51.4	16.2	23.0	9.0	7.1	11.3	11.5	17.0	95.2
D. Neuro-psychiatric	599.8	36.1	71.5	37.0	48.4	54.1	37.4	60.2	344.5	37.5	48.9	32.1	24.2	21.9	24.8	65.9	255.3
D1. Psychoses	42.3	—	—	3.1	6.6	5.7	3.6	6.3	25.5	—	—	1.8	2.7	2.8	2.4	6.2	16.7
D2. Epilepsy	102.5	4.0	16.5	10.8	12.6	9.2	3.9	3.1	60.1	3.8	10.6	12.1	7.2	4.0	2.4	2.4	42.4
D3. Alcohol dependence	31.0	—	—	1.3	7.5	9.7	3.0	3.4	26.9	—	—	—	1.5	1.5	—	—	4.0
D4. Alzheimer & other dementias	99.8	—	—	—	2.6	6.9	8.6	19.1	50.0	—	—	—	1.5	3.2	6.6	26.7	49.8
D5. Parkinson disease	31.5	—	—	—	—	1.0	4.5	13.6	19.3	—	—	—	—	—	2.6	9.0	12.3
D6. Multiple sclerosis	24.8	—	—	—	2.8	4.0	2.4	1.6	11.4	—	—	1.6	4.0	3.7	2.6	1.9	13.4
E. Cardiovascular diseases	9,016.7	63.5	31.0	64.4	229.1	768.1	1,133.2	2,209.8	4,499.0	58.7	48.8	76.5	169.8	598.9	967.3	2,597.7	4,517.7
E1. Rheumatic diseases	440.2	1.8	2.2	11.5	15.6	32.0	34.9	49.8	146.7	1.9	4.0	14.0	26.0	72.7	84.8	90.2	293.5
E2. Ischaemic heart disease	2,469.0	1.8	1.1	9.2	62.1	253.8	368.6	653.5	1,350.1	—	—	6.1	22.6	115.8	250.8	722.3	1,118.9
E3. Cerebrovascular diseases	3,181.2	7.8	6.4	12.6	49.3	222.4	390.9	834.4	1,523.8	5.8	8.4	16.7	49.0	212.0	360.9	1,004.8	1,657.4
E4. Inflammatory cardiac disease	1,228.7	31.7	14.8	21.2	68.1	139.9	148.6	228.0	652.2	36.2	25.7	20.7	39.5	95.0	113.0	246.4	576.4
F. Respiratory	2,336.3	77.5	31.2	13.6	29.9	122.4	282.8	692.2	1,249.7	78.6	18.6	17.5	28.9	99.6	182.8	660.6	1,086.6
F1. Chronic obstructive lung disease	1,714.0	10.9	3.4	1.1	13.0	91.7	239.8	588.9	949.0	9.0	2.3	1.5	12.4	70.5	152.6	516.6	764.9
F2. Asthma	147.2	4.7	15.2	5.1	5.6	8.7	9.5	16.5	65.3	4.5	9.7	7.3	7.6	12.8	11.2	28.6	81.9
G. Digestive	1,415.7	87.4	20.3	29.2	130.8	217.1	161.8	178.7	825.3	106.2	25.5	27.9	67.3	118.7	96.2	148.5	590.4
G1. Peptic ulcer disease	194.3	—	1.4	5.0	17.7	33.5	27.1	36.1	121.7	1.2	—	5.3	9.9	15.9	12.2	27.4	72.6
G2. Cirrhosis	563.0	4.1	2.9	10.4	83.7	138.9	90.7	53.1	383.7	3.2	4.1	8.0	29.2	58.4	39.7	36.8	179.3
H. Genito-urinary	535.2	12.1	24.4	14.7	22.0	43.9	47.3	111.6	276.1	7.7	20.5	20.8	22.7	54.5	57.0	75.8	259.1
H1. Nephritis/nephrosis	327.3	5.7	22.3	13.3	17.4	32.6	31.2	54.2	176.7	4.4	19.0	13.9	16.4	27.2	31.0	38.8	150.6
I. Musculo-skeletal	105.9	—	2.6	1.8	1.3	3.8	10.0	21.6	41.5	1.2	3.1	5.7	7.0	8.8	9.5	29.1	64.4
J. Congenital	595.0	271.0	20.8	12.0	4.6	1.1	—	—	311.3	231.9	20.9	15.0	11.4	3.6	—	—	283.7

A dash (-) indicates less than 1000 deaths.

Estimated deaths (in thousands) by age, sex and cause, 1990: Established Market Economies

No. of deaths (in thousands)

Cause of Death (ICD 9)	Both sexes	Males 0-4	5-14	15-29	30-44	45-59	60-69	70+	All ages	Females 0-4	5-14	15-29	30-44	45-59	60-69	70+	All ages
Population (in millions)	797.8	26.4	53.3	93.7	90.4	66.1	34.2	26.4	390.5	25.1	50.7	90.0	89.2	67.8	40.5	44.0	407.3
All Causes	7,121.2	60.2	13.8	113.9	186.6	467.6	741.9	2,075.5	3,659.3	45.3	8.8	39.3	87.3	243.7	447.7	2,589.8	3,461.9
I. Communicable, maternal & perinatal	438.8	34.9	-	7.7	24.4	17.3	20.6	127.2	232.6	25.2	-	2.6	5.4	6.1	12.2	154.3	206.3
A. Infectious & parasitic	111.0	2.7	-	6.7	21.7	11.2	7.6	20.6	70.7	2.1	-	1.5	3.6	3.2	4.9	24.7	40.3
A1. Tuberculosis	14.6	-	-	-	-	1.6	2.3	5.3	9.9	-	-	-	-	-	-	3.0	4.6
A2. Syphilis	-	-	-	-	-	-	-	-	-	-	-	-	-	-	-	-	-
A3. HIV	41.8	-	-	5.5	18.3	8.7	-	1.2	35.1	-	-	1.4	3.2	-	-	-	6.7
A4. Diarrhoeal diseases	2.7	-	-	-	-	-	-	1.2	1.2	-	-	-	-	-	-	1.3	1.6
a. Acute watery	2.6	-	-	-	-	-	-	1.1	1.1	-	-	-	-	-	-	1.2	1.5
b. Persistent	-	-	-	-	-	-	-	-	-	-	-	-	-	-	-	-	-
c. Dysentery	-	-	-	-	-	-	-	-	-	-	-	-	-	-	-	-	-
A5. Pertussis	-	-	-	-	-	-	-	-	-	-	-	-	-	-	-	-	-
A6. Measles	-	-	-	-	-	-	-	-	-	-	-	-	-	-	-	-	-
A7. Tetanus	-	-	-	-	-	-	-	-	-	-	-	-	-	-	-	-	-
A8. Meningitis	4.8	-	-	-	-	-	-	-	2.6	-	-	-	-	-	-	-	2.2
A9. Malaria	-	-	-	-	-	-	-	-	-	-	-	-	-	-	-	-	-
A10. Trypanosomiasis	-	-	-	-	-	-	-	-	-	-	-	-	-	-	-	-	-
A11. Chagas disease	-	-	-	-	-	-	-	-	-	-	-	-	-	-	-	-	-
A12. Schistosomiasis	-	-	-	-	-	-	-	-	-	-	-	-	-	-	-	-	-
A13. Leishmaniasis	-	-	-	-	-	-	-	-	-	-	-	-	-	-	-	-	-
A14. Onchocerciasis	-	-	-	-	-	-	-	-	-	-	-	-	-	-	-	-	-
B. Respiratory infections	275.3	2.2	-	-	2.7	6.1	13.1	106.6	131.8	1.5	-	-	1.4	2.9	7.3	129.6	143.5
C. Maternal causes	-	-	-	-	-	-	-	-	-	-	-	-	-	-	-	-	-
C1. Haemorrhage	-	-	-	-	-	-	-	-	-	-	-	-	-	-	-	-	-
C2. Sepsis	-	-	-	-	-	-	-	-	-	-	-	-	-	-	-	-	-
C3. Eclampsia	-	-	-	-	-	-	-	-	-	-	-	-	-	-	-	-	-
C4. Hypertension	-	-	-	-	-	-	-	-	-	-	-	-	-	-	-	-	-
C5. Obstructed labour	-	-	-	-	-	-	-	-	-	-	-	-	-	-	-	-	-
C6. Abortion	-	-	-	-	-	-	-	-	-	-	-	-	-	-	-	-	-
D. Perinatal causes	51.8	30.0	-	-	-	-	-	-	30.0	21.7	-	-	-	-	-	-	21.7
III. Injuries	444.8	5.9	7.1	80.3	65.5	51.6	31.0	56.8	298.3	4.0	3.5	20.4	19.0	18.2	15.3	66.2	146.5
A. Unintentional	301.9	5.3	6.3	53.2	36.9	30.3	20.1	42.3	194.3	3.5	3.0	13.6	9.9	9.6	9.8	58.1	107.6
A1. Road traffic accidents	131.4	1.4	3.4	38.3	19.0	13.2	7.8	10.9	94.0	1.0	1.9	10.9	6.1	5.1	4.3	8.1	37.4
A2. Poisoning	12.9	-	-	2.2	3.8	1.5	-	-	9.1	-	-	-	1.0	-	-	1.0	3.8
A3. Falls	69.1	-	-	1.6	2.7	4.3	3.8	17.2	30.1	-	-	-	-	1.1	2.0	35.0	39.0
A4. Fires	10.5	-	-	-	1.1	1.0	-	1.5	6.2	-	-	-	-	-	-	1.7	4.3
A5. Drowning	12.9	1.0	2.3	1.3	1.7	1.4	-	1.3	9.7	-	-	-	-	-	-	1.2	3.2
A6. Occupational	8.6	-	-	-	-	-	-	-	7.4	-	-	-	-	-	-	-	1.3
B. Intentional	142.8	-	-	27.2	28.7	21.3	11.0	14.4	104.0	-	-	6.8	9.0	8.5	5.5	8.1	38.9
B1. Self-inflicted	112.1	-	-	17.3	21.2	18.4	9.9	13.7	80.9	-	-	4.3	6.8	7.5	5.0	7.5	31.3
B2. Homicide and violence	30.6	-	-	9.9	7.5	2.9	-	-	23.0	-	-	2.5	2.2	-	-	-	7.6
B3. War	-	-	-	-	-	-	-	-	-	-	-	-	-	-	-	-	-

A dash (-) indicates less than 1000 deaths.

Estimated deaths (in thousands) by age, sex and cause, 1990: Established Market Economies

No. of deaths (in thousands)

Cause of Death (ICD 9)	Both sexes	Males								Females							
		0-4	5-14	15-29	30-44	45-59	60-69	70+	All ages	0-4	5-14	15-29	30-44	45-59	60-69	70+	All ages
II. Noncommunicable	6,237.6	19.4	6.0	25.9	96.7	398.7	690.2	1,891.5	3,128.5	16.1	4.8	16.3	62.9	219.5	420.3	2,369.3	3,109.1
A. Malignant neoplasms	1,763.8	1.0	2.2	7.7	30.2	162.4	274.4	498.6	976.5	–	1.7	5.6	33.8	118.5	179.6	447.3	787.3
A1. Mouth and oropharynx	32.8	–	–	–	1.5	8.2	7.6	7.3	24.7	–	–	–	–	1.4	1.9	4.3	8.1
A2. Oesophagus	42.3	–	–	–	–	7.9	10.5	12.5	31.8	–	–	–	–	1.2	2.3	6.8	10.5
A3. Stomach	140.1	–	–	–	2.5	13.6	22.3	44.6	83.2	–	–	–	2.3	6.2	10.1	38.1	56.9
A4. Colorectal	209.2	–	–	–	2.6	15.2	27.2	58.1	103.3	–	–	–	2.3	11.3	20.6	71.6	105.9
A5. Liver	37.6	–	–	–	–	7.0	9.8	9.3	27.0	–	–	–	–	1.3	3.0	6.0	10.5
A6. Pancreas	85.5	–	–	–	1.2	7.6	12.8	21.6	43.1	–	–	–	–	5.2	9.4	28.0	42.4
A7. Lung	379.9	–	–	–	5.6	49.6	93.0	130.6	279.0	–	–	–	2.5	16.5	30.8	51.0	100.9
A8. Breast	134.2	–	–	–	–	–	–	–	–	–	–	–	11.0	32.3	30.8	58.1	134.2
A9. Cervix	15.7	–	–	–	–	–	–	–	–	–	–	–	2.5	3.8	3.5	5.7	15.7
A10. Ovary	41.2	–	–	–	–	–	–	–	–	–	–	–	1.9	8.8	11.4	18.8	41.2
A11. Prostate	92.5	–	–	–	–	3.0	15.6	73.8	92.5	–	–	–	–	–	–	–	–
A12. Bladder	46.5	–	–	–	–	2.8	7.5	22.6	33.2	–	–	–	–	–	2.1	10.5	13.3
A13. Lymphoma	79.4	–	–	1.4	2.9	7.2	10.4	19.4	41.6	–	–	–	1.5	4.4	8.3	22.7	37.8
A14. Leukemia	57.2	–	–	1.9	2.3	4.2	6.6	15.0	31.2	–	–	1.2	1.7	3.2	4.5	14.5	26.0
B. Diabetes mellitus	145.4	–	–	–	2.2	7.3	12.9	34.5	57.3	–	–	–	1.3	5.2	14.4	66.8	88.0
C. Nutritional/endocrine	66.3	–	–	–	1.2	3.0	5.2	16.8	28.4	–	–	–	1.0	2.5	4.2	27.9	37.9
C1. Protein-energy malnutrition	6.1	–	–	–	–	–	–	1.8	2.2	–	–	–	–	–	–	3.6	3.9
C2. Anaemia	14.6	–	–	–	–	–	–	4.2	6.1	–	–	–	–	–	–	6.7	8.5
D. Neuro-psychiatric	203.0	1.4	–	5.4	8.6	12.3	13.8	53.4	95.8	1.1	–	2.1	3.4	6.2	9.9	83.7	107.2
D1. Psychoses	12.5	–	–	–	–	–	–	3.5	5.3	–	–	–	–	–	–	6.5	7.3
D2. Epilepsy	7.4	–	–	–	–	–	–	–	4.5	–	–	–	–	–	–	–	2.9
D3. Alcohol dependence	15.8	–	–	–	2.7	5.1	2.9	1.6	12.6	–	–	–	–	1.3	–	–	3.3
D4. Alzheimer & other dementias	92.5	–	–	–	–	2.2	4.9	26.3	34.9	–	–	–	–	1.6	4.5	50.3	57.6
D5. Parkinson disease	29.1	–	–	–	–	–	1.5	13.3	15.0	–	–	–	–	–	–	13.1	14.2
D6. Multiple sclerosis	5.6	–	–	–	–	–	–	–	2.2	–	–	–	–	1.1	–	–	3.4
E. Cardiovascular diseases	3,174.7	1.5	–	6.2	35.1	156.2	292.2	1,000.3	1,492.0	1.3	–	3.3	13.3	57.6	156.7	1,449.9	1,682.7
E1. Rheumatic diseases	20.3	–	–	–	–	1.0	1.6	3.0	6.2	–	–	–	–	1.6	3.2	8.8	14.1
E2. Ischaemic heart disease	1,561.6	–	–	1.2	15.6	91.3	178.1	512.8	798.8	–	–	–	3.0	23.5	79.3	656.7	762.8
E3. Cerebrovascular diseases	782.0	–	–	1.2	6.2	24.3	47.3	239.5	319.0	–	–	–	4.4	15.5	35.7	406.2	462.9
E4. Inflammatory cardiac disease	91.8	–	–	1.4	3.3	7.2	9.4	25.5	47.0	–	–	–	1.1	2.7	4.8	35.2	44.7
F. Respiratory	341.6	–	–	1.4	2.6	12.7	39.1	151.3	208.1	–	–	–	1.7	7.6	20.3	102.2	133.5
F1. Chronic obstructive lung disease	242.4	–	–	–	–	7.8	29.5	117.3	155.5	–	–	–	–	4.5	14.7	67.2	87.0
F2. Asthma	21.9	–	–	–	–	1.4	2.1	5.4	10.3	–	–	–	–	1.4	2.0	6.9	11.6
G. Digestive	305.2	–	–	1.5	13.2	36.4	37.8	73.5	163.1	–	–	–	5.0	14.2	21.1	100.3	142.1
G1. Peptic ulcer disease	31.1	–	–	–	–	1.8	2.9	10.6	15.9	–	–	–	–	–	1.5	12.9	15.2
G2. Cirrhosis	117.1	–	–	–	9.2	26.3	22.3	19.2	77.7	–	–	–	3.3	9.2	10.6	16.0	39.5
H. Genito-urinary	123.0	–	–	–	1.4	3.9	8.1	43.9	58.0	–	–	–	–	2.9	6.7	53.9	65.0
H1. Nephritis/nephrosis	79.8	–	–	–	1.1	3.0	6.0	27.9	38.5	–	–	–	–	2.0	4.7	33.6	41.3
I. Musculo-skeletal	32.0	–	–	–	–	–	1.6	5.8	8.8	–	–	–	–	1.7	3.1	17.0	23.1
J. Congenital	34.2	12.8	1.4	1.4	–	–	–	–	18.3	10.8	–	–	–	–	–	1.2	15.9

A dash (-) indicates less than 1000 deaths.

Estimated deaths (in thousands) by age, sex and cause, 1990: Formerly Socialist Economies

No. of deaths (in thousands)

Cause of Death (ICD 9)	Both sexes	Males 0-4	5-14	15-29	30-44	45-59	60-69	70+	All ages	Females 0-4	5-14	15-29	30-44	45-59	60-69	70+	All ages
Population (in millions)	346.2	13.8	27.3	36.3	40.0	27.0	14.2	6.8	165.3	13.1	26.4	35.0	40.0	30.0	20.1	16.3	180.9
All Causes	3,761.9	63.0	14.9	76.7	170.9	419.3	439.9	706.6	1,891.3	45.2	8.3	22.5	55.7	179.2	319.4	1,240.4	1,870.6
I. Communicable, maternal & perinatal	135.9	38.5	-	2.3	7.8	13.6	8.7	11.6	83.3	26.8	-	2.2	2.9	3.1	3.9	12.9	52.6
A. Infectious & parasitic	42.0	5.8	-	1.4	5.7	8.8	4.6	2.9	29.6	4.4	-	-	1.1	1.7	1.7	2.6	12.4
A1. Tuberculosis	22.9	-	-	-	4.8	7.3	3.7	2.2	19.0	-	-	-	-	-	-	1.4	3.9
A2. Syphilis	-	-	-	-	-	-	-	-	-	-	-	-	-	-	-	-	-
A3. HIV	-	-	-	-	-	-	-	-	-	-	-	-	-	-	-	-	-
A4. Diarrhoeal diseases	4.2	1.9	-	-	-	-	-	-	2.2	1.6	-	-	-	-	-	-	2.0
a. Acute watery	4.0	1.8	-	-	-	-	-	-	2.1	1.6	-	-	-	-	-	-	1.9
b. Persistent	-	-	-	-	-	-	-	-	-	-	-	-	-	-	-	-	-
c. Dysentery	-	-	-	-	-	-	-	-	-	-	-	-	-	-	-	-	-
A5. Pertussis	-	-	-	-	-	-	-	-	-	-	-	-	-	-	-	-	-
A6. Measles	-	-	-	-	-	-	-	-	-	-	-	-	-	-	-	-	-
A7. Tetanus	-	-	-	-	-	-	-	-	-	-	-	-	-	-	-	-	-
A8. Meningitis	5.4	1.6	-	-	-	-	-	-	3.2	1.1	-	-	-	-	-	-	2.2
A9. Malaria	-	-	-	-	-	-	-	-	-	-	-	-	-	-	-	-	-
A10. Trypanosomiasis	-	-	-	-	-	-	-	-	-	-	-	-	-	-	-	-	-
A11. Chagas disease	-	-	-	-	-	-	-	-	-	-	-	-	-	-	-	-	-
A12. Schistosomiasis	-	-	-	-	-	-	-	-	-	-	-	-	-	-	-	-	-
A13. Leishmaniasis	-	-	-	-	-	-	-	-	-	-	-	-	-	-	-	-	-
A14. Onchocerciasis	-	-	-	-	-	-	-	-	-	-	-	-	-	-	-	-	-
B. Respiratory infections	54.7	10.2	-	-	2.1	4.8	4.1	8.7	31.3	7.9	-	-	-	1.4	2.2	10.3	23.5
C. Maternal causes	2.2	-	-	-	-	-	-	-	-	-	-	1.1	1.1	-	-	-	2.2
C1. Haemorrhage	-	-	-	-	-	-	-	-	-	-	-	-	-	-	-	-	-
C2. Sepsis	-	-	-	-	-	-	-	-	-	-	-	-	-	-	-	-	-
C3. Eclampsia	-	-	-	-	-	-	-	-	-	-	-	-	-	-	-	-	-
C4. Hypertension	-	-	-	-	-	-	-	-	-	-	-	-	-	-	-	-	-
C5. Obstructed labour	-	-	-	-	-	-	-	-	-	-	-	-	-	-	-	-	-
C6. Abortion	1.0	-	-	-	-	-	-	-	-	-	-	-	-	-	-	-	1.0
D. Perinatal causes	36.9	22.4	-	-	-	-	-	-	22.4	14.6	-	-	-	-	-	-	14.6
III. Injuries	361.9	6.6	9.2	58.8	84.3	70.4	24.9	19.0	273.1	4.4	3.8	10.2	14.4	17.9	12.3	25.7	88.7
A. Unintentional	255.8	6.4	8.5	42.1	56.6	48.8	17.0	13.0	192.5	4.2	3.5	6.9	8.8	11.7	8.1	20.1	63.3
A1. Road traffic accidents	87.4	-	2.8	21.8	20.4	13.7	5.2	3.5	68.3	-	1.4	3.7	3.3	3.6	2.6	3.9	19.1
A2. Poisoning	42.9	-	-	3.2	11.3	12.7	3.3	1.1	32.9	-	-	-	1.9	3.3	1.6	1.5	10.0
A3. Falls	27.6	-	-	1.7	3.3	3.5	2.0	4.0	15.2	-	-	-	-	-	1.1	9.6	12.4
A4. Fires	7.4	-	-	-	1.2	1.3	-	-	4.8	-	-	-	-	-	-	-	2.6
A5. Drowning	22.7	-	2.4	4.9	5.7	3.6	1.1	-	19.1	-	-	-	-	-	-	-	3.6
A6. Occupational	13.3	-	-	1.6	5.6	4.1	-	-	11.5	-	-	-	-	-	-	-	1.8
B. Intentional	106.1	-	-	16.6	27.7	21.7	7.9	5.9	80.6	-	-	3.4	5.6	6.3	4.2	5.6	25.4
B1. Self-inflicted	77.4	-	-	10.4	19.1	17.5	6.7	5.4	59.5	-	-	2.1	3.2	4.6	3.4	4.6	17.8
B2. Homicide and violence	28.7	-	-	6.2	8.6	4.2	1.1	-	21.1	-	-	1.3	2.4	1.7	-	-	7.6
B3. War	-	-	-	-	-	-	-	-	-	-	-	-	-	-	-	-	-

A dash (-) indicates less than 1000 deaths.

Estimated deaths (in thousands) by age, sex and cause, 1990: Formerly Socialist Economies

No. of deaths (in thousands)

Cause of Death (ICD 9)	Both sexes	Males 0-4	5-14	15-29	30-44	45-59	60-69	70+	All ages	Females 0-4	5-14	15-29	30-44	45-59	60-69	70+	All ages
II. Noncommunicable	3,264.2	17.9	4.8	15.7	78.8	335.2	406.4	676.1	1,534.9	14.0	3.7	10.0	38.3	158.2	303.2	1,201.9	1,729.3
A. Malignant neoplasms	666.9	1.3	2.1	4.6	20.0	117.3	127.3	104.8	377.4	-	1.4	3.6	18.2	62.7	84.1	118.6	289.5
A1. Mouth and oropharynx	17.6	-	-	-	1.3	6.6	4.2	2.3	14.6	-	-	-	-	-	-	1.5	3.1
A2. Oesophagus	15.4	-	-	-	-	4.4	4.0	2.7	11.5	-	-	-	-	-	-	2.3	3.9
A3. Stomach	103.9	-	-	-	3.1	18.4	20.0	18.4	60.2	-	-	-	1.9	7.5	12.3	21.7	43.7
A4. Colorectal	71.2	-	-	-	1.4	7.3	10.7	13.1	32.8	-	-	-	1.3	6.4	10.9	19.6	38.4
A5. Liver	6.3	-	-	-	-	-	1.3	1.2	3.4	-	-	-	-	-	-	1.5	2.9
A6. Pancreas	10.7	-	-	-	-	1.5	2.0	2.0	6.0	-	-	-	-	-	1.5	2.4	4.8
A7. Lung	146.6	-	-	-	4.3	44.1	47.2	27.3	123.1	-	-	-	-	4.7	7.9	9.8	23.4
A8. Breast	40.7	-	-	-	-	-	-	-	-	-	-	-	4.5	13.4	11.4	11.2	40.7
A9. Cervix	15.8	-	-	-	-	-	-	-	-	-	-	-	2.0	4.0	4.5	5.1	15.8
A10. Ovary	14.5	-	-	-	-	-	-	-	-	-	-	-	-	3.8	4.7	5.0	14.5
A11. Prostate	15.2	-	-	-	-	1.3	4.0	9.8	15.2	-	-	-	-	-	-	-	-
A12. Bladder	24.4	-	-	-	-	4.2	5.9	6.9	17.7	-	-	-	-	1.1	2.0	3.2	6.7
A13. Lymphoma	16.8	-	-	-	1.3	2.7	2.5	1.7	9.5	-	-	-	-	1.5	2.1	2.3	7.3
A14. Leukemia	19.5	-	-	-	1.0	2.3	2.7	2.4	10.6	-	-	-	-	1.7	2.2	2.7	8.9
B. Diabetes mellitus	31.2	-	-	-	-	2.4	3.7	4.0	11.3	-	-	-	-	2.5	6.6	9.8	19.8
C. Nutritional/endocrine	7.3	-	-	-	-	-	-	-	3.3	-	-	-	-	-	-	1.1	4.0
C1. Protein-energy malnutrition	2.1	-	-	-	-	-	-	-	-	-	-	-	-	-	-	-	-
C2. Anaemia	2.1	-	-	-	-	-	-	-	-	-	-	-	-	-	-	-	-
D. Neuro-psychiatric	29.1	-	-	1.8	4.0	5.5	2.5	1.9	17.5	-	-	1.2	2.0	2.6	1.7	2.8	11.6
D1. Psychoses	3.1	-	-	-	-	-	-	-	1.5	-	-	-	-	-	-	-	1.6
D2. Epilepsy	5.2	-	-	-	1.1	-	-	-	3.3	-	-	-	-	-	-	-	2.0
D3. Alcohol dependence	6.0	-	-	-	1.3	2.4	-	-	5.0	-	-	-	-	-	-	-	1.2
D4. Alzheimer & other dementias	2.3	-	-	-	-	-	-	-	-	-	-	-	-	-	-	-	-
D5. Parkinson disease	1.0	-	-	-	-	-	-	-	-	-	-	-	-	-	-	-	-
D6. Multiple sclerosis	2.8	-	-	-	-	-	-	-	1.2	-	-	-	-	-	-	-	1.6
E. Cardiovascular diseases	2,153.3	-	-	4.9	39.3	162.6	218.1	482.7	908.7	-	-	2.0	10.6	68.2	177.2	985.7	1,244.6
E1. Rheumatic diseases	25.5	-	-	-	2.0	4.6	2.4	1.8	10.5	-	-	-	1.4	5.9	4.8	2.5	15.0
E2. Ischaemic heart disease	1,116.3	-	-	1.5	23.0	99.4	120.7	239.9	484.5	-	-	-	3.0	26.4	83.9	518.2	631.8
E3. Cerebrovascular diseases	665.9	-	-	-	6.6	36.8	62.3	139.5	246.4	-	-	-	3.2	25.1	65.2	325.3	419.6
E4. Inflammatory cardiac disease	43.9	-	-	-	2.0	4.2	4.9	11.7	23.7	-	-	-	-	1.7	3.0	14.4	20.2
F. Respiratory	167.1	-	-	1.1	2.4	17.9	28.0	51.3	100.6	-	-	-	1.1	5.0	11.2	48.5	66.5
F1. Chronic obstructive lung disease	115.9	-	-	-	-	11.0	21.1	39.8	72.6	-	-	-	-	3.0	8.1	31.9	43.3
F2. Asthma	12.2	-	-	-	-	1.9	1.5	-	6.2	-	-	-	-	-	1.1	3.3	6.0
G. Digestive	122.0	1.1	-	1.3	8.4	21.9	19.0	17.5	69.4	-	-	-	2.8	9.5	13.6	25.2	52.5
G1. Peptic ulcer disease	15.2	-	-	-	1.1	3.2	3.0	3.0	10.4	-	-	-	-	-	1.2	2.8	4.8
G2. Cirrhosis	29.2	-	-	-	2.8	7.5	5.8	3.4	19.8	-	-	-	-	2.7	2.8	2.8	9.4
H. Genito-urinary	45.9	-	-	-	2.1	4.8	5.7	12.0	25.7	-	-	-	1.6	4.3	5.6	7.8	20.2
H1. Nephritis/nephrosis	20.1	-	-	-	1.6	2.9	2.4	3.0	10.7	-	-	-	-	2.1	2.5	3.2	9.4
I. Musculo-skeletal	5.2	-	-	-	-	-	-	-	1.6	-	-	-	-	-	1.0	-	3.6
J. Congenital	26.6	12.5	-	-	-	-	-	-	14.8	9.9	-	-	-	-	-	-	11.8

A dash (-) indicates less than 1000 deaths.

Estimated deaths (in thousands) by age, sex and cause, 1990: India

No. of deaths (in thousands)

		Males								Females							
Cause of Death (ICD 9)	Both sexes	0-4	5-14	15-29	30-44	45-59	60-69	70+	All ages	0-4	5-14	15-29	30-44	45-59	60-69	70+	All ages
Population (in millions)	849.5	59.8	101.8	121.5	79.0	47.6	19.1	10.6	439.4	56.7	95.3	111.3	72.0	46.0	18.5	10.4	410.1
All Causes	9,371.0	1,600.0	256.0	251.0	343.0	665.0	738.0	1,022.0	4,875.0	1,650.0	294.0	306.0	261.0	479.0	569.0	937.0	4,496.0
I. Communicable, maternal & perinatal	4,059.7	1,357.5	132.8	81.9	113.7	148.9	91.9	127.5	2,054.2	1,354.9	163.9	141.5	117.8	89.6	52.1	85.8	2,005.5
A. Infectious & parasitic	2,188.4	655.5	102.8	66.9	103.6	133.1	39.4	50.2	1,151.4	696.8	124.1	55.7	60.1	70.6	12.4	17.1	1,036.9
A1. Tuberculosis	451.8	6.6	10.9	28.9	67.4	103.2	30.2	44.4	291.7	11.2	21.2	25.9	38.2	43.0	7.5	13.0	160.1
A2. Syphilis	25.8	3.4	-	5.8	3.9	1.4	-	-	14.7	3.6	-	3.6	2.7	1.1	-	-	11.1
A3. HIV	-	-	-	-	-	-	-	-	-	-	-	-	-	-	-	-	-
A4. Diarrhoeal diseases	825.2	348.6	26.5	12.3	8.4	5.4	1.1	-	402.9	366.5	31.4	10.2	6.9	6.0	-	-	422.4
a. Acute watery	448.9	177.7	20.0	9.8	6.6	4.0	-	-	219.4	186.9	23.7	8.1	5.5	4.4	-	-	229.5
b. Persistent	248.2	119.6	1.3	-	-	-	-	-	120.9	125.8	1.5	-	-	-	-	-	127.3
c. Dysentery	128.2	51.3	5.2	2.5	1.7	1.5	-	-	62.6	53.9	6.2	2.1	1.4	1.6	-	-	65.6
A5. Pertussis	81.6	34.5	4.9	-	-	-	-	-	39.4	36.3	5.9	-	-	-	-	-	42.2
A6. Measles	276.3	116.8	16.7	-	-	-	-	-	133.4	122.8	20.0	-	-	-	-	-	142.8
A7. Tetanus	160.4	69.2	3.9	1.1	2.4	1.7	-	-	78.1	73.1	4.7	2.5	1.3	1.9	-	-	82.3
A8. Meningitis	61.8	16.9	10.1	3.7	2.4	2.8	-	-	37.5	14.6	4.5	2.5	1.3	1.9	-	-	24.2
A9. Malaria	27.5	1.6	3.6	3.5	2.3	2.1	1.4	-	13.9	1.7	4.2	2.9	1.9	2.3	-	-	13.7
A10. Trypanosomiasis	-	-	-	-	-	-	-	-	-	-	-	-	-	-	-	-	-
A11. Chagas disease	-	-	-	-	-	-	-	-	-	-	-	-	-	-	-	-	-
A12. Schistosomiasis	13.4	-	-	-	-	-	-	-	7.8	-	-	-	-	-	-	-	5.6
A13. Leishmaniasis	36.1	2.3	8.4	5.3	3.6	1.1	-	-	20.9	1.7	7.1	3.1	2.1	1.0	-	-	15.2
A14. Onchocerciasis	-	-	-	-	-	-	-	-	-	-	-	-	-	-	-	-	-
B. Respiratory infections	1,096.1	348.2	30.0	14.9	10.1	15.8	52.5	77.3	548.9	366.1	35.5	12.3	8.4	16.6	39.6	68.7	547.2
C. Maternal causes	129.4	-	-	-	-	-	-	-	-	-	4.2	73.4	49.3	2.4	-	-	129.4
C1. Haemorrhage	38.8	-	-	-	-	-	-	-	-	-	1.3	22.0	14.8	-	-	-	38.8
C2. Sepsis	25.9	-	-	-	-	-	-	-	-	-	-	14.7	9.9	-	-	-	25.9
C3. Eclampsia	12.9	-	-	-	-	-	-	-	-	-	-	7.3	4.9	-	-	-	12.9
C4. Hypertension	6.5	-	-	-	-	-	-	-	-	-	-	3.7	2.5	-	-	-	6.5
C5. Obstructed labour	12.9	-	-	-	-	-	-	-	-	-	-	7.3	4.9	-	-	-	12.9
C6. Abortion	25.9	-	-	-	-	-	-	-	-	-	-	14.7	9.9	-	-	-	25.9
D. Perinatal causes	645.9	353.8	-	-	-	-	-	-	353.8	292.0	-	-	-	-	-	-	292.0
III. Injuries	611.3	39.2	61.9	90.2	77.3	44.9	16.8	23.6	353.9	45.0	53.3	78.2	37.2	21.0	8.5	14.1	257.4
A. Unintentional	506.6	38.1	57.9	64.0	58.3	38.7	15.2	21.3	293.5	44.5	49.2	54.3	26.7	18.3	7.6	12.5	213.1
A1. Road traffic accidents	115.4	5.9	8.9	24.2	22.4	12.5	4.5	6.3	84.7	6.0	9.1	6.2	3.6	2.3	1.4	2.2	30.8
A2. Poisoning	10.4	1.5	-	1.4	2.4	1.3	-	-	8.1	-	-	-	-	-	-	-	2.4
A3. Falls	29.7	3.2	2.6	2.9	2.6	3.6	1.3	1.8	18.0	4.0	1.8	-	-	1.6	1.2	1.9	11.7
A4. Fires	19.6	5.9	1.3	-	-	-	-	-	9.4	3.3	3.7	1.8	-	-	-	-	10.2
A5. Drowning	57.0	5.5	10.4	6.7	3.1	2.1	1.7	1.2	29.8	6.5	8.2	6.5	2.3	2.0	-	1.0	27.3
A6. Occupational	35.5	-	-	4.6	10.4	5.4	-	-	20.8	-	-	4.6	7.0	2.8	-	-	14.6
B. Intentional	104.7	1.2	4.0	26.2	19.0	6.1	1.7	2.3	60.4	-	4.1	23.9	10.5	2.8	-	1.5	44.3
B1. Self-inflicted	78.0	-	3.2	18.8	12.5	4.3	1.2	1.7	41.7	-	3.9	20.6	8.9	1.8	-	-	36.3
B2. Homicide and violence	19.9	-	-	5.2	5.1	1.7	-	-	14.1	-	-	2.5	1.1	-	-	-	5.8
B3. War	6.7	-	-	2.2	1.4	-	-	-	4.6	-	-	-	-	-	-	-	2.1

A dash (-) indicates less than 1000 deaths.

Estimated deaths (in thousands) by age, sex and cause, 1990: India

No. of deaths (in thousands)

Cause of Death (ICD 9)	Both sexes	Males								Females							
		0-4	5-14	15-29	30-44	45-59	60-69	70+	All ages	0-4	5-14	15-29	30-44	45-59	60-69	70+	All ages
II. Noncommunicable	4,700.0	203.3	61.4	78.9	152.0	471.3	629.2	870.9	2,466.9	250.1	76.8	86.3	106.0	368.4	508.4	837.2	2,233.1
A. Malignant neoplasms	775.8	3.2	9.3	13.3	19.6	111.8	149.9	143.2	450.2	9.8	1.2	10.4	31.1	99.5	89.6	83.9	325.6
A1. Mouth and oropharynx	157.1	-	-	2.2	3.2	12.6	45.9	43.8	108.0	-	-	-	2.6	7.4	19.5	18.3	49.1
A2. Oesophagus	83.2	-	-	-	1.1	13.7	18.4	17.5	51.5	-	-	-	1.5	8.9	10.7	10.0	31.7
A3. Stomach	63.4	-	-	1.1	1.7	12.4	14.2	13.6	43.0	-	-	-	1.3	6.1	6.5	6.1	20.4
A4. Colorectal	39.6	-	-	-	1.2	3.3	8.9	8.5	22.7	-	-	-	1.2	2.1	6.8	6.3	16.8
A5. Liver	19.7	-	-	-	-	4.9	4.3	4.1	14.3	-	-	-	-	1.4	1.7	1.6	5.3
A6. Pancreas	12.3	-	-	-	-	2.1	2.9	2.7	8.0	-	-	-	-	1.1	1.4	1.3	4.2
A7. Lung	54.4	-	-	-	1.3	13.0	16.0	15.3	46.4	-	-	-	-	1.9	2.9	2.7	7.9
A8. Breast	40.7									-	-	1.9	5.6	14.9	9.5	8.9	40.7
A9. Cervix	63.0									-	-	2.3	6.9	27.0	13.9	13.0	63.0
A10. Ovary	14.0									-	-	-	2.4	3.7	3.5	3.3	14.0
A11. Prostate	25.0	-	-	-	-	2.3	11.6	11.1	25.0								
A12. Bladder	12.4	-	-	-	-	1.7	4.2	4.0	10.3								
A13. Lymphoma	29.5	-	1.9	1.2	1.8	2.3	5.6	5.3	18.8	-	-	-	-	1.2	4.0	3.7	10.7
A14. Leukaemia	25.7	1.2	3.5	1.1	1.7	1.3	3.4	3.2	15.5	-	1.4	-	-	-	1.8	1.7	10.2
B. Diabetes mellitus	144.5	-	-	3.6	2.4	15.3	26.7	15.1	63.0	-	-	2.9	2.0	20.1	36.9	19.6	81.5
C. Nutritional/endocrine	187.5	35.6	2.1	13.7	15.7	6.4	4.8	7.1	85.3	46.5	8.0	10.3	4.4	10.9	9.9	12.1	102.1
C1. Protein-energy malnutrition	61.8	18.8	1.4	1.7	-	-	-	2.2	25.0	29.6	1.7	-	-	-	-	2.6	36.8
C2. Anaemia	44.3	6.4	1.3	1.7	-	1.5	1.4	1.7	14.4	5.3	7.2	3.5	1.0	4.1	4.2	4.6	29.9
D. Neuro-psychiatric	178.9	11.6	18.9	11.8	12.6	19.6	13.4	15.5	103.3	17.0	16.0	11.3	4.8	5.5	7.0	14.0	75.6
D1. Psychoses	12.1	-	-	1.7	1.0	2.4	1.6	2.0	7.4	-	-	-	-	-	-	2.7	4.7
D2. Epilepsy	31.2	1.3	4.3	3.4	3.4	3.7	1.6	1.5	18.3	1.7	3.4	4.2	1.4	-	-	-	12.9
D3. Alcohol dependence	6.8	-	-	-	1.5	2.9	-	-	5.9								
D4. Alzheimer & other dementias	29.8	1.9	-	1.0	-	2.9	3.4	5.0	15.9	3.3	1.3	-	-	-	1.9	5.7	13.8
D5. Parkinson disease	8.4	-	-	-	-	-	1.6	3.5	5.6	-	-	-	-	-	-	1.9	2.8
D6. Multiple sclerosis	7.6	-	-	-	-	1.7	-	-	4.1	-	-	-	-	1.0	-	-	3.5
E. Cardiovascular diseases	2,385.9	16.5	5.9	15.6	58.2	222.7	344.7	553.0	1,216.6	22.2	14.4	19.7	32.7	159.9	299.2	621.1	1,169.3
E1. Rheumatic diseases	141.3	-	-	-	3.5	10.1	13.8	12.6	41.5	-	1.1	2.6	4.8	25.5	39.1	26.1	99.8
E2. Ischaemic heart disease	783.2	-	-	1.1	14.5	87.2	142.4	201.7	447.0	-	-	-	3.7	35.4	92.5	203.8	336.3
E3. Cerebrovascular diseases	619.2	1.5	-	1.9	8.1	34.0	67.1	166.1	279.6	1.8	1.9	4.1	8.3	38.7	74.7	210.0	339.6
E4. Inflammatory cardiac disease	527.5	11.1	3.7	9.6	25.2	64.6	77.3	97.5	288.9	16.5	9.3	8.9	11.5	39.7	55.8	97.0	238.7
F. Respiratory	272.4	22.3	8.8	4.2	6.1	19.9	30.5	60.5	152.3	29.3	6.3	7.7	5.2	19.9	17.7	34.0	120.1
F1. Chronic obstructive lung disease	140.8	3.2	-	1.6	1.4	12.3	23.0	46.9	88.0	3.3	-	-	2.0	11.9	12.9	22.4	52.7
F2. Asthma	32.6	1.4	4.3	8.4	1.6	2.2	1.6	2.2	14.8	1.7	3.3	3.2	2.0	3.6	1.8	2.3	17.9
G. Digestive	353.3	24.9	4.0	8.4	30.6	59.1	41.0	37.8	205.8	43.1	7.3	8.1	15.4	30.2	22.5	20.8	147.5
G1. Peptic ulcer disease	41.8	-	-	1.3	4.6	8.9	6.1	5.7	26.8	-	-	1.2	2.3	4.5	3.4	3.1	15.0
G2. Cirrhosis	135.7	-	-	2.8	18.7	39.0	24.1	10.0	96.0	-	-	2.5	6.7	14.7	8.1	5.1	39.7
H. Genito-urinary	144.5	3.4	6.1	2.5	3.8	11.9	13.1	29.9	70.7	2.4	6.5	6.9	3.4	16.8	19.7	18.0	73.8
H1. Nephritis/nephrosis	74.6	1.4	5.6	2.0	2.7	8.8	7.7	11.9	40.1	-	6.1	3.9	2.1	6.7	8.7	6.0	34.5
I. Musculo-skeletal	24.4	-	-	-	-	-	2.3	4.1	8.9	-	-	1.8	1.4	2.4	2.8	5.8	15.5
J. Congenital	181.3	83.1	4.3	3.6	1.4	-	-	-	93.3	75.0	4.4	4.0	3.2	1.2	-	-	88.0

A dash (-) indicates less than 1000 deaths.

Estimated deaths (in thousands) by age, sex and cause, 1990: China

No. of deaths (in thousands)

Cause of Death (ICD 9)	Both sexes	Males 0-4	5-14	15-29	30-44	45-59	60-69	70+	All ages	Females 0-4	5-14	15-29	30-44	45-59	60-69	70+	All ages
Population (in millions)	1,133.7	60.2	97.0	184.1	122.2	72.7	31.4	17.6	585.2	57.9	90.4	171.6	112.5	64.4	30.1	21.5	548.5
All Causes	8,885.0	505.0	86.0	279.0	347.0	746.0	1,061.0	1,805.0	4,829.0	565.0	63.0	231.0	233.0	462.0	695.0	1,807.0	4,056.0
I. Communicable, maternal & perinatal	1,342.5	333.1	12.1	23.0	38.3	81.8	78.0	121.8	688.2	377.7	11.8	36.9	33.9	41.0	48.9	104.1	654.4
A. Infectious & parasitic	612.9	58.1	8.0	21.0	37.3	77.6	70.1	89.7	361.8	62.1	8.4	15.8	25.0	37.0	40.4	62.5	251.1
A1. Tuberculosis	356.1	3.6	-	8.7	23.2	59.7	58.7	67.4	222.1	3.9	2.5	9.3	18.8	30.2	31.2	38.1	134.0
A2. Syphilis	1.5	-	-	-	-	-	-	-	-	-	-	-	-	-	-	-	-
A3. HIV	-	-	-	-	-	-	-	-	-	-	-	-	-	-	-	-	-
A4. Diarrhoeal diseases	95.3	22.9	1.5	1.6	1.3	1.7	5.1	11.3	45.5	29.6	1.3	-	1.2	1.2	2.3	13.5	49.8
a. Acute watery	59.4	11.5	1.1	1.3	1.0	1.4	4.1	9.1	29.4	14.8	-	-	-	-	1.7	10.1	30.0
b. Persistent	19.5	8.0	-	-	-	-	-	-	8.1	10.4	-	-	-	-	-	-	11.4
c. Dysentery	16.4	3.4	-	-	-	-	1.0	2.3	7.9	4.4	-	-	-	-	-	2.7	8.5
A5. Pertussis	12.9	5.9	-	-	-	-	-	-	6.6	5.7	-	-	-	-	-	-	6.3
A6. Measles	8.7	4.0	-	-	-	-	-	-	4.4	3.8	-	-	-	-	-	-	4.3
A7. Tetanus	21.9	8.7	-	-	-	-	-	-	11.9	7.0	-	-	-	-	-	-	9.9
A8. Meningitis	22.4	6.5	2.0	1.5	-	-	1.1	-	12.9	3.7	-	1.6	-	-	-	-	9.5
A9. Malaria	-	-	-	-	-	-	-	-	-	-	-	-	-	-	-	-	-
A10. Trypanosomiasis	-	-	-	-	-	-	-	-	-	-	-	-	-	-	-	-	-
A11. Chagas disease	-	-	-	-	-	-	-	-	-	-	-	-	-	-	-	-	-
A12. Schistosomiasis	1.3	-	-	-	-	-	-	-	1.2	-	-	-	-	-	-	-	-
A13. Leishmaniasis	-	-	-	-	-	-	-	-	-	-	-	-	-	-	-	-	-
A14. Onchocerciasis	3.0	-	-	-	-	-	-	-	1.8	-	-	-	-	-	-	-	1.1
B. Respiratory infections	410.7	136.1	4.2	2.1	1.0	4.2	7.9	32.0	187.4	165.0	3.5	1.4	1.0	2.3	8.5	41.6	223.3
C. Maternal causes	29.3	-	-	-	-	-	-	-	-	-	-	19.7	7.9	1.7	-	-	29.3
C1. Haemorrhage	14.4	-	-	-	-	-	-	-	-	-	-	9.7	3.9	-	-	-	14.4
C2. Sepsis	1.8	-	-	-	-	-	-	-	-	-	-	1.2	-	-	-	-	1.8
C3. Eclampsia	2.1	-	-	-	-	-	-	-	-	-	-	1.4	-	-	-	-	2.1
C4. Hypertension	-	-	-	-	-	-	-	-	-	-	-	-	-	-	-	-	-
C5. Obstructed labour	-	-	-	-	-	-	-	-	-	-	-	-	-	-	-	-	-
C6. Abortion	2.9	-	-	-	-	-	-	-	-	-	-	2.0	-	-	-	-	2.9
D. Perinatal causes	289.5	138.9	-	-	-	-	-	-	138.9	150.6	-	-	-	-	-	-	150.6
III. Injuries	1,023.3	77.1	43.3	151.1	112.7	81.2	54.1	70.6	590.0	72.4	28.3	114.0	58.2	49.9	35.8	74.9	433.3
A. Unintentional	629.8	72.2	39.8	97.2	69.1	51.2	29.6	42.1	401.2	63.4	25.0	36.0	21.4	22.3	17.1	43.3	228.6
A1. Road traffic accidents	135.4	4.0	6.1	26.5	27.9	16.5	8.8	6.9	96.7	2.9	5.8	9.5	6.1	7.6	3.4	3.5	38.7
A2. Poisoning	65.4	5.1	1.6	6.4	6.9	9.0	3.5	5.5	38.0	1.6	2.3	9.2	5.3	2.3	2.6	4.1	27.4
A3. Falls	65.0	2.4	-	5.9	3.7	4.5	5.1	9.7	32.2	3.7	-	-	1.0	3.3	4.9	18.1	32.8
A4. Fires	24.1	2.7	1.1	2.3	1.7	1.1	-	4.8	13.6	1.9	-	-	-	1.0	1.1	4.0	10.5
A5. Drowning	149.0	31.0	22.7	20.0	6.2	4.4	2.7	5.1	92.2	26.2	11.3	7.4	2.8	2.1	2.1	4.9	56.8
A6. Occupational	23.9	-	-	5.8	8.6	4.6	-	-	19.4	-	-	-	2.0	1.4	-	-	4.5
B. Intentional	393.5	4.9	3.5	53.9	43.6	29.9	24.5	28.5	188.9	9.0	3.2	77.9	36.7	27.6	18.7	31.6	204.7
B1. Self-inflicted	342.7	-	2.5	41.4	36.5	27.3	22.9	28.1	158.6	-	1.8	75.6	33.0	26.0	17.6	30.2	184.1
B2. Homicide and violence	50.8	4.9	1.0	12.5	7.1	2.7	1.6	-	30.3	9.0	1.4	2.3	3.7	1.6	1.1	1.4	20.6
B3. War	-	-	-	-	-	-	-	-	-	-	-	-	-	-	-	-	-

A dash (-) indicates less than 1000 deaths.

Estimated deaths (in thousands) by age, sex and cause, 1990: China

No. of deaths (in thousands)

Cause of Death (ICD 9)	Both sexes	Males								Females							
		0-4	5-14	15-29	30-44	45-59	60-69	70+	All ages	0-4	5-14	15-29	30-44	45-59	60-69	70+	All ages
II. Noncommunicable	6,519.2	94.8	30.6	104.9	196.0	583.0	928.9	1,612.6	3,550.8	114.9	22.9	80.1	141.0	371.1	610.3	1,628.0	2,968.4
A. Malignant neoplasms	1,408.0	4.8	10.2	28.2	80.6	231.9	284.9	245.2	885.9	6.2	5.1	19.3	48.8	122.8	147.5	172.3	522.1
A1. Mouth and oropharynx	34.8	-	-	1.1	4.8	6.2	6.3	4.9	23.8	-	-	-	1.7	3.2	3.0	2.3	11.0
A2. Oesophagus	182.7	-	-	-	6.1	29.2	44.9	42.9	123.9	-	-	-	-	11.1	24.0	22.4	58.8
A3. Stomach	307.9	-	-	1.1	8.7	51.5	74.9	64.9	201.2	-	-	2.1	8.4	20.9	32.9	42.0	106.7
A4. Colorectal	80.1	-	-	2.2	4.1	9.9	13.1	15.1	44.3	-	-	-	3.2	8.4	10.5	12.6	35.8
A5. Liver	279.4	-	-	5.2	38.1	71.6	53.6	33.0	202.3	-	-	1.5	8.9	21.7	21.1	23.5	77.0
A6. Pancreas	31.1	-	-	-	-	3.8	6.6	7.1	18.9	-	-	-	-	1.7	4.5	5.5	12.2
A7. Lung	210.7	-	-	1.9	3.0	32.7	58.1	50.2	146.6	-	-	-	1.8	14.7	19.7	27.2	64.1
A8. Breast	24.9	-	-	-	-	-	-	-	-	-	-	-	5.8	7.8	5.0	6.0	24.9
A9. Cervix	20.6	-	-	-	-	-	-	-	-	-	-	-	2.3	6.3	6.0	5.4	20.6
A10. Ovary	10.1	-	-	-	-	-	-	-	-	-	-	-	1.8	2.9	1.8	2.2	10.1
A11. Prostate	4.7	-	-	-	-	-	2.1	2.2	4.7	-	-	-	-	-	-	-	-
A12. Bladder	18.2	-	-	-	-	1.9	5.7	6.2	14.3	-	-	-	-	2.6	1.5	1.8	3.9
A13. Lymphoma	21.8	-	-	2.4	-	3.3	4.7	2.8	14.5	-	-	-	-	5.1	1.5	1.9	7.3
A14. Leukemia	63.4	2.7	5.1	7.7	5.6	5.7	3.0	2.9	32.8	2.9	2.7	7.1	4.5	6.3	3.2	3.8	30.7
B. Diabetes mellitus	59.5	-	-	-	2.6	5.7	8.0	9.2	26.6	-	-	1.1	1.8	1.5	11.0	12.4	33.0
C. Nutritional/endocrine	79.0	10.4	1.5	2.7	1.2	1.8	3.0	5.4	26.0	24.5	3.0	3.0	-	-	4.3	12.2	53.0
C1. Protein-energy malnutrition	37.4	8.0	-	-	-	-	-	1.5	11.2	18.3	-	-	-	-	-	5.8	26.1
C2. Anaemia	26.9	1.6	1.9	1.9	-	-	1.4	1.8	8.8	4.8	2.3	1.5	3.0	-	2.4	3.3	18.1
D. Neuro-psychiatric	97.5	2.1	-	13.2	10.0	5.4	5.1	14.4	52.1	1.7	-	6.8	6.8	4.9	6.3	18.1	45.4
D1. Psychoses	15.4	-	-	2.5	3.6	-	-	2.5	10.0	-	-	1.1	1.4	-	-	1.0	5.3
D2. Epilepsy	16.0	-	-	3.8	2.7	-	-	-	9.1	-	-	2.5	2.0	-	-	-	6.9
D3. Alcohol dependence	6.5	-	-	1.0	1.4	2.0	1.2	-	5.7	-	-	-	-	-	-	-	-
D4. Alzheimer & other dementias	19.0	-	-	-	-	-	-	4.7	8.0	-	-	-	-	-	-	-	11.0
D5. Parkinson disease	7.2	-	-	-	-	-	-	3.2	3.9	-	-	-	-	-	-	-	3.3
D6. Multiple sclerosis	5.5	-	-	-	-	-	-	-	1.9	-	-	-	1.2	-	-	-	3.6
E. Cardiovascular diseases	2,566.2	9.8	4.1	27.9	46.7	191.3	338.0	704.4	1,322.1	7.2	2.3	25.3	42.6	143.1	253.2	770.4	1,244.1
E1. Rheumatic diseases	162.8	-	-	9.5	7.0	12.7	12.4	26.0	68.3	-	-	8.5	11.6	19.4	16.8	36.8	94.5
E2. Ischaemic heart disease	441.8	1.4	-	5.3	13.2	36.4	57.4	119.8	234.2	-	-	3.0	5.8	16.3	16.3	139.3	207.6
E3. Cerebrovascular disease	1,271.1	2.1	1.7	6.8	18.2	97.5	186.3	358.8	671.4	1.3	-	5.1	13.8	71.2	136.6	370.6	599.6
E4. Inflammatory cardiac disease	92.0	1.5	-	2.0	2.2	8.6	12.2	22.9	49.8	-	-	1.9	2.4	5.8	7.5	23.1	42.3
F. Respiratory	1,584.9	10.8	3.9	5.2	11.5	71.2	207.3	521.7	828.8	14.9	-	1.5	11.1	47.8	135.5	544.6	756.2
F1. Chronic obstructive lung disease	1,320.3	1.5	-	-	8.9	60.1	182.8	456.8	710.7	1.7	-	-	9.6	39.7	118.2	440.2	609.6
F2. Asthma	56.2	-	-	1.9	-	3.2	5.4	10.4	22.9	-	-	-	-	3.6	6.4	20.8	33.3
G. Digestive	414.9	16.0	-	10.1	32.5	57.4	57.4	65.6	242.9	18.0	3.3	8.7	12.6	30.3	33.1	65.9	171.9
G1. Peptic ulcer disease	81.2	-	-	2.5	4.8	11.9	12.6	19.5	52.5	-	-	2.8	2.4	3.6	3.6	15.6	28.7
G2. Cirrhosis	187.0	-	-	3.8	23.8	37.2	33.6	22.6	123.3	-	-	2.4	6.0	17.6	17.6	19.5	63.7
H. Genito-urinary	123.5	1.2	1.7	8.7	8.6	11.3	13.6	27.7	73.2	1.7	1.1	4.8	7.9	8.2	11.0	15.5	50.3
H1. Nephritis/nephrosis	98.2	1.5	1.7	8.6	7.9	9.6	10.9	17.0	56.8	1.7	1.1	4.5	7.4	6.6	8.4	11.7	41.4
I. Musculo-skeletal	36.0	1.2	-	-	-	1.1	4.6	10.3	17.3	-	-	1.1	1.9	1.9	2.3	11.0	18.7
J. Congenital	99.4	37.0	4.7	5.3	-	-	-	-	48.0	38.2	5.0	6.5	1.3	-	-	-	51.4

A dash (-) indicates less than 1000 deaths.

Estimated deaths (in thousands) by age, sex and cause, 1990: Other Asia and Islands

No. of deaths (in thousands)

Cause of Death (ICD 9)	Both sexes	Males								Females							
		0-4	5-14	15-29	30-44	45-59	60-69	70+	All ages	0-4	5-14	15-29	30-44	45-59	60-69	70+	All ages
Population (in millions)	682.5	43.8	84.0	99.2	61.6	34.1	13.1	7.1	343.0	42.0	80.2	98.0	61.6	35.1	14.0	8.7	339.6
All Causes	5,519.0	899.0	229.0	205.0	246.0	398.0	421.0	637.0	3,035.0	714.0	171.0	156.0	183.0	278.0	314.0	668.0	2,484.0
I. Communicable, maternal & perinatal	2,306.4	778.0	124.4	51.6	57.2	86.7	75.8	74.5	1,248.2	617.8	101.1	85.7	81.3	45.3	49.6	77.5	1,058.3
A. Infectious & parasitic	1,217	352.1	97.9	44.9	52.6	80.4	41.3	22.5	691.8	291.3	75.7	46.2	44.2	38.3	18.4	11.5	525.7
A1. Tuberculosis	353.2	5.6	16.7	30.3	41.8	70.8	36.8	19.8	221.9	4.8	15.9	30.4	28.9	29.1	13.8	8.4	131.3
A2. Syphilis	-	-	-	-	-	-	-	-	-	-	-	-	-	-	-	-	-
A3. HIV	-	-	-	-	-	-	-	-	-	-	-	-	-	-	-	-	-
A4. Diarrhoeal diseases	432.3	199.5	19.9	4.8	3.3	2.6	-	-	231.5	170.3	17.3	4.6	4.4	2.7	-	-	200.8
a. Acute watery	232.9	98.7	15.8	3.9	2.7	2.0	-	-	124.3	84.2	13.6	3.8	3.6	2.1	-	-	108.7
b. Persistent	132.4	70.6	-	-	-	-	-	-	71.4	60.3	-	-	-	-	-	-	61.0
c. Dysentery	66.9	30.3	3.3	-	-	-	-	-	35.8	25.8	2.9	-	-	-	-	-	31.1
A5. Pertussis	33.0	15.9	2.7	-	-	-	-	-	18.7	12.2	2.1	-	-	-	-	-	14.4
A6. Measles	122.8	56.5	9.7	-	-	-	-	-	66.1	48.2	8.4	-	-	-	-	-	56.6
A7. Tetanus	64.5	30.7	2.3	-	-	-	-	-	34.7	26.0	2.0	-	-	-	-	-	29.8
A8. Meningitis	39.8	11.9	14.0	-	-	-	-	-	27.8	6.7	3.1	-	-	-	-	-	12.0
A9. Malaria	74.3	4.9	14.4	7.2	5.0	3.8	1.5	-	37.5	4.2	12.5	7.0	6.6	3.9	1.6	-	36.7
A10. Trypanosomiasis	-	-	-	-	-	-	-	-	-	-	-	-	-	-	-	-	-
A11. Chagas disease	-	-	-	-	-	-	-	-	-	-	-	-	-	-	-	-	-
A12. Schistosomiasis	-	-	-	-	-	-	-	-	-	-	-	-	-	-	-	-	-
A13. Leishmaniasis	1.6	-	-	-	-	-	-	-	-	-	-	-	-	-	-	-	-
A14. Onchocerciasis	-	-	-	-	-	-	-	-	-	-	-	-	-	-	-	-	-
B. Respiratory infections	691.3	227.6	26.5	6.6	4.6	6.3	34.5	52.1	358.2	194.3	22.9	6.5	6.1	6.2	31.2	66.0	333.2
C. Maternal causes	67.3									-	2.4	33.0	31.0	-	-	-	67.3
C1. Haemorrhage	20.2									-	-	9.9	9.3	-	-	-	20.2
C2. Sepsis	13.5									-	-	6.6	6.2	-	-	-	13.5
C3. Eclampsia	6.7									-	-	3.3	3.1	-	-	-	6.7
C4. Hypertension	8.7									-	-	4.3	4.0	-	-	-	8.7
C5. Obstructed labour	6.7									-	-	3.3	3.1	-	-	-	6.7
C6. Abortion	3.4									-	-	1.7	1.6	-	-	-	3.4
D. Perinatal causes	330.4	198.2	-	-	-	-	-	-	198.2	132.2	-	-	-	-	-	-	132.2
III. Injuries	476.8	27.9	43.9	127.0	88.0	47.4	18.3	15.5	368.1	20.9	16.0	25.4	15.6	11.9	7.0	12.0	108.7
A. Unintentional	343.3	26.0	40.0	83.9	56.4	33.0	13.0	11.7	263.9	18.9	14.3	15.0	8.9	7.7	4.9	9.7	79.4
A1. Road traffic accidents	122.3	4.2	12.4	38.9	23.7	11.7	4.4	3.0	98.3	2.9	5.4	6.8	3.3	2.6	1.5	1.5	24.0
A2. Poisoning	20.9	1.5	-	3.6	5.0	3.4	-	-	16.0	-	-	1.0	-	-	-	-	4.9
A3. Falls	24.1	1.2	1.4	3.6	3.1	3.0	1.6	2.8	16.5	-	-	-	-	-	-	3.9	7.5
A4. Fires	11.3	2.3	1.2	-	-	-	-	-	7.3	1.6	-	-	-	-	-	-	4.0
A5. Drowning	43.8	5.5	11.0	9.9	4.2	2.1	-	-	34.2	3.5	3.0	-	-	-	-	-	9.6
A6. Occupational	18.0	-	-	4.3	7.4	3.5	-	-	15.3	-	-	-	1.3	-	-	-	2.6
B. Intentional	133.5	1.9	3.9	43.1	31.6	14.5	5.4	3.8	104.1	2.0	1.7	10.4	6.7	4.2	2.1	2.3	29.3
B1. Self-inflicted	81.5	-	2.0	23.2	19.0	10.5	4.3	3.3	62.4	-	-	7.1	4.5	3.2	1.7	1.8	19.1
B2. Homicide and violence	43.1	1.3	1.6	17.0	10.8	3.7	-	-	35.8	1.3	-	2.2	1.6	-	-	-	7.4
B3. War	8.8	-	-	2.8	1.7	-	-	-	5.9	-	-	1.0	-	-	-	-	2.9

A dash (-) indicates less than 1000 deaths.

Estimated deaths (in thousands) by age, sex and cause, 1990: Other Asia and Islands

No. of deaths (in thousands)

Cause of Death (ICD 9)	Both sexes	Males 0-4	5-14	15-29	30-44	45-59	60-69	70+	All ages	Females 0-4	5-14	15-29	30-44	45-59	60-69	70+	All ages
II. Noncommunicable	2,735.8	93.1	60.6	26.5	100.8	263.9	326.9	547.0	1,418.8	75.3	53.9	44.9	86.0	220.9	257.4	578.5	1,317.0
A. Malignant neoplasms	540.6	2.0	10.4	4.8	16.9	75.4	92.9	108.7	311.0	2.8	1.7	7.0	26.5	67.0	54.9	69.8	229.6
A1. Mouth and oropharynx	63.2	-	-	-	1.9	4.8	14.9	17.5	40.0	-	-	-	2.0	2.8	7.8	9.9	23.2
A2. Oesophagus	21.0	-	-	-	-	3.6	4.8	5.7	14.5	-	-	-	-	1.7	1.9	2.4	6.4
A3. Stomach	52.0	-	-	-	1.4	9.1	10.5	12.3	33.7	-	-	-	1.3	4.7	5.2	6.6	18.3
A4. Colorectal	37.3	-	-	-	1.0	2.3	7.5	8.7	19.9	-	-	-	1.3	2.6	5.8	7.3	17.4
A5. Liver	57.8	-	-	-	2.9	15.2	10.5	12.3	42.2	-	-	-	1.1	4.3	4.3	5.5	15.7
A6. Pancreas	8.9	-	-	-	-	1.2	1.8	2.2	5.5	-	-	-	-	-	1.1	1.3	3.3
A7. Lung	79.9	-	-	-	1.4	14.5	20.4	23.9	60.7	-	-	-	-	4.5	6.0	7.6	19.1
A8. Breast	24.8	-	-	-	-	-	-	-	-	-	-	1.1	4.0	9.8	4.4	5.6	24.8
A9. Cervix	29.8	-	-	-	-	-	-	-	-	-	-	1.0	3.9	13.1	5.2	6.6	29.8
A10. Ovary	9.0	-	-	-	-	-	-	-	-	-	-	-	2.3	2.6	1.5	1.9	9.0
A11. Prostate	13.0	-	-	-	-	-	5.5	6.5	13.0	-	-	-	-	-	-	-	-
A12. Bladder	10.4	-	-	-	-	1.2	2.9	3.4	7.7	-	-	-	-	1.0	-	1.2	2.7
A13. Lymphoma	20.4	-	1.4	1.2	1.2	1.5	3.4	3.9	12.1	-	-	-	1.0	1.0	2.5	3.2	8.3
A14. Leukemia	19.8	-	3.9	-	1.6	-	1.9	2.2	11.6	-	-	-	1.8	-	1.5	1.9	8.2
B. Diabetes mellitus	87.0	-	-	-	1.4	8.4	14.2	8.5	33.6	-	-	-	1.3	13.2	22.9	14.3	53.4
C. Nutritional/endocrine	82.8	15.9	2.0	3.8	8.5	3.2	2.5	4.7	40.4	11.7	5.3	1.7	3.3	5.5	4.2	7.7	42.4
C1. Protein-energy malnutrition	23.4	8.3	1.4	-	-	-	-	1.3	12.2	7.3	1.1	-	-	-	-	1.5	11.2
C2. Anaemia	22.4	2.9	1.2	-	-	-	-	1.3	7.6	1.4	4.6	-	-	2.0	1.7	2.8	14.9
D. Neuro-psychiatric	119.2	5.7	18.2	3.7	7.8	10.3	8.1	14.5	68.3	4.7	11.0	4.7	4.0	4.3	4.9	16.4	50.9
D1. Psychoses	4.3	-	-	-	-	-	-	-	2.3	-	-	-	-	-	-	-	2.0
D2. Epilepsy	19.6	-	4.2	1.1	2.2	-	-	-	11.7	-	2.3	1.6	1.2	-	-	-	7.9
D3. Alcohol dependence	2.9	-	-	-	-	2.0	-	-	2.5	-	-	-	-	-	-	-	-
D4. Alzheimer & other dementias	22.6	-	-	-	-	-	-	4.8	11.5	-	-	-	-	-	-	-	11.0
D5. Parkinson disease	7.5	-	-	-	-	-	-	3.3	4.6	-	-	-	-	-	-	-	2.9
D6. Multiple sclerosis	5.3	-	-	-	-	-	-	-	2.5	-	-	-	-	-	-	-	2.8
E. Cardiovascular diseases	1,351.6	8.1	6.9	6.5	38.4	114.8	163.2	327.0	665.0	6.3	10.8	5.7	27.3	90.6	137.3	403.0	686.7
E1. Rheumatic diseases	33.6	-	-	-	1.1	2.1	2.4	2.9	9.2	-	-	-	2.3	6.5	7.1	6.9	24.5
E2. Ischaemic heart disease	589.2	-	-	2.5	16.1	59.5	82.4	156.8	316.0	-	-	2.1	5.8	30.1	56.4	179.8	273.2
E3. Cerebrovascular diseases	350.4	-	1.2	1.1	5.0	21.6	39.5	86.0	155.2	-	2.0	1.3	6.6	26.4	40.9	116.3	195.2
E4. Inflammatory cardiac disease	129.6	3.4	3.1	2.8	8.4	13.2	13.4	22.7	66.8	3.3	4.7	4.0	5.5	10.1	10.2	25.7	62.8
F. Respiratory	138.1	8.7	7.2	2.5	3.2	8.8	13.8	34.6	77.5	6.6	3.7	1.2	3.6	9.6	8.6	25.4	60.7
F1. Chronic obstructive lung disease	76.3	-	-	-	-	5.5	10.4	26.8	45.6	-	-	-	-	5.7	6.3	16.7	30.8
F2. Asthma	17.5	1.2	3.5	-	-	-	-	1.2	8.2	-	1.9	-	1.4	1.7	-	1.7	9.3
G. Digestive	203.6	11.3	4.1	1.9	20.3	34.3	22.7	25.9	121.4	10.7	5.0	3.3	12.0	18.4	12.5	19.5	82.2
G1. Peptic ulcer disease	26.3	-	-	-	3.0	5.2	3.4	3.9	16.1	-	-	-	1.8	2.8	1.9	2.9	10.2
G2. Cirrhosis	83.0	-	-	-	12.4	22.5	12.9	7.4	57.1	-	-	-	5.2	9.1	4.8	4.5	25.9
H. Genito-urinary	84.6	1.6	5.9	-	2.6	6.2	6.7	17.8	41.8	-	4.3	1.9	2.9	9.2	9.0	13.4	42.8
H1. Nephritis/nephrosis	50.1	-	5.4	-	2.0	4.7	4.3	8.4	26.3	-	4.0	-	1.9	4.4	4.7	6.6	23.8
I. Musculo-skeletal	15.0	-	-	-	-	-	1.2	2.6	5.3	-	-	-	1.1	1.4	1.4	4.0	9.7
J. Congenital	84.5	38.7	4.0	-	-	-	-	-	45.0	30.6	4.0	1.9	2.3	-	-	-	39.6

A dash (-) indicates less than 1000 deaths.

Estimated deaths (in thousands) by age, sex and cause, 1990: Sub-Saharan Africa

No. of deaths (in thousands)

Cause of Death (ICD 9)	Both sexes	Males								Females							
		0-4	5-14	15-29	30-44	45-59	60-69	70+	All ages	0-4	5-14	15-29	30-44	45-59	60-69	70+	All ages
Population (in millions)	510.3	47.5	70.3	66.8	37.0	20.3	7.0	3.5	252.3	47.0	69.8	67.4	38.8	22.1	8.1	4.6	258.0
All Causes	7,937.0	2,142.0	369.0	391.0	321.0	332.0	258.0	359.0	4,172.0	1,834.0	344.0	324.0	293.0	283.0	251.0	436.0	3,765.0
I. Communicable, maternal & perinatal	5,414.7	1,955.6	261.2	198.2	116.8	118.9	86.2	69.3	2,806.2	1,683.6	264.1	274.1	181.7	75.8	59.0	70.2	2,608.5
A. Infectious & parasitic	3,759.5	1,265.9	227.1	188.0	111.6	113.4	56.5	27.9	1,990.3	1,127.9	224.5	185.6	120.4	67.7	27.6	15.6	1,769.2
A1. Tuberculosis	535.5	12.7	27.5	71.2	52.9	83.5	44.4	21.9	314.1	11.5	31.5	66.2	42.9	41.1	18.0	10.1	221.4
A2. Syphilis	152.7	35.2	-	27.3	14.0	3.4	-	-	80.8	31.4	-	22.0	14.4	3.1	-	-	71.8
A3. HIV	217.8	27.8	4.5	42.0	21.4	6.5	2.0	1.0	105.3	25.4	4.7	45.7	29.6	5.2	1.1	-	112.4
A4. Diarrhoeal diseases	887.1	417.5	34.1	5.0	2.5	1.6	-	-	461.5	378.4	35.6	5.3	3.4	1.9	-	-	425.6
a. Acute watery	471.3	210.4	25.9	4.0	2.0	1.2	-	-	244.3	190.7	27.1	4.2	2.7	1.5	-	-	227.1
b. Persistent	279.0	144.6	1.6	-	-	-	-	-	146.3	131.1	1.7	-	-	-	-	-	132.8
c. Dysentery	136.8	62.5	6.6	1.0	-	-	-	-	71.0	56.6	6.8	1.1	-	-	-	-	65.8
A5. Pertussis	133.7	62.7	10.2	-	-	-	-	-	72.9	51.2	9.5	-	-	-	-	-	60.7
A6. Measles	472.7	211.2	34.3	-	-	-	-	-	245.6	191.4	35.7	-	-	-	-	-	227.2
A7. Tetanus	174.5	85.6	4.2	-	-	-	-	-	92.4	74.6	4.4	-	-	-	-	-	82.1
A8. Meningitis	49.6	15.0	14.1	2.0	-	-	-	-	32.0	9.2	4.1	2.8	1.2	-	-	-	17.6
A9. Malaria	805.3	323.5	55.1	19.6	10.0	3.3	1.3	-	413.6	293.2	57.5	20.9	13.6	4.1	1.5	-	391.7
A10. Trypanosomiasis	55.1	1.5	10.2	7.1	3.6	4.8	-	-	28.2	2.7	9.1	6.8	4.4	3.2	-	-	26.8
A11. Chagas disease																	
A12. Schistosomiasis	21.0	-	4.5	4.2	2.1	1.4	-	-	13.6	-	1.9	2.3	1.5	-	-	-	7.4
A13. Leishmaniasis	10.4	-	3.1	1.0	-	-	-	-	5.0	-	3.3	1.1	-	-	-	-	5.4
A14. Onchocerciasis	29.7	-	-	2.7	1.4	6.1	4.8	2.4	17.3	-	-	1.9	1.2	4.6	3.1	1.7	12.4
B. Respiratory infections	1,028.8	396.7	34.1	10.3	5.2	5.5	29.7	41.4	522.9	359.5	35.5	10.9	7.1	6.8	31.4	54.6	505.9
C. Maternal causes	137.2										4.0	77.6	54.2	1.4			137.2
C1. Haemorrhage	41.2										1.2	23.3	16.2				41.2
C2. Sepsis	27.4											15.5	10.8				27.4
C3. Eclampsia	13.7											7.8	5.4				13.7
C4. Hypertension	6.9											3.9	2.7				6.9
C5. Obstructed labour	13.7											7.8	5.4				13.7
C6. Abortion	20.6											11.6	8.1				20.6
D. Perinatal causes	489.3	293.0							293.0	196.2							196.2
III. Injuries	623.8	58.7	51.4	178.8	109.8	35.2	10.5	2.1	446.5	53.3	29.0	33.9	27.6	13.5	7.4	12.4	177.2
A. Unintentional	335.3	41.2	38.7	85.2	52.4	21.3	6.0	-	245.6	35.3	20.7	6.5	8.2	5.8	3.9	9.2	89.7
A1. Road traffic accidents	113.9	6.7	12.0	39.5	22.0	7.6	2.0	-	90.0	5.5	7.9	2.9	3.0	2.0	1.2	1.4	23.9
A2. Poisoning	19.5	2.4	-	3.7	4.7	2.2	-	-	14.4	1.8	-	-	-	-	-	-	5.1
A3. Falls	20.4	1.9	1.4	3.6	2.9	1.9	-	-	12.6	1.8	1.2	-	-	-	-	3.7	7.8
A4. Fires	13.0	3.7	1.1	-	-	-	-	-	7.7	3.0	-	-	-	-	-	-	5.4
A5. Drowning	48.3	8.8	10.7	10.1	3.9	1.4	-	-	35.2	6.5	4.4	-	-	-	-	-	13.0
A6. Occupational	15.5	-	-	4.3	6.8	2.3	-	-	13.5	-	-	-	1.2	-	-	-	2.0
B. Intentional	288.5	17.5	12.7	93.6	57.4	13.9	4.5	1.3	200.9	18.0	8.3	27.4	19.4	7.7	3.6	3.2	87.6
B1. Self-inflicted	66.0	-	1.9	23.6	17.7	6.8	2.0	-	52.2	-	-	3.1	4.2	2.5	1.3	1.7	13.8
B2. Homicide and violence	41.0	2.0	1.5	17.3	10.0	2.4	-	-	33.7	2.5	1.1	-	1.2	1.5	-	-	7.2
B3. War	181.6	15.5	9.3	52.8	29.7	4.6	2.1	1.0	115.0	15.5	6.2	23.4	13.7	4.6	2.0	1.1	66.6

A dash (-) indicates less than 1000 deaths.

Estimated deaths (in thousands) by age, sex and cause, 1990: Sub-Saharan Africa

No. of deaths (in thousands)

Cause of Death (ICD 9)	Both sexes	Males								Females							
		0-4	5-14	15-29	30-44	45-59	60-69	70+	All ages	0-4	5-14	15-29	30-44	45-59	60-69	70+	All ages
II. Noncommunicable	1,898.5	127.6	56.4	13.9	94.4	178.0	161.3	287.6	919.2	97.1	50.9	16.0	83.7	193.7	184.6	353.4	979.3
A. Malignant neoplasms	305.2	2.1	9.1	1.7	7.8	46.2	45.1	50.5	162.5	3.3		1.7	21.0	48.8	33.7	33.9	142.6
A1. Mouth and oropharynx	20.1					1.7	4.5	5.1	12.0					1.1	2.9	2.9	8.1
A2. Oesophagus	19.9					5.4	3.8	4.2	14.0					1.8	1.8	1.8	5.9
A3. Stomach	27.8					5.1	4.6	5.1	15.4				1.2	4.9	3.1	3.1	12.4
A4. Colorectal	13.1					1.0	2.4	2.7	6.5					1.0	2.4	2.4	6.6
A5. Liver	43.8				3.3	12.1	6.0	6.7	29.2				2.8	4.7	3.4	3.4	14.7
A6. Pancreas	6.0					1.2			3.2					1.1			2.8
A7. Lung	16.9					4.2	3.7	4.2	12.5					1.7	1.2	1.2	4.4
A8. Breast	16.7												2.8	6.4	3.6	3.6	16.7
A9. Cervix	31.9												4.3	12.4	7.4	7.4	31.9
A10. Ovary	7.1												1.4	2.6	1.5	1.5	7.1
A11. Prostate	29.9					3.3	12.5	14.0	29.9								
A12. Bladder	12.1					1.9	2.6	3.0	7.7					1.3	1.3	1.3	4.4
A13. Lymphoma	21.3	1.1	5.0			1.7	2.6	2.9	14.2	1.1			1.5	1.2	1.5	1.5	7.0
A14. Leukemia	7.2								3.7								3.5
B. Diabetes mellitus	24.6					2.2	3.5	2.1	8.2					4.3	7.4	4.1	16.4
C. Nutritional/endocrine	89.3	23.6	1.6	3.5	11.8	2.3	1.2	2.1	46.0	16.5	5.3	2.0	3.8	6.5	3.8	5.2	43.2
C1. Protein-energy malnutrition	29.8	12.6	1.4						15.8	10.6	1.2					1.1	14.0
C2. Anaemia	22.1	4.3	1.1						7.6	1.9	4.9		2.5				14.6
D. Neuro-psychiatric	83.6	7.3	17.6	2.0	7.8	7.5	3.4	4.5	50.1	5.9	10.7	2.2	3.8	2.7	2.6	5.6	33.6
D1. Psychoses	4.5								2.5								1.9
D2. Epilepsy	15.1		4.1		2.1	1.3			9.4		2.3		1.1			1.1	5.7
D3. Alcohol dependence	3.8					1.3			3.2								
D4. Alzheimer & other dementias	12.1	1.2	1.6			1.0		1.3	6.4	1.1						2.3	5.7
D5. Parkinson disease	2.6								1.5								1.1
D6. Multiple sclerosis	3.2								1.5								1.7
E. Cardiovascular diseases	933.9	10.7	5.3	2.3	36.7	83.8	86.1	186.1	411.0	7.8	9.7	3.8	27.6	91.6	113.1	269.4	522.9
E1. Rheumatic diseases	64.6				2.6	4.4	3.7	5.0	16.3				4.4	14.6	14.9	13.0	48.4
E2. Ischaemic heart disease	109.1				3.6	12.5	12.8	26.4	55.4				1.1	6.8	11.7	34.0	53.7
E3. Cerebrovascular diseases	389.1				6.7	27.4	36.8	86.9	160.1				7.5	35.7	51.1	131.8	229.0
E4. Inflammatory cardiac disease	234.3	1.2	3.4	1.5	18.6	27.9	20.8	38.3	117.6	5.8	6.1	1.8	10.6	22.7	21.3	48.5	116.7
F. Respiratory	102.6	13.5	7.7		3.8	6.9	7.1	17.2	56.7	9.0	3.7	1.4	3.8	9.9	5.8	12.4	45.9
F1. Chronic obstructive lung disease	47.0	1.9				4.2	5.4	13.3	26.6	1.0				5.9	4.2	8.1	20.4
F2. Asthma	15.2								7.5		1.9		1.5	1.8			7.7
G. Digestive	159.9	16.7	3.8	2.1	21.9	22.7	10.3	12.3	89.8	15.3	4.9	1.6	14.0	17.2	8.5	8.5	70.1
G1. Peptic ulcer disease	18.3					3.4	1.5	1.8	10.6				2.1	2.6	1.3	1.3	7.7
G2. Cirrhosis	60.4				13.3	14.9	6.0	3.2	39.4				5.9	8.1	3.1	2.2	21.0
H. Genito-urinary	64.6	2.2	5.9		2.6	4.7	3.3	10.1	29.2		4.4		2.9	9.9	7.5	8.5	35.4
H1. Nephritis/nephrosis	34.1		5.4		1.8	3.5	2.0	3.5	17.5		4.1		1.7	3.8	3.3	2.6	16.6
I. Musculo-skeletal	10.1								3.2				1.1	1.2	1.0	2.5	6.9
J. Congenital	100.1	50.0	3.6					1.4	55.4	36.7	3.4		3.0				44.6

A dash (-) indicates less than 1000 deaths.

Estimated deaths (in thousands) by age, sex and cause, 1990: Latin America and the Caribbean

No. of deaths (in thousands)

Cause of Death (ICD 9)	Both sexes	Males								Females							
		0-4	5-14	15-29	30-44	45-59	60-69	70+	All ages	0-4	5-14	15-29	30-44	45-59	60-69	70+	All ages
Population (in millions)	444.3	28.7	52.1	64.1	40.2	22.2	8.8	5.4	221.6	27.7	50.7	63.2	40.9	23.4	9.9	7.0	222.7
All Causes	2,992.0	401.0	72.0	150.0	165.0	227.0	218.0	411.0	1,644.0	304.0	54.0	96.0	111.0	170.0	176.0	437.0	1,348.0
I. Communicable, maternal & perinatal	966.1	328.1	34.7	38.9	35.9	35.2	17.6	39.6	530.0	245.5	30.1	50.7	39.7	23.2	11.8	35.1	436.1
A. Infectious & parasitic	490.2	117.4	24.8	35.2	31.8	30.7	12.8	21.9	274.7	96.4	21.7	28.7	26.0	18.5	7.9	16.2	215.5
A1. Tuberculosis	111.5	1.7	2.9	13.5	14.8	19.8	6.0	11.2	69.9	1.6	3.1	9.8	11.6	8.3	2.1	5.0	41.6
A2. Syphilis	11.5	1.6	–	–	–	–	–	–	6.2	1.5	–	2.0	1.4	–	–	–	5.2
A3. HIV	28.9	1.0	–	11.5	7.5	2.3	1.3	–	23.6	1.0	–	2.3	1.5	–	–	–	5.3
A4. Diarrhoeal diseases	170.8	73.6	7.4	2.5	1.2	1.4	1.1	4.0	90.4	59.6	6.8	3.5	2.2	1.9	1.5	4.9	80.4
a. Acute watery	96.0	36.8	5.6	1.4	–	–	–	3.2	49.9	29.8	5.1	2.8	1.8	1.5	1.2	3.9	46.1
b. Persistent	47.3	25.8	–	–	–	–	–	–	26.1	20.9	–	–	–	–	–	–	21.2
c. Dysentery	27.5	11.0	1.5	1.1	–	–	–	–	14.4	8.9	1.4	–	–	–	–	–	13.1
A5. Pertussis	17.9	8.7	–	–	–	–	–	–	9.6	7.5	–	–	–	–	–	–	8.3
A6. Measles	11.1	4.3	1.2	–	–	–	–	–	5.6	3.9	1.2	–	–	–	–	–	5.5
A7. Tetanus	7.6	2.7	–	–	–	–	–	–	4.0	2.6	–	–	–	–	–	–	3.6
A8. Meningitis	21.4	7.1	2.5	–	–	–	–	–	11.6	5.3	2.1	1.2	1.1	–	–	–	9.8
A9. Malaria	11.9	–	1.4	1.7	1.1	–	–	–	5.9	–	1.4	1.7	–	–	–	–	6.0
A10. Trypanosomiasis	–	–	–	–	–	–	–	–	–	–	–	–	–	–	–	–	–
A11. Chagas disease	23.1	–	–	–	2.7	3.4	2.3	2.2	11.5	–	–	–	3.2	3.6	1.9	1.8	11.6
A12. Schistosomiasis	1.3	–	–	–	–	–	–	–	–	–	–	–	–	–	–	–	–
A13. Leishmaniasis	–	–	–	–	–	–	–	–	–	–	–	–	–	–	–	–	–
A14. Onchocerciasis	–	–	–	–	–	–	–	–	–	–	–	–	–	–	–	–	–
B. Respiratory infections	211.1	66.8	9.8	3.7	4.1	4.5	4.7	17.7	111.3	52.2	8.2	1.1	5.1	4.6	3.9	18.8	99.9
C. Maternal causes	23.8	–	–	–	–	–	–	–	–	–	–	14.9	8.5	–	–	–	23.8
C1. Haemorrhage	4.8	–	–	–	–	–	–	–	–	–	–	3.0	1.7	–	–	–	4.8
C2. Sepsis	2.4	–	–	–	–	–	–	–	–	–	–	1.5	–	–	–	–	2.4
C3. Eclampsia	5.0	–	–	–	–	–	–	–	–	–	–	3.3	1.6	–	–	–	5.0
C4. Hypertension	2.4	–	–	–	–	–	–	–	–	–	–	1.5	–	–	–	–	2.4
C5. Obstructed labour	2.4	–	–	–	–	–	–	–	–	–	–	1.5	–	–	–	–	2.4
C6. Abortion	3.4	–	–	–	–	–	–	–	–	–	–	2.3	1.0	–	–	–	3.4
D. Perinatal causes	240.9	143.9	–	–	–	–	–	–	144.0	96.9	–	–	–	–	–	–	96.9
III. Injuries	293.0	14.0	18.3	82.0	57.3	29.8	13.0	13.9	228.4	10.4	7.3	14.3	9.9	7.5	4.9	10.3	64.6
A. Unintentional	207.3	12.6	16.4	48.8	35.9	21.1	9.9	11.7	156.5	9.1	6.4	9.3	6.6	5.8	4.0	9.6	50.9
A1. Road traffic accidents	80.0	2.6	6.4	21.1	16.1	9.0	3.9	3.2	62.3	1.7	2.8	4.2	3.1	2.7	1.6	1.6	17.7
A2. Poisoning	3.1	–	–	–	1.6	1.3	–	–	1.9	–	–	–	–	–	–	–	1.2
A3. Falls	14.0	–	1.7	1.7	–	–	–	–	8.7	–	–	–	–	–	–	3.7	5.3
A4. Fires	5.7	–	–	–	–	–	–	–	3.5	–	–	–	–	–	–	–	2.3
A5. Drowning	19.9	2.0	3.1	6.3	2.9	1.3	–	–	16.4	1.2	–	–	–	–	–	–	3.5
A6. Occupational	13.3	–	–	3.0	5.5	2.6	–	–	11.2	–	–	–	–	–	–	–	2.0
B. Intentional	85.7	1.4	1.9	33.2	21.3	8.7	3.1	2.2	71.9	1.3	–	4.9	3.4	1.7	–	–	13.7
B1. Self-inflicted	17.2	–	–	4.5	3.4	2.3	1.3	1.2	13.0	–	–	1.5	1.1	–	–	–	4.3
B2. Homicide and violence	55.0	–	1.1	24.4	15.2	6.1	1.6	–	49.8	–	–	2.0	1.4	–	–	–	5.2
B3. War	13.4	–	–	4.3	2.8	–	–	–	9.2	–	–	1.4	–	–	–	–	4.3

A dash (–) indicates less than 1000 deaths.

Estimated deaths (in thousands) by age, sex and cause, 1990: Latin America and the Caribbean

No. of deaths (in thousands)

Cause of Death (ICD 9)	Both sexes, All ages	M 0-4	M 5-14	M 15-29	M 30-44	M 45-59	M 60-69	M 70+	M All ages	F 0-4	F 5-14	F 15-29	F 30-44	F 45-59	F 60-69	F 70+	F All ages
II. Noncommunicable	1,732.9	58.8	19.0	29.0	71.8	162.0	187.5	357.5	885.6	48.1	16.6	31.0	61.3	139.2	159.3	391.7	847.3
A. Malignant neoplasms	341.0	1.8	4.9	5.6	10.7	35.6	44.6	65.5	168.8	1.5	3.8	6.0	18.5	44.3	41.5	56.6	172.2
A1. Mouth and oropharynx	12.7	–	–	–	–	3.2	2.1	3.1	9.4	–	–	–	–	–	–	1.3	3.3
A2. Oesophagus	9.0	–	–	–	–	1.8	1.8	2.6	6.5	–	–	–	–	–	–	1.1	2.4
A3. Stomach	36.4	–	–	–	–	5.2	6.7	9.8	23.0	–	–	–	–	2.6	4.2	5.7	13.4
A4. Colorectal	22.8	–	–	–	–	2.3	3.2	4.7	11.1	–	–	–	–	2.5	3.6	4.8	11.7
A5. Liver	4.8	–	–	–	–	–	–	–	2.5	–	–	–	–	–	–	–	2.2
A6. Pancreas	6.5	–	–	–	–	–	1.1	1.6	3.6	–	–	–	–	–	–	1.3	2.8
A7. Lung	28.2	–	–	–	–	5.4	6.2	9.1	21.8	–	–	–	–	1.5	1.9	2.6	6.4
A8. Breast	31.1									–	–	1.5	4.6	11.1	5.9	8.0	31.1
A9. Cervix	25.5									–	–	1.7	5.2	9.1	4.0	5.5	25.5
A10. Ovary	5.0									–	–	–	–	1.6	–	1.2	5.0
A11. Prostate	22.8	–	–	–	–	1.4	8.6	12.7	22.8								
A12. Bladder	9.7	–	–	–	–	1.3	2.4	3.6	7.5	–	–	–	–	–	–	–	2.2
A13. Lymphoma	15.4	–	–	–	1.3	1.7	1.5	2.2	8.7	–	–	–	–	1.3	1.4	1.9	6.7
A14. Leukemia	10.3	–	1.7	–	–	–	–	–	5.9	–	1.2	–	–	–	–	–	4.4
B. Diabetes mellitus	85.2	–	–	1.8	2.5	7.4	9.6	13.0	33.5	–	–	–	2.1	10.6	15.2	22.6	51.7
C. Nutritional/endocrine	79.6	16.2	2.3	2.3	2.4	2.8	3.2	10.3	39.1	13.4	2.1	2.2	2.3	3.3	3.5	13.9	40.6
C1. Protein-energy malnutrition	33.6	9.7	–	–	–	–	–	4.2	17.3	7.9	–	–	–	–	–	5.4	16.3
C2. Anaemia	15.7	1.5	–	–	–	–	–	2.4	7.3	1.1	–	–	–	–	–	3.0	8.5
D. Neuro-psychiatric	51.6	3.0	3.1	4.2	6.5	6.5	3.6	5.2	32.1	2.4	2.5	3.1	2.5	2.4	1.8	4.7	19.5
D1. Psychoses	3.9	–	–	–	1.1	–	–	–	2.2	–	–	–	–	–	–	–	1.7
D2. Epilepsy	8.8	–	–	–	–	–	–	–	4.8	–	–	–	–	–	–	–	4.0
D3. Alcohol dependence	9.9	–	–	1.4	2.9	3.1	1.3	–	8.7	–	–	–	–	–	–	–	1.2
D4. Alzheimer & other dementias	4.4	–	–	–	–	–	–	1.2	2.1	–	–	–	–	–	–	1.8	2.3
D5. Parkinson disease	2.7	–	–	–	–	–	–	1.2	1.7								
D6. Multiple sclerosis																	
E. Cardiovascular diseases	786.7	4.0	2.6	7.6	26.4	71.2	90.0	193.2	394.9	3.1	2.4	8.7	21.3	53.6	70.9	231.9	391.8
E1. Rheumatic diseases	8.2	–	–	–	–	–	–	–	2.8	–	–	–	1.1	1.4	–	–	5.4
E2. Ischaemic heart disease	269.1	–	–	1.3	8.8	28.7	36.1	71.2	146.3	–	–	–	4.0	15.2	23.7	78.8	122.8
E3. Cerebrovascular diseases	224.1	–	–	1.9	7.6	20.5	25.2	51.6	107.7	–	–	–	7.7	19.0	22.4	64.0	116.4
E4. Inflammatory cardiac disease	121.9	2.5	–	3.7	7.5	12.4	12.6	24.1	64.3	2.7	–	–	5.3	8.7	9.4	27.4	57.6
F. Respiratory	118.2	8.9	–	1.9	3.2	7.8	12.5	31.0	66.7	7.4	–	–	2.9	6.0	8.1	23.9	51.5
F1. Chronic obstructive lung disease	67.4	–	–	–	–	4.8	9.4	24.0	40.6	–	–	–	–	3.5	5.9	15.7	26.8
F2. Asthma	11.9	1.3	–	–	–	–	–	1.1	5.4	1.1	–	–	1.1	1.1	–	1.6	6.6
G. Digestive	147.7	3.1	1.5	4.2	16.6	25.1	17.3	22.0	89.7	2.2	1.2	3.2	6.4	12.0	11.3	21.6	58.0
G1. Peptic ulcer disease	11.8	–	–	–	–	1.4	1.5	3.0	7.0	–	–	–	–	–	–	2.7	4.8
G2. Cirrhosis	60.5	–	–	1.7	10.9	16.1	8.7	6.4	44.1	–	–	–	2.7	5.3	3.9	3.5	16.4
H. Genito-urinary	55.4	1.4	–	1.3	2.2	3.1	5.0	13.6	28.3	1.1	–	2.4	3.1	4.3	4.5	10.8	27.1
H1. Nephritis/nephrosis	38.6	–	–	1.2	1.8	–	3.6	8.1	19.4	–	–	1.6	2.0	3.2	3.4	7.6	19.2
I. Musculo-skeletal	10.1	–	–	–	–	–	–	1.5	3.1	–	–	–	–	1.1	–	2.8	7.0
J. Congenital	42.0	19.3	1.4	1.2	1.8	3.1	–	–	22.6	16.2	1.3	–	–	–	–	–	19.4

A dash (–) indicates less than 1000 deaths.

Estimated deaths (in thousands) by age, sex and cause, 1990: Middle Eastern Crescent

No. of deaths (in thousands)

Cause of Death (ICD 9)	Both sexes	Males								Females							
		0-4	5-14	15-29	30-44	45-59	60-69	70+	All ages	0-4	5-14	15-29	30-44	45-59	60-69	70+	All ages
Population (in millions)	503.1	41.2	65.3	70.2	43.7	22.3	9.0	4.7	256.4	39.7	62.0	66.1	41.1	22.3	9.6	5.9	246.7
All Causes	4,384.0	938.0	148.0	124.0	142.0	247.0	267.0	436.0	2,302.0	891.0	134.0	108.0	107.0	169.0	206.0	467.0	2,082.0
I. Communicable, maternal & perinatal	2,025.6	786.2	67.5	19.9	23.5	38.6	37.5	39.6	1,012.7	758.6	77.4	54.4	35.7	19.3	25.0	42.4	1,012.9
A. Infectious & parasitic	1,032	365.1	52.1	17.3	21.6	36.0	19.7	10.8	522.5	376.1	57.9	27.2	18.1	16.3	8.6	6.0	510.2
A1. Tuberculosis	170.0	4.1	8.1	13.1	17.1	32.0	17.7	9.0	101.2	4.2	10.4	18.9	11.9	12.7	6.6	4.0	68.8
A2. Syphilis	–	–	–	–	–	–	–	–	–	–	–	–	–	–	–	–	–
A3. HIV	–	–	–	–	–	–	–	–	–	–	–	–	–	–	–	–	–
A4. Diarrhoeal diseases	455.0	200.6	13.3	2.4	2.9	1.8	–	–	222.2	206.9	15.5	3.5	3.7	1.8	–	–	232.8
a. Acute watery	238.2	99.6	9.7	1.7	2.4	1.4	–	–	115.9	102.8	11.3	2.6	3.1	1.4	–	–	122.3
b. Persistent	144.9	70.5	2.9	–	–	–	–	–	71.3	72.8	3.4	–	–	–	–	–	73.6
c. Dysentery	72.0	30.4	2.5	–	–	–	–	–	35.0	31.4	3.0	–	–	–	–	–	36.9
A5. Pertussis	41.9	17.9	6.9	–	–	–	–	–	20.4	18.5	8.1	–	–	–	–	–	21.5
A6. Measles	114.7	49.1	1.6	–	–	–	–	–	55.9	50.6	1.9	–	–	–	–	–	58.7
A7. Tetanus	75.7	34.7	7.3	–	–	–	–	–	37.3	35.3	3.1	–	–	–	–	–	38.4
A8. Meningitis	36.7	13.2	1.2	–	–	–	–	–	21.4	10.7	1.4	–	–	–	–	–	15.4
A9. Malaria	7.1	–	–	–	–	–	–	–	3.2	–	–	–	–	–	–	–	3.8
A10. Trypanosomiasis	–	–	–	–	–	–	–	–	–	–	–	–	–	–	–	–	–
A11. Chagas disease	–	–	–	–	–	–	–	–	–	–	–	–	–	–	–	–	–
A12. Schistosomiasis	–	–	–	–	–	–	–	–	–	–	–	–	–	–	–	–	–
A13. Leishmaniasis	1.9	–	–	–	–	–	–	–	1.1	–	–	–	–	–	–	–	–
A14. Onchocerciasis	–	–	–	–	–	–	–	–	–	–	–	–	–	–	–	–	–
B. Respiratory infections	546.3	195.8	15.4	2.6	1.9	2.6	17.8	28.8	264.8	202.0	17.9	3.8	2.4	2.6	16.4	36.4	281.5
C. Maternal causes	40.7	–	–	–	–	–	–	–	–	–	–	23.4	15.2	–	–	–	40.7
C1. Haemorrhage	10.2	–	–	–	–	–	–	–	–	–	–	5.9	3.8	–	–	–	10.2
C2. Sepsis	8.1	–	–	–	–	–	–	–	–	–	–	4.7	3.0	–	–	–	8.1
C3. Eclampsia	4.1	–	–	–	–	–	–	–	–	–	–	2.3	1.5	–	–	–	4.1
C4. Hypertension	6.1	–	–	–	–	–	–	–	–	–	–	3.5	2.3	–	–	–	6.1
C5. Obstructed labour	4.1	–	–	–	–	–	–	–	–	–	–	2.3	1.5	–	–	–	4.1
C6. Abortion	4.1	–	–	–	–	–	–	–	–	–	–	2.3	1.5	–	–	–	4.1
D. Perinatal causes	405.9	225.4	–	–	–	–	–	–	225.4	180.5	–	–	–	–	–	–	180.5
III. Injuries	392.0	37.0	38.0	87.6	63.1	28.8	11.9	10.3	276.7	31.4	16.0	26.7	17.3	9.9	5.7	8.4	115.3
A. Unintentional	214.4	26.8	29.9	36.0	27.5	18.3	7.7	7.3	153.4	21.0	11.3	8.6	5.6	4.9	3.3	6.3	61.0
A1. Road traffic accidents	70.0	4.3	9.2	16.7	11.5	6.5	2.6	1.9	52.8	3.3	4.3	3.9	2.1	1.6	1.0	–	17.2
A2. Poisoning	12.7	1.6	1.1	1.6	2.5	1.9	–	–	9.1	1.1	–	–	–	–	–	–	3.6
A3. Falls	15.0	1.2	1.6	1.5	1.5	1.6	–	1.7	9.6	1.1	–	–	–	–	–	2.6	5.4
A4. Fires	8.6	2.4	–	–	–	–	–	–	5.2	1.8	–	–	–	–	–	–	3.4
A5. Drowning	30.5	5.7	8.2	4.3	2.0	1.2	–	–	22.3	3.9	2.4	1.3	–	–	–	–	8.2
A6. Occupational	9.1	–	–	1.8	3.6	2.0	–	–	7.5	–	–	–	–	–	–	–	1.6
B. Intentional	177.5	10.2	8.2	51.6	35.6	10.5	4.2	2.9	123.3	10.4	4.6	18.1	11.7	5.0	2.4	2.1	54.3
B1. Self-inflicted	43.1	–	1.5	9.9	9.3	5.9	2.6	2.1	31.2	–	–	4.1	2.9	2.0	1.1	1.2	11.9
B2. Homicide and violence	23.3	1.3	1.2	7.3	5.3	2.1	–	–	17.9	1.5	–	1.3	1.0	–	–	–	5.3
B3. War	111.2	8.9	5.6	34.4	21.1	2.5	1.1	–	74.1	8.9	3.5	12.7	7.8	2.5	1.0	–	37.1

A dash (–) indicates less than 1000 deaths.

Estimated deaths (in thousands) by age, sex and cause, 1990: Middle Eastern Crescent

No. of deaths (in thousands)

Cause of Death (ICD 9)	Both sexes	Males								Females							
		0-4	5-14	15-29	30-44	45-59	60-69	70+	All ages	0-4	5-14	15-29	30-44	45-59	60-69	70+	All ages
II. Noncommunicable	1,966.5	114.8	42.5	16.5	55.5	179.7	217.6	386.1	1,012.6	101.0	40.6	26.9	54.0	139.8	175.3	416.2	953.8
A. Malignant neoplasms	327.4	2.3	7.1	2.9	10.1	46.0	55.1	64.8	188.2	3.3	1.3	3.7	15.9	37.6	34.7	42.7	139.1
A1. Mouth and oropharynx	27.4	–	–	–	–	2.5	6.6	7.7	18.2	–	–	–	–	1.4	2.9	3.6	9.2
A2. Oesophagus	16.2	–	–	–	–	2.7	3.1	3.6	9.8	–	–	–	–	1.8	1.8	2.2	6.3
A3. Stomach	34.6	–	–	–	–	5.5	6.5	7.7	20.9	–	–	–	–	3.1	4.2	5.2	13.7
A4. Colorectal	22.1	–	–	–	–	1.5	4.2	4.9	11.4	–	–	–	–	1.3	3.8	4.7	10.7
A5. Liver	14.0	–	–	–	–	2.3	2.7	3.2	8.8	–	–	–	–	1.4	1.5	1.9	5.2
A6. Pancreas	7.8	–	–	–	–	1.3	1.4	1.7	4.6	–	–	–	–	–	–	1.2	3.2
A7. Lung	50.4	–	–	–	1.1	11.5	12.8	15.0	41.0	–	–	–	–	–	2.9	3.5	9.5
A8. Breast	19.3	–	–	–	–	–	–	–	–	–	–	2.3	3.3	6.9	3.7	4.6	19.3
A9. Cervix	12.5	–	–	–	–	–	–	–	–	–	–	–	1.7	4.8	2.5	3.1	12.5
A10. Ovary	5.5	–	–	–	–	–	–	–	–	–	–	–	1.2	1.8	–	1.2	5.5
A11. Prostate	9.4	–	–	–	–	–	3.9	4.6	9.4	–	–	–	–	–	–	–	–
A12. Bladder	16.9	–	–	–	–	2.8	4.7	5.6	13.8	–	–	–	–	–	–	1.1	3.1
A13. Lymphoma	12.9	–	1.3	1.2	1.0	1.1	2.1	2.5	8.7	–	–	1.5	1.3	–	1.1	1.3	4.2
A14. Leukemia	16.3	–	2.4	1.8	1.3	–	1.8	2.1	9.2	1.1	1.5	2.5	1.3	–	1.5	1.8	7.1
B. Diabetes mellitus	82.3	–	–	–	3.5	8.9	14.1	8.1	33.6	–	–	–	1.8	12.3	20.4	13.3	48.8
C. Nutritional/endocrine	59.5	16.8	1.3	1.8	1.3	1.9	1.4	2.6	29.4	13.9	–	–	–	2.5	1.9	3.6	30.1
C1. Protein-energy malnutrition	20.7	8.4	–	–	–	–	–	–	10.3	8.4	–	–	–	–	–	–	10.4
C2. Anaemia	15.1	3.3	–	–	–	–	–	–	5.8	1.8	–	–	–	–	–	1.2	9.2
D. Neuro-psychiatric	68.9	6.4	11.7	2.0	3.7	4.8	3.7	6.2	38.5	5.7	7.8	3.1	2.3	2.1	2.2	7.1	30.4
D1. Psychoses	2.1	–	–	–	–	–	–	–	1.1	–	–	–	–	–	–	–	1.1
D2. Epilepsy	11.7	–	2.7	–	1.1	–	–	–	6.7	1.1	1.7	1.1	–	–	–	–	4.9
D3. Alcohol dependence	1.1	–	–	–	–	–	–	–	–	–	–	–	–	–	–	–	–
D4. Alzheimer & other dementias	12.0	–	–	–	–	–	–	2.1	6.1	–	–	–	–	–	–	2.9	5.9
D5. Parkinson disease	3.3	–	–	–	–	–	–	1.4	2.0	–	–	–	–	–	–	–	1.3
D6. Multiple sclerosis	2.6	–	–	–	–	–	–	–	1.2	–	–	–	–	–	–	–	1.4
E. Cardiovascular diseases	992.3	14.5	6.2	4.5	22.7	84.3	111.2	246.1	489.4	12.2	9.2	7.6	18.4	60.1	93.5	301.9	502.0
E1. Rheumatic diseases	29.7	–	1.1	–	–	2.1	2.2	2.9	8.6	–	1.5	1.7	1.7	5.2	6.1	6.7	21.1
E2. Ischaemic heart disease	276.6	–	–	–	6.0	29.5	37.5	77.6	151.2	–	–	–	2.2	12.0	24.2	86.7	125.4
E3. Cerebrovascular diseases	327.4	–	–	–	3.7	21.4	36.0	85.1	149.8	–	–	–	5.0	21.0	35.1	112.1	177.6
E4. Inflammatory cardiac disease	123.3	1.7	–	1.9	6.3	13.1	12.2	27.1	64.9	1.0	–	1.8	4.2	8.0	8.8	24.8	58.5
F. Respiratory	120.0	13.2	–	–	2.0	7.8	11.7	27.1	67.8	11.4	–	–	2.3	6.4	7.1	20.3	52.2
F1. Chronic obstructive lung disease	62.1	–	–	–	–	4.8	8.8	21.0	37.6	–	–	–	–	3.8	5.1	13.4	24.5
F2. Asthma	13.7	–	–	–	–	–	–	–	6.6	–	–	–	–	1.1	–	1.4	7.1
G. Digestive	136.3	15.4	3.0	1.6	8.9	18.6	13.1	15.1	75.6	16.8	3.7	2.3	6.8	10.7	8.2	12.2	60.7
G1. Peptic ulcer disease	15.0	–	–	–	1.3	2.8	2.0	2.3	8.7	–	–	–	1.0	1.6	1.2	1.8	6.2
G2. Cirrhosis	36.5	–	–	–	4.6	9.1	5.4	3.4	23.8	–	–	–	2.7	4.1	2.2	2.0	12.6
H. Genito-urinary	62.7	2.0	3.9	–	2.3	5.9	5.5	12.5	32.9	1.0	3.2	2.1	2.4	6.1	5.4	9.6	29.8
H1. Nephritis/nephrosis	31.6	–	3.4	–	1.1	2.8	2.7	5.3	16.6	–	2.9	1.1	1.2	2.5	2.5	4.3	15.0
I. Musculo-skeletal	10.3	–	–	–	–	–	–	1.8	3.7	–	–	–	–	–	–	2.9	6.7
J. Congenital	87.7	42.9	2.8	–	–	–	–	–	47.0	35.1	2.9	1.0	1.2	–	–	–	40.7

A dash (-) indicates less than 1000 deaths.

Estimated deaths (in thousands) by age, sex and cause, 1990: World

No. of deaths (in thousands)

Cause of Death (ICD 9)	Both sexes	Males 0-4	5-14	15-29	30-44	45-59	60-69	70+	All ages	Females 0-4	5-14	15-29	30-44	45-59	60-69	70+	All ages
Population (in millions)	5,267.4	321.3	551.2	735.9	514.0	312.4	136.8	82.0	2,653.7	309.3	525.5	702.7	496.0	311.1	150.9	118.3	2,613.7
All Causes	49,971.1	6,608.1	1,188.7	1,590.6	1,921.5	3,501.5	4,144.8	7,452.1	26,407.6	6,048.5	1,077.1	1,282.8	1,331.0	2,263.9	2,978.1	8,582.2	23,563.5
I. Communicable, maternal & perinatal	16,689.7	5,611.9	634.1	423.5	417.5	541.0	416.2	611.0	8,655.3	5,090.1	649.7	648.1	498.3	303.5	262.5	582.2	8,034.5
A. Infectious & parasitic	9,454.1	2,822.6	513.4	381.5	385.8	491.1	252.0	246.5	5,092.9	2,657.0	513.0	361.4	298.5	253.1	122.0	156.2	4,361.2
A1. Tuberculosis	2,015.5	34.4	66.8	166.7	222.7	378.1	199.8	181.3	1,249.8	37.3	84.6	160.9	153.0	165.7	81.0	83.1	765.7
A2. Syphilis	193.4	40.5	-	35.9	19.7	5.2	-	-	103.0	36.7	5.0	28.1	19.6	4.5	1.3	-	90.4
A3. HIV	290.8	30.2	4.8	59.4	47.5	17.7	3.2	2.7	165.5	27.8	5.0	49.5	34.3	6.4	1.3	-	125.4
A4. Diarrhoeal diseases	2,872.7	1,264.9	102.7	27.4	19.7	14.7	9.7	18.2	1,457.3	1,213.1	107.8	27.9	21.9	15.6	7.0	22.1	1,415.3
a. Acute watery	1,553.3	636.7	78.1	21.8	15.9	11.3	7.8	14.7	786.3	610.8	81.8	22.0	17.6	11.9	5.5	17.3	767.0
b. Persistent	871.5	439.3	4.9	-	-	-	-	-	444.2	421.2	5.2	-	-	-	-	-	427.3
c. Dysentery	447.9	188.9	19.8	5.6	3.8	3.4	1.9	3.4	226.9	181.1	20.9	5.8	4.2	3.6	1.4	4.1	221.1
A5. Pertussis	321.2	145.8	21.9	-	-	-	-	-	167.7	131.5	22.0	-	-	-	-	-	153.5
A6. Measles	1,006.4	441.9	69.2	-	-	-	-	-	511.3	420.8	74.0	-	-	-	-	-	495.1
A7. Tetanus	505.0	231.6	13.9	2.9	2.2	3.8	2.3	1.8	258.5	218.6	14.1	2.9	2.4	4.2	2.2	2.0	246.5
A8. Meningitis	241.8	73.1	50.2	9.2	4.8	5.8	3.6	2.1	148.	51.9	17.9	10.3	5.0	2.9	2.7	2.2	93.0
A9. Malaria	926.4	331.5	75.7	32.5	19.1	10.2	3.6	1.9	474.5	300.5	77.0	33.2	23.7	11.3	3.9	2.3	451.9
A10. Trypanosomiasis	55.1	1.5	10.2	7.1	3.6	4.8	-	-	28.2	2.7	9.1	6.8	4.4	3.2	-	-	26.8
A11. Chagas disease	23.1	-	-	-	2.7	3.4	2.3	2.2	11.5	-	-	1.1	3.2	3.6	1.9	1.8	11.6
A12. Schistosomiasis	37.6	-	4.7	4.6	9.1	2.5	1.8	-	23.8	-	2.0	2.5	1.6	6.6	-	-	13.8
A13. Leishmaniasis	53.7	4.1	13.0	7.0	4.6	1.2	-	-	30.2	3.1	11.4	4.6	3.1	1.1	-	-	23.5
A14. Onchocerciasis	29.8	-	-	2.7	1.4	6.1	4.8	2.4	17.4	-	-	1.9	1.2	4.6	3.1	1.7	12.4
B. Respiratory infections	4,314.4	1,383.6	120.7	42.0	31.7	49.8	164.3	364.5	2,156.6	1,348.4	124.3	43.1	32.2	43.2	140.5	426.0	2,157.8
C. Maternal causes	430.7	-	-	-	-	-	-	-		-	12.4	243.5	167.7	7.1	-	-	430.7
C1. Haemorrhage	129.6	-	-	-	-	-	-	-		-	3.6	73.8	49.8	2.4	-	-	129.6
C2. Sepsis	79.2	-	-	-	-	-	-	-		-	2.5	44.2	31.3	1.2	-	-	79.2
C3. Eclampsia	44.6	-	-	-	-	-	-	-		-	1.3	25.5	17.2	-	-	-	44.6
C4. Hypertension	31.7	-	-	-	-	-	-	-		-	-	17.6	12.7	-	-	-	31.7
C5. Obstructed labour	40.4	-	-	-	-	-	-	-		-	1.2	22.6	16.0	-	-	-	40.4
C6. Abortion	61.3	-	-	-	-	-	-	-		-	1.8	35.1	23.5	-	-	-	61.3
D. Perinatal causes	2,490.5	1,405.7	-	-	-	-	-	-	1,405.7	1,084.7	-	-	-	-	-	-	1,084.7
III. Injuries	4,226.7	266.5	273.2	855.9	657.9	389.2	180.5	211.7	2,835.0	241.7	157.2	323.1	199.3	149.8	96.8	223.9	1,391.7
A. Unintentional	2,794.4	228.5	237.5	510.4	393.0	262.7	118.4	150.3	1,900.9	199.8	133.6	150.2	96.3	86.1	58.6	168.9	893.5
A1. Road traffic accidents	855.8	30.0	61.1	227.1	163.0	90.5	39.3	35.9	647.1	23.8	38.7	48.0	30.5	27.5	16.9	23.3	208.7
A2. Poisoning	187.7	13.5	5.7	22.6	37.0	32.0	9.8	8.7	129.2	7.2	5.6	13.3	11.1	7.9	5.5	7.9	58.4
A3. Falls	264.8	10.8	8.5	22.5	21.4	23.7	16.3	39.7	143.0	12.2	4.6	3.1	3.5	8.4	11.6	78.5	121.9
A4. Fires	100.3	19.0	6.1	7.4	7.6	5.9	3.1	8.7	57.7	13.2	8.2	4.4	2.8	2.7	2.8	8.4	42.6
A5. Drowning	384.1	60.5	69.6	64.5	29.7	17.5	7.6	9.5	258.9	48.8	31.1	18.0	7.7	6.4	4.2	9.0	125.2
A6. Occupational	137.2	-	-	26.6	51.1	27.0	2.0	-	106.6	-	-	7.6	14.7	7.6	-	-	30.6
B. Intentional	1,432.3	37.9	35.8	345.5	264.9	126.5	62.1	61.4	934.1	41.9	23.6	172.9	103.0	63.7	38.2	55.0	498.2
B1. Self-inflicted	818.0	-	12.1	149.2	138.6	93.0	51.0	55.7	499.5	-	8.3	48.0	64.5	48.4	30.9	48.0	318.5
B2. Homicide and violence	292.4	11.4	7.5	99.9	69.7	25.7	7.6	3.9	225.7	15.3	4.8	15.1	14.9	7.5	4.0	5.1	66.7
B3. War	321.9	26.5	16.1	96.5	56.6	7.9	3.5	1.8	208.9	26.6	10.5	39.3	23.6	7.8	3.3	1.9	113.0

A dash (-) indicates less than 1000 deaths.

Estimated deaths (in thousands) by age, sex and cause, 1990: World

No. of deaths (in thousands)

Cause of Death (ICD 9)	Both sexes	Males								Females							
		0-4	5-14	15-29	30-44	45-59	60-69	70+	All ages	0-4	5-14	15-29	30-44	45-59	60-69	70+	All ages
II. Noncommunicable	29,054.7	729.8	281.3	311.3	846.0	2,571.7	3,548.0	6,629.3	14,917.4	716.6	270.2	311.6	633.4	1,810.7	2,618.7	7,776.2	14,137.3
A. Malignant neoplasms	6,128.7	18.6	55.3	68.7	195.8	826.7	1,074.3	1,281.3	3,520.6	28.8	16.4	57.1	213.6	601.2	665.7	1,025.2	2,608.1
A1. Mouth and oropharynx	365.7	-	1.0	4.7	14.8	45.9	92.2	91.8	250.7	-	-	2.7	9.0	18.7	39.7	44.0	115.0
A2. Oesophagus	389.4	-	-	1.7	9.8	68.8	91.2	91.8	263.6	-	-	1.3	3.8	27.4	44.2	49.1	125.8
A3. Stomach	766.1	-	-	3.9	19.6	120.7	159.7	176.4	480.7	-	-	3.9	18.2	56.1	78.5	128.4	285.4
A4. Colorectal	495.5	-	-	4.3	11.8	42.7	77.1	115.8	252.1	-	-	2.3	11.3	35.6	64.4	129.4	243.4
A5. Liver	463.4	-	1.7	7.4	46.3	114.4	88.8	70.7	329.8	-	-	2.3	13.9	35.6	36.5	44.3	133.6
A6. Pancreas	168.7	-	-	-	3.3	19.5	29.5	39.8	93.1	-	-	-	1.9	11.1	20.5	41.8	75.7
A7. Lung	966.9	-	-	4.4	17.7	175.1	257.4	275.5	731.1	-	1.5	6.3	7.6	47.8	73.1	105.5	235.8
A8. Breast	332.4									-	-	6.6	41.7	102.7	75.7	106.0	332.4
A9. Cervix	215.0									-	-	3.4	28.9	80.4	47.0	51.8	215.0
A10. Ovary	106.4									-	-	-	12.7	27.9	26.4	35.1	106.4
A11. Prostate	212.5					13.3	63.8	134.7	212.5								
A12. Bladder	150.5	-	-	-	2.2	17.8	36.1	55.2	112.2	-	-	1.3	1.3	5.3	10.3	20.9	38.2
A13. Lymphoma	217.5	3.1	12.1	7.3	10.8	21.3	32.7	40.8	128.1	-	1.2	3.0	7.8	13.8	22.3	38.6	89.4
A14. Leukemia	219.4	7.0	19.3	13.0	14.4	16.0	20.9	29.8	120.4	10.2	6.5	10.3	14.5	13.7	16.0	27.9	99.0
B. Diabetes mellitus	659.7	-	-	8.4	13.6	57.5	92.6	94.5	267.1	-	-	9.0	10.5	74.3	134.9	162.9	392.5
C. Nutritional/endocrine	651.3	119.9	11.4	28.5	44.7	22.0	21.8	49.6	298.0	127.7	28.2	25.9	21.5	33.5	32.8	83.8	353.3
C1. Protein-energy malnutrition	212.9	65.8	5.9	2.2	2.3	2.7	3.0	12.2	94.1	82.1	5.6	2.1	1.4	1.7	5.1	20.8	118.8
C2. Anaemia	163.3	20.1	6.2	5.8	2.8	4.9	5.9	12.6	58.4	16.4	23.2	9.3	7.5	11.8	12.5	24.3	104.8
D. Neuro-psychiatric	831.9	38.4	73.3	44.1	61.0	71.8	53.7	115.5	457.8	39.3	50.2	35.4	29.6	30.7	36.5	152.4	374.1
D1. Psychoses	57.9	-	-	3.2	7.2	6.9	4.6	10.2	32.3	-	-	1.9	2.9	3.3	3.1	13.6	25.6
D2. Epilepsy	115.2	4.2	16.8	12.3	14.9	11.0	4.7	4.0	67.9	4.0	10.8	13.1	8.3	4.9	2.9	3.4	47.3
D3. Alcohol dependence	52.8	-	-	3.6	11.6	17.3	6.7	5.3	44.5	-	-	1.8	1.9	3.2	1.4	1.1	8.3
D4. Alzheimer & other dementias	194.6	5.9	6.4	1.6	3.3	9.3	13.8	45.7	86.0	7.2	3.8	1.8	1.9	5.0	11.4	77.5	108.6
D5. Parkinson disease	61.7	-	-	-	-	1.2	6.1	27.2	34.8	-	-	-	-	-	3.7	22.4	26.9
D6. Multiple sclerosis	33.2	-	-	-	3.5	5.1	3.2	2.1	14.8	-	-	1.1	5.0	5.4	3.8	2.9	18.4
E. Cardiovascular diseases	14,344.7	65.6	32.0	75.4	303.5	1,086.9	1,643.5	3,692.8	6,899.7	60.6	49.6	81.8	193.8	724.7	1,301.2	5,033.3	7,445.0
E1. Rheumatic diseases	486.0	1.8	2.3	12.1	18.0	37.6	38.9	53.7	163.3	1.9	4.1	14.3	27.8	80.2	92.8	101.5	322.6
E2. Ischaemic heart disease	5,147.0	1.2	1.2	11.6	100.8	444.5	667.4	1,406.2	2,633.5	1.0	-	6.6	28.6	165.6	414.0	1,897.2	2,513.5
E3. Cerebrovascular diseases	4,629.1	8.2	6.7	14.9	62.1	283.5	500.4	1,213.5	2,089.2	6.0	8.6	18.2	56.6	252.6	461.7	1,736.3	2,539.9
E4. Inflammatory cardiac disease	1,364.3	32.1	15.0	23.0	73.4	151.3	162.9	265.2	723.0	36.7	25.9	21.3	41.2	99.4	120.8	296.0	641.4
F. Respiratory	2,844.9	78.5	31.7	15.6	34.9	152.9	349.9	894.8	1,558.4	79.3	18.9	18.8	31.7	112.3	214.2	811.3	1,286.5
F1. Chronic obstructive lung disease	2,072.2	11.1	3.5	1.3	14.2	110.6	290.5	746.0	1,177.1	9.0	2.4	1.7	12.9	78.1	175.5	615.7	895.1
F2. Asthma	181.3	4.8	15.4	5.8	6.9	12.1	13.1	23.8	81.8	4.5	9.9	7.9	8.7	15.1	14.4	38.9	99.4
G. Digestive	1,842.9	89.1	20.7	32.0	152.3	275.4	218.6	269.8	1,057.9	107.3	25.8	29.4	75.1	142.4	130.9	274.0	785.0
G1. Peptic ulcer disease	240.6	-	1.4	5.3	19.3	38.5	33.0	49.7	148.0	1.2	-	5.4	10.3	17.1	14.9	43.1	92.6
G2. Cirrhosis	709.3	4.2	2.9	11.1	95.8	172.7	118.8	75.7	481.1	3.2	4.2	8.4	33.4	70.3	53.2	55.5	228.2
H. Genito-urinary	704.0	12.5	24.6	16.0	25.5	52.6	61.1	167.5	359.8	8.0	20.6	21.8	25.2	61.7	69.3	137.5	344.2
H1. Nephritis/nephrosis	427.1	6.1	22.4	14.3	20.0	38.5	39.6	85.1	225.9	4.6	19.1	14.5	17.9	31.3	38.1	75.6	201.2
I. Musculo-skeletal	143.0	-	2.7	2.1	1.8	5.1	12.0	27.6	51.9	1.2	3.2	6.4	8.2	11.5	13.6	47.0	91.2
J. Congenital	655.8	296.3	22.4	14.0	5.9	2.3	1.7	1.8	344.4	252.6	22.3	16.4	12.4	4.7	1.4	1.7	311.5

A dash (-) indicates less than 1000 deaths.

Quantifying disability: data, methods and results

C.J.L. Murray[1] & A.D. Lopez[2]

Conventional methods for collecting, analysing and disseminating data and information on disability in populations have relied on cross-sectional censuses and surveys which measure prevalence in a given period. While this may be relevant for defining the extent and demographic pattern of disabilities in a population, and thus indicating the need for rehabilitative services, prevention requires detailed inform-ation on the underlying diseases and injuries that cause disabilities. The Global Burden of Disease methodology described in this paper provides a mechanism for quantifying the health consequences of the years of life lived with disabilities by first estimating the age-sex-specific incidence rates of under-lying conditions, and then mapping these to a single disability index which collectively reflects the pro-bability of progressing to a disability, the duration of life lived with the disability, and the approximate severity of the disability in terms of activity restriction. Detailed estimates of the number of disability-adjusted life years (DALYs) lived are provided in this paper, for eight geographical regions. The results should be useful to those concerned with planning health services for the disabled and, more particular-ly, with determining policies to prevent the underlying conditions which give rise to serious disabling sequelae.

Introduction

This paper is one of four in this issue of the *Bulletin of the World Health Organization* on the Global Burden of Disease study (*1–3*). Through the study, a new measure, the disability-adjusted life year (DALY), was developed and applied to estimating the burden of disease due to more than 100 causes, for five age groups and the two sexes in eight regions of the world. The conceptual underpinnings of the strategy used to measure the time lived with a disability in a manner that can be meaningfully com-pared with the time lost due to premature mortality have been described (*1*). This article focuses on the methods, sources and results for the measurement of time lived with a disability. DALYs require for their computation extensive age- and sex-specific infor-mation for regions on the incidence of disease, the proportion of disease incidence leading to a disabling outcome, the average age of disability onset, the duration of disability, and the distribution of disabili-ty across the six classes of disability severity.

For some regions, there are minimal data on the epidemiology of important health problems. Few community studies, for example, are available on heart disease in sub-Saharan Africa. Knowledge of the disabling sequelae even of well-studied diseases is missing for large parts of the developing and sur-prisingly the industrialized worlds. Nevertheless, choices between competing health priorities are made every day by decision-makers in the public and private sectors. These choices reflect their implicit understanding of the epidemiological profile as well as opportunities for intervention. The philosophy of the Global Burden of Disease study is that assump-tions about the burden of disease should be made explicit. In other words, it is preferable to make an informed estimate of disability flowing from a par-ticular condition than to have no estimate at all. No estimate often leads to the tacit assumption that there is no problem. Perhaps, the continued neglect of pri-mary and secondary prevention and rehabilitation of disability is related to the lack of data on its magni-tude that is comparable with life lost due to prema-ture mortality.

Materials and methods

Study design

To calculate DALYs, detailed estimates of the age- and sex-specific epidemiology of each disease are required. Table 1 illustrates the worksheet developed for each disease for each of the eight regions; the sample provides results for cataract-related blindness in sub-Saharan Africa. Estimates of disease inciden-ce, proportion becoming disabled, average age of

[1] Assistant Professor of International Health Economics, Har-vard Center for Population and Development Studies, 9 Bow Street, Cambridge, MA 02138, USA. Requests for reprints should be sent to this author.

[2] Scientist, Tobacco or Health Programme, World Health Organ-ization, Geneva, Switzerland.

Reprinted from *Bulletin of the World Health Organization*, 1994, **72** (3): 481–494.

Table 1: **Sample worksheet for estimating years of life lived with a disability (blindness due to cataract) in sub-Saharan Africa, disability only, 1990**

Sex and age group (years)	Inci-dence (cases)	Age of onset (years)	Dura-tion (years)	Disa-bility weight	YLD incidence age[a]	YLD age lived[b]	Inci-dence (per 1000)	Preva-lence (per 1000)	Popu-lation (x 1000)	Preva-lence (cases)	YLD preva-lence[c]
Male											
0–4	1 899	0.5	23.28	0.583	18 448	1 791	0.04	0.08	47 484	3 989	355
5–14	0	0	0	0	0	8 718	0.00	0.16	70 258	11 031	7 097
15–44	5 188	35	13.42	0.583	42 882	42 286	0.05	0.76	103 764	79 276	63 461
45–59	74 124	55	8.48	0.583	292 583	196 725	3.65	23.40	20 308	475 288	267 288
60+	111 805	70	4.89	0.583	192 771	297 164	10.64	90.46	10 508	950 596	372 690
Total	193 017				546 684	546 684			252 322	1 520 179	710 891
Female											
0–4	1 881	0.5	20.37	0.583	15 810	1 774	0.04	0.09	47 030	3 998	356
5–14	0	0	0	0	0	8 634	0.00	0.16	69 818	11 031	7 097
15–44	6 375	35	13.46	0.583	52 808	47 610	0.06	0.78	106 257	82 349	65 922
45–59	78 073	55	8.86	0.583	318 972	208 816	3.53	22.35	22 117	494 381	278 026
60+	110 751	70	5.02	0.583	195 347	316 104	8.70	77.69	12 730	988 994	387 744
Total	197 081				582 938	582 938			257 952	1 580 753	739 145

[a] DALYs attributed to the age of onset of a disability.
[b] DALYs attributed to the age at which a disability would be lived.
[c] DALYs calculated using prevalence of a disability times a duration of 1 year.

onset of the disability, duration of the disability, and distribution of disabilities across the six classes of severity are required. In addition, information on prevalence, remission, and case fatality were used in checking for internal consistency and calculating the duration and mortality. Valid community-based epidemiological studies for information on these estimates do not exist for many of the variables in many regions. To both identify all useful sources and supplement empirical data with informed judgment, we used an iterative process that was implemented over a period of 9 months. The following eight steps are a summary of the actual mechanism used to generate estimates for each disease.

(1) More than 100 conditions were chosen to be included in the Global Burden of Disease study. The set which is organized in a tree structure begins with three large groups: communicable, maternal and perinatal; noncommunicable; and injuries. Group I (communicable, maternal and perinatal) are all causes that decline dramatically with the epidemiological transition (4, 5). The remaining causes have been divided into noncommunicable diseases and injuries because injuries appear to be largely unrelated to the total level of mortality and noncommunicable disease patterns (6). This basic structure was first developed in the World Bank study on adult health (5) and has been modified by adding conditions that were known to be large causes of mortality and significant contributors to disability, or for which significant resources are spent in the health sector.

(2) Disease experts, or groups of experts in some cases, were identified for each of the more than 100 conditions in the Global Burden of Disease study. Study participants were drawn from the World Health Organization, the International Agency for Research on Cancer, the World Bank, the U.S. Centers for Disease Control, and academic institutions in several countries including China, France, India, New Zealand, Sri Lanka, United Kingdom and USA.

(3) First-round estimates were made by experts on the basis of published and unpublished studies of disease and disability incidence, remission, case fatality, prevalence, and the distribution by severity class of the disability. Where no data for a region were available, experts were encouraged to make informed estimates. Frequently, age patterns of incidence of remission were based on regions thought to have similar epidemiological profiles. In the worst case, when no information was available, all rates would be imputed from other regions.

(4) These estimates were reviewed critically by the authors. Internal consistency between incidence, remission, case-fatality rates, duration, and prevalence estimates was ascertained using the Harvard incidence-prevalence model described below. These checks identified major inconsistencies with many estimates. Disease experts then revised their estimates, in consultation with us, to make them internally consistent.

(5) Revised estimates were used to produce the Version 1 results. These estimates were extensively reviewed by a large group of international health

experts at a WHO meeting on 8–11 December 1992. Disease experts subsequently revised their estimates, taking the discussions at this conference into account. These revisions were subjected again to internal consistency validation and then used to generate Version 2 results.

(6) The mapping from disease to disability and the distribution of disabling sequelae across the six severity classes was independently reviewed. A group of public health practitioners, meeting in Atlanta on 15 March 1993, were charged with modifying these distributions as required to make each disability class homogeneous with respect to severity.

(7) Version 3 results, based on these revisions of the mapping of disease to disabling sequelae by class, were published recently (7).

(8) Selected disease experts have subsequently revised their estimates based on wider critical review and recently collected data, and these modifications have been incorporated into the Version 4 results presented here.

From prevalence to incidence and back

Three clear needs were appreciated early in the exercise.

(1) Results of studies have been reported using different indicators. Prevalence results differed in the age groups used and the indicators used such as point, period or lifetime cumulative prevalence. A simple method to convert between measures was needed to facilitate comparisons of study results.

(2) When estimates of incidence, duration and prevalence were made, internal consistency between the two had to be established.

(3) Data on prevalence were available frequently, but none on incidence.

Estimates of incidence consistent with observed prevalence had to be developed.

The relationship between epidemiological variables is not simple. The oft-cited relationship:

$$P = ID$$

(where P is prevalence, I is incidence and D is duration) is an oversimplification. It holds true for the population on average only if the incidence has been constant over time. For calculating DALYs, we need to know the average duration of a disability at different ages of onset. When the equality $P = ID$ is extended to determining the duration by age of onset, it no longer works under most circumstances. Fig. 1 shows the average duration estimated using prevalence, divided by the incidence within an age group and the true duration for the same age group for a disease with a constant incidence of 1 per 1000 across all ages and no case-fatality rate. With rising age, true duration is lower because of increasing gen-

Fig. 1. **Comparison of estimated durations: prevalence/ incidence and life-table methods.**

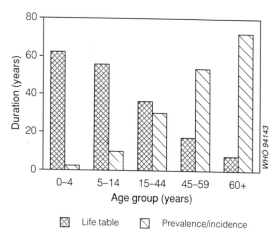

eral mortality and thus declining life expectancy, whereas duration estimated by age-specific prevalence divided by incidence is increasing because of the accumulation of prevalence cases.

In order to address these needs, we developed a model formalizing the relationship between incidence, remission, case fatality, and prevalence. Fig. 2 illustrates the basic relationships. Susceptibles in the population can get a disease or disability at rate i and can die at a general mortality rate m. Cases of disease or disability can remit at rate r, die from general causes at the same rate as the susceptibles m, and die from cause-specific mortality at rate f. If these rates can be approximated as constant over a short interval such as a year, we can define a set of linear differential equations that characterize movement between the three states shown. Using matrix algebra, this is a simple problem to solve. In fact, a general eigenvector/eigenvalue solution can be conveniently written in a spreadsheet such as Lotus 123. We then follow a cohort from birth onwards exposed

Fig. 2. **Schema for the Harvard incidence-prevalence model.**

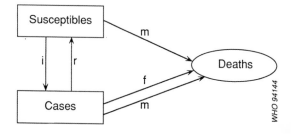

to a set of age-specific incidence, remission, case fatality, and general mortality risks using a life-table approach. For each year in the life-table, a new solution is calculated for the set of differential equations and this solution is used to calculate the number of susceptibles, cases and deaths for the beginning of the next year. This process is repeated until a competing-risks life-table has been fully constructed until age 85 years.

More specifically, the model input is a set of instantaneous incidence, remission, and cause-specific mortality risks for the age groups 0–4, 5–14, 15–44, 45–59 and 60+ years. Within each age group, we have made the simplifying assumption that the various instantaneous risks are constant. General mortality rates for the eight regions for males and females are built into the programme and are selected through a menu. The output of the model (shown in Table 2) provides prevalence rates and numbers by age, deaths attributable to that condition, incidence rates, and duration by age of onset. The data in the Table are for asthma in Indian women.

This model, named the Harvard incidence prevalence model, now in its sixth revision has been used primarily for three purposes. First, when prevalence is known and reasonable assumptions about remission and case fatality can be made, the model can be used iteratively to define incidence and duration by age. Second, when incidence is known we can simply estimate the expected prevalence. This is useful in establishing internal consistency between the estimates of incidence and prevalence. Third, for diseases such as diabetes where there is a relative risk from all causes or a group of important causes, like cardiovascular diseases, attributable deaths rather than directly coded cause-specific mortality can be easily estimated.

Mapping disease to disability and adjusting for treatment

A major obstacle to linking public health studies on particular diseases with research on disability has been the absence of a probability map extending from disease to impairments and disabilities. While on paper, arrows may be drawn from disease all the way to handicap, even those who work on disability can rarely provide concrete information on the probability that someone with a particular disease will go on to suffer disabilities of particular severities. For the Global Burden of Disease (GBD) study, such a mapping from disease through impairment to disability was required. As described in the section on study design, this map was developed in an iterative fashion based on inputs from disease experts and then independently reviewed.

Table 3 provides the distribution, by severity class, of disabilities stemming from selected diseases in the GBD list for one region (Latin America and the Caribbean). The full detail is too extensive to present here but is available, on request, to those who are interested. Some diseases may cause several disabilities and consequently have more than one entry in the Table. The Table provides the proportion of disease incidence cases that go on to develop a disability, which varies by region and age group, and the distribution of disabling sequelae by class. For some conditions, the percentage becoming disabled is better interpreted as the proportion of time the individuals with this condition are disabled, such as for bipolar affective (manic-depressive) disease or asthma. The proportion going on to develop a disability is also a function of the definition of incidence; a restricted definition of incidence means a higher proportion will go on to develop a disability, a loose definition means a lower proportion will develop a disability. The definition of incidence used in the study often depends on the definitions used in extant datasets. For example, the data on motor vehicle accidents in Mexico, based on police records, refer only to those injuries that lead to hospitaliza-

Table 2: **Harvard disease model output for asthma for females in India**

Inputs to model	Instantaneous rates		
Age groups (years)	Incidence	Remission	Cause-specific mortality
0–4	0.00675	0.430	0.00325
5–14	0.00377	0.440	0.00368
15–44	0.00155	0.335	0.00580
45–59	0.00223	0.138	0.00700
60+	0.00259	0.268	0.01400

Output from model		Annual incidence rate (per 1000)	Annual cause-specific mortality rate
Prevalence rate (per 1000)	Expected duration (years)		
8.984	1.92	6.69	0.029
9.583	2.21	3.73	0.035
4.914	3.55	1.54	0.029
10.761	3.77	2.21	0.075
10.125	2.33	2.56	0.142

Population (x 1000)	Prevalence	Annual incidence	Annual cause-specific deaths
56 679	509 228	378 966	1 655
95 263	912 931	355 445	3 360
183 242	900 483	281 772	5 223
46 005	495 075	101 583	3 466
28 924	292 863	74 029	4 100

Table 3: **An estimated proportion of incident cases developing a disability and the distribution of these disabilities by severity class for a few illustrative conditions in LAC males**

Disease/injury	Age group (years)	Proportion of incident cases developing a disability	I 0.096[b]	II 0.220[b]	III 0.400[b]	IV 0.600[b]	V 0.810[b]	VI 0.920[b]
Communicable, maternal and perinatal:								
Meningitis								
Acute	0–4	100	0	0	0	50	35	15
	5–14	100	0	0	0	50	35	15
	15–44	100	0	0	0	50	35	15
	45–59	100	0	0	0	50	35	15
	60+	100	0	0	0	50	35	15
Retardation	0–4	8	0	50	50	0	0	0
	5–14	8	0	50	50	0	0	0
	15–44	8	0	50	50	0	0	0
	45–59	8	0	50	50	0	0	0
	60+	8	0	50	50	0	0	0
Deafness	0–4	2	0	0	100	0	0	0
	5–14	2	0	0	100	0	0	0
	15–44	2	0	0	100	0	0	0
	45–59	2	0	0	100	0	0	0
	60+	2	0	0	100	0	0	0
Noncommunicable:								
Lung cancer:								
Terminal	0–4	100				40	30	30
	5–14	100				40	30	30
	15–44	100				40	30	30
	45–59	100				40	30	30
	60+	100				40	30	30
Preterminal	0–4	50		100				
	5–14	50		100				
	15–44	50		100				
	45–59	50		100				
	60+	50		100				
Psychoses	0–4	100			60	25	15	
	5–14	100			60	25	15	
	15–44	100			60	25	15	
	45–59	100			60	25	15	
	60+	100			60	25	15	
Cerebrovascular	0–4	100	35	30	15	10	5	5
	5–14	100	35	30	15	10	5	5
	15–44	100	35	30	15	10	5	5
	45–59	100	35	30	15	10	5	5
	60+	100	35	30	15	10	5	5
Periodontal disease	0–4	10		100				
	5–14	10		100				
	15–44	10		100				
	45–59	10		100				
	60+	10		100				
Injuries:								
Motor vehicle accidents	0–4	10		30	30	30	10	
	5–14	10		30	30	30	10	
	15–44	10		30	30	30	10	
	45–59	10		30	30	30	10	
	60+	10		30	30	30	10	
Falls	0–4	50		50	40	10		
	5–14	50		50	40	10		
	15–44	50		50	40	10		
	45–59	50		50	40	10		
	60+	80			40	40		30

[a] Note distributions across the six classes of disability sum to 100 percent.
[b] Weight for time spent in each disability class.

tion whereas in other countries they refer to all motor vehicle accidents in which a vehicle is damaged.

The mapping in Table 3 is preliminary; undoubtedly, it will be substantially revised as more attention is directed to the disabling sequelae of disease and definitions of incidence are altered. More detail on a the map and its empirical basis will be provided in a forthcoming book on the global burden of disease and injury (8). Another important improvement to previous approaches to assessing disability is the inclusion of short-term consequences of disease such as diarrhoeal diseases which have not traditionally been considered as a cause of disability although, by virtue of the volume of cases, they represent a significant proportion of the overall disease burden.

A final issue in the calculation of DALYs due to disability must be addressed: the effects of treatment or rehabilitation on disability. The objective of measuring DALYs is to quantify the current burden of disease, taking into account current activities including preventive and curative health care. Medical intervention can affect disability in four ways: changing the disease incidence, the probability of developing a disabling sequelae, the duration of disability, and the severity of disability. The first three treatment effects are already captured in the calculation of DALYs as described here and by Murray (1). When the proportion progressing to a disability is less than 100%, an adjustment is made to the disability weight itself. Changes in the severity of disability or the distribution of disabilities across the six classes owing to treatment has not so far been captured. In the case of certain disabling sequelae, such as those due to angina, cerebrovascular disease, conditions causing near-blindness, schizophrenia and others, interventions can reduce their severity. We have tried to capture this treatment effect by introducing a series of adjustments to the disability weight for each region and age-sex group, reflecting the likely impact of treatment on the distribution of disabilities across the six classes.

Results

The overall magnitude of disability by cause group and its distribution by age and region are summarized in Table 4, in which YLD refers to DALYs due to years of life lived with a disability. The Established Market Economies (EME) and the Former Socialist Economies of Europe (FSE) together account for only 15% of the global burden of disability (85% is in the developing world). However, as noted earlier (1), the proportion of total burden which is due to disability within EME and FSE is higher than in other regions. Owing to the combination of

population size and high disease and injury rates, India and China together account for nearly 40% of the total years lived with a disability (YLD). Sub-Saharan Africa (SSA) and Other Asia and Islands (OAI) each account for about 15% of the global total.

Globally, only about one-quarter of the total disability burden is due to Group I conditions (communicable, maternal and perinatal), over 60% arise from noncommunicable diseases, and the remaining 13% from injuries and poisonings. The distribution of YLD, by broad causal group, across regions is particularly revealing. While Sub-Saharan Africa and India together account for almost half of the global total due to Group I conditions, our estimates suggest that in terms of numbers or years lived with a disability, there is more noncommunicable disability in India than in the Established Market Economies. As countries pass through the health transition, the distribution of YLD shifts away from Group I (which accounts for 44% in SSA but less than 10% in EME and FSE). The absolute and relative variation in the share of YLD due to Group III (injuries) is smaller—from 8% in EME to 18% in Latin America and the Caribbean.

The age pattern of disability DALYs by region, summarized in Table 4, suggests the need for much greater emphasis on health protection among young adults. Almost one-quarter of the global total of YLD are because of diseases and injuries occurring among young children, but significantly more (36%) arise from conditions incurred at ages 15–44. Another 15% or so is due to the incidence of disease and injury at older adult ages (45–59), and a comparable amount among the elderly (60 years and over). The largest number of YLD at ages 15–44, partly reflecting the population size, occurs in China and India. The contribution in other regions of the developing world is at least as great as in the EME region, emphasizing that, irrespective of the stage of the health transition, the prevention of disease and injury among young adults is a global priority.

Comparative rates of disability across the three groups of causes are summarized in Fig. 3 (females) and Fig. 4 (males). The top histogram presents the YLD rates per 1000 population per year by region for the age group 0–14 years, the middle histogram those for ages 15–59 years, and the bottom graph those aged 60 and above. While there will be some effect of differences in age structure within these three broad age groups, much of the effect of age structure across regions is controlled for in this disaggregation. Each bar for each region distinguishes YLD due to Group I, Group II and Group III. Although less so than for mortality, there is still more than a fivefold variation in the rates of disability in children aged 0–14 across regions. Disability

Table 4: **Percentage distribution of YLD[a] according to region, by broad cause group and age group, 1990**

Region	Cause group			All causes	Age group (years)					All ages
	I	II	III		0–4	5–14	15–44	45–59	60+	
EME	0.9	8.0	0.7	9.6	0.6	0.3	3.3	1.8	3.5	9.6
FSE	0.4	4.1	0.5	5.0	0.4	0.2	1.8	1.1	1.5	5.0
CHN	4.1	12.1	2.2	18.4	3.1	2.3	6.9	2.4	3.6	18.4
LAC	2.7	5.2	1.7	9.6	1.9	1.6	4.0	1.1	1.0	9.6
OAI	3.9	8.0	1.6	13.6	2.8	2.5	5.1	1.6	1.5	13.6
MEC	2.4	5.7	1.7	9.8	2.9	1.5	3.5	1.0	0.9	9.8
IND	5.3	12.2	2.2	19.7	6.1	2.6	6.5	2.3	2.1	19.7
SSA	6.3	6.1	2.0	14.4	5.0	2.4	5.0	1.2	0.8	14.4
All regions	26.0	61.4	12.6	100.0	22.8	13.4	36.2	12.6	15.0	100.0

[a] YLD are expressed as a percent of the global YLD.

in children arises from all three groups, although perinatal causes in Group I and congenital causes in Group II predominate. Disability rates in this age group are only slightly higher in males than in females. Below age 60, much of the difference between regions in YLD for females is due to Group I disability, particularly from sexually transmitted diseases and maternal causes.

The significantly larger contribution from Group III causes (injuries) in Latin American women at ages 15–59 is particularly notable, and consistent with the higher death rates from these causes compared to other regions. The main cause of Group II YLD among women at these ages is neuropsychiatric illness, for which the rates are very nearly equal in all regions. Among the elderly, noncommunicable diseases, as expected, are the main cause of YLD, with overall rates being similar in all developing regions, but markedly lower (about one-third less) in the developed world.

The matching histograms for males (Fig. 4) demonstrate the greater regional heterogeneity and variation across age groups than for females. The highest overall YLD rates are in SSA, followed by LAC, India and FSE. Group I is much more prominent as a cause of disability in adult women than in men. Group III is the greatest determinant of the difference between regions in male DALY rates. The extremely high Group III YLD rates in LAC, exceeding even those for SSA, are particularly notable. These estimates also confirm the significance of injuries as a major public health problem in Latin America, with the impact concentrated among young adult men.

Another representation of years of life lived with a disability (YLD) is based on the impact not at the age of onset, but at the age at which the disability would be lived. YLD attributed to the age lived can be considered as a form of projected future prevalence of YLD if current incidence rates were to hold

constant. The age-sex-region specific rates using this alternative approach are given in Table 5. As expected, this perspective reveals higher rates of YLD lost at older ages because the disabling effect of disease and injury at earlier ages accumulates in a cohort. This effect is less apparent in EME and FSE, however, owing to a lower incidence of disabling conditions at younger ages compared with the developing world. The age pattern, however, is similar across all regions with monotonically rising rates, distinct from the J-shaped curve seen when analysing the rates by age of onset.

The sex ratio of YLD rates for the five age groups for each region is given in Table 6. In general, males have higher rates of disability. The notable exception is in the reproductive age group 15–44 years, where in most regions the rates are higher for women. Higher YLD rates in this age group reflect the substantial contribution of Group I causes in women. In older age groups, the situation is reversed although the excess in males is small except in FSE and EME.

More detail on the leading causes of YLD is given in Table 7, which shows within each age group and for each sex separately the percentage distribution of causes at the broad (Groups I, II and III) level of disaggregation and the next level down. Consider, first, the developed regions, EME and FSE. Congenital anomalies are by far the leading cause of YLD at younger ages (0–4 years), followed by perinatal conditions and injuries. Neuropsychiatric causes emerge as a major cause of disability at ages 5–14, with a further 20% of the burden in males and 13% in females because of injuries. This pattern is preserved for men aged 15–44 but diseases of the musculoskeletal system emerge as a major cause of disability in young women. Among adults aged 45–59, cardiovascular diseases and cancer each account for 15–20% of the disability burden with cardiovascular diseases rising to one-third of all

Fig. 3. **YLD rates for females within broad age ranges, by region, 1990 (rates/1000 population).**

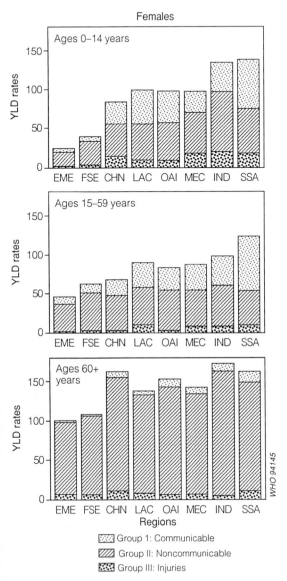

Fig. 3. **YLD rates for females within broad age ranges, by region, 1990 (rates/1000 population).**

ies are the major contributors to YLD at ages 0–4 and again at ages 5–14 years. In young adult males, injuries (30.2%), neuropsychiatric disease (26%), and infectious and parasitic diseases (13.3%) are the most important causes of disability. In young females (15–44), disability is dominated by neuropsychiatric disease (21%), causes related to pregnancy (20%), and infectious and parastic diseases (24.5%) including a large component due to sexually

Fig. 4. **YLD rates for males within broad age ranges, by region, 1990 (rates/1000 population).**

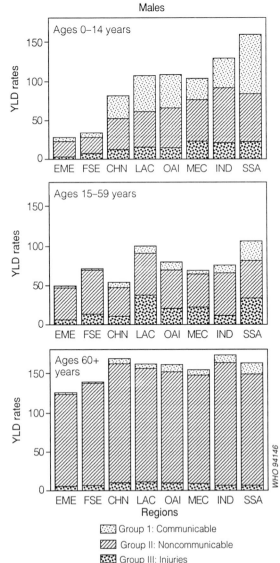

YLD in both men and women at ages 60 and over. The Table also illustrates the importance of non-fatal conditions as contributors to the disease burden in these regions, with almost 10% of the YLD among women aged 45–59 being due to poor oral health.

A very different pattern of YLD is apparent for the developing regions. Infectious and parasitic diseases, nutritional and endocrine disorders, and injur-

Table 5: **Rates of YLD age lived by region, sex and age group (per thousand population)**[a]

Region	Males in age group (years):					Females in age group (years):				
	0–4	5–14	15–44	45–59	60+	0–4	5–14	15–44	45–59	60+
EME	8	17	37	76	161	8	16	37	53	128
FSE	11	22	49	117	198	10	20	43	71	152
CHN	17	40	54	116	233	17	41	71	119	230
LAC	18	51	103	234	307	17	47	105	155	240
OAI	18	49	94	188	278	17	45	100	148	258
MEC	21	55	87	193	283	20	51	111	166	243
IND	31	65	101	175	256	34	68	136	158	237
SSA	66	78	158	257	289	64	71	173	205	252

[a] Please see text for a definition of YLD age lived.

transmitted diseases, especially pelvic inflammatory disease (PID). In older adult men and women the pattern of disability, by causes, shifts increasingly to cardiovascular diseases including ischaemic heart disease and stroke, chronic respiratory diseases, and other noncommunicable causes but neuropsychiatric disease, particularly the component due to dementia, remains a major factor.

Discussion

The estimates of the burden of disability represent an enormous effort on the part of nearly 100 disease experts to try and define the disabilities caused by most diseases and injuries. While the analysis provides an overall picture of disability by cause and is provocative in many details, we remain painfully aware of the limitations of the empirical database. Where no information is available, the results go beyond the database to speculate in a systematic fashion on the likely patterns of disability by cause, age and sex. Without this information, however, disability will continue to be underappreciated as a contributor to the burden of disease. The detailed review of each disease reveals the extraordinary dearth of data on disability from most diseases. We hope this

study will stimulate interest in describing the burden of disability by cause, age, sex and location.

Most work on disability or impairment has been general in nature, measuring prevalence in the population of moderate and severe disability (9–17). These studies are important in their own right; but they do not identify the causes of disability and consequently have little influence on the allocation of health resources to specific interventions, except perhaps for rehabilitation services. The work reported here on disability linked to specific health problems and, by inference, specific health interventions should be seen as a complement and not a substitute to the efforts at defining and quantifying the general level of disability in the community.

Many of the estimates presented are uncertain. Indeed, for most we cannot even define statistically a 95% confidence interval. The degree of uncertainty also varies from disease to disease, across age groups, and between regions. How should uncertainty alter the way in which decision-makers analyse these results? According to economic theory, the response to uncertainty depends on whether utility as a function of the magnitude of a problem is linear or non-linear. The shape of the utility function depends on how risk-averse or risk-taking a society chooses to be. For most diseases, we cannot even speculate whether the utility or consequences for society as a function of the disease burden magnitude are likely to be linear or non-linear.

The issue can be simplified; decision-makers can treat very uncertain estimates with wide confidence intervals as the same as, or less or more important than an equal estimate with a narrow confidence interval. At the extreme, one can ignore the uncertain, an all too common response. For a few infectious diseases such as HIV, tuberculosis and some epidemic diseases, there is a potential for a secondary effect of increased transmission in the future if the true incidence is at the higher end of the confidence interval. In these cases, one might choose

Table 6: **Ratio of male to female YLD rates**

Region	Age group (years):				
	0–4	5–14	15–44	45–59	60+
EME	1.04	1.21	0.94	1.43	1.26
FSE	1.06	1.23	1.07	1.53	1.26
CHN	0.92	1.04	0.70	1.11	1.03
LAC	1.07	1.09	1.04	1.41	1.17
OAI	1.04	1.17	0.89	1.17	1.05
MEC	1.03	1.13	0.70	1.29	1.09
IND	0.90	1.07	0.65	1.32	1.09
SSA	1.05	1.31	0.81	1.17	0.97

Table 7: Percentage distribution within each age group of YLD for developed and developing regions

	Males in age group (years):						Females in age group (years):						Both sexes
	0–14	5–14	15–44	45–59	60+	All ages	0–4	5–14	15–44	45–59	60+	All ages	
Developed regions													
I. Communicable, maternal and perinatal	23.0	9.5	5.3	1.9	1.4	4.7	23.9	11.4	29.0	2.9	1.6	13.3	8.9
A. Infectious & parasitic	2.8	4.7	2.4	0.6	0.4	1.5	2.6	5.5	18.0	0.7	0.4	7.0	4.2
B. Respiratory infections	9.2	4.8	2.9	1.3	0.9	2.4	9.6	5.9	3.1	2.0	1.2	2.7	2.6
C. Maternal conditions	-[a]	-	-	-	-	-	-	-	7.9	0.2	-	2.8	1.4
D. Perinatal conditions	11.0	-	-	-	-	0.8	11.7	-	-	-	-	0.8	0.8
II. Noncommunicable	67.0	70.1	75.2	92.5	94.2	84.4	67.9	75.4	65.4	94.4	92.3	81.0	82.7
A. Malignant neoplasms	1.6	5.6	5.3	17.6	18.1	11.9	1.4	6.0	4.6	18.9	12.6	9.9	10.9
B. Other neoplasm	-	-	-	-	-	-	-	-	-	-	-	-	-
C. Diabetes mellitus	-	-	0.8	1.8	0.7	0.9	-	-	0.8	2.9	0.9	1.1	1.0
D. Nutritional/endocrine	9.1	10.1	1.1	1.2	1.0	2.0	9.3	11.9	2.8	1.7	1.0	2.7	2.3
E. Neuropsychiatric	4.9	30.5	42.6	27.3	21.5	29.4	4.2	30.9	29.1	23.1	23.1	24.2	26.8
F. Sense organ	0.1	-	-	0.2	0.2	0.1	0.1	-	-	0.6	0.4	0.3	0.2
G. Cardiovascular diseases	1.9	1.6	6.7	17.6	33.0	16.9	1.7	1.6	2.8	11.1	36.6	16.9	16.9
H. Chronic respiratory diseases	2.0	12.6	3.7	3.7	6.3	4.7	1.7	13.1	3.4	3.4	3.8	3.7	4.2
I. Diseases of the digestive system	2.2	1.1	4.0	6.6	4.7	4.6	1.6	1.1	2.0	4.7	4.0	3.2	3.9
J. Diseases of the genito-urinary system	0.3	0.4	0.9	3.6	4.0	2.4	0.2	0.5	0.7	1.7	2.7	1.6	2.0
K. Skin disease	-	-	-	-	-	-	-	-	-	-	-	-	-
L. Diseases of the musculo-skeletal system	-	6.2	5.3	7.7	2.9	4.8	-	7.1	14.4	17.6	4.8	10.1	7.4
M. Congenital abnormalities	44.1	-	-	-	-	3.1	47.0	-	-	-	-	3.1	3.1
N. Oral health	0.5	2.0	4.8	5.1	1.8	3.5	0.5	3.1	4.9	8.4	2.5	4.2	3.9
III. Injuries	10.0	20.4	19.5	5.6	4.5	11.0	8.2	13.2	5.6	2.8	6.1	5.7	8.4
A. Unintentional	8.6	17.8	10.5	4.2	4.3	7.2	6.7	10.6	3.1	2.0	5.9	4.5	5.9
B. Intentional	1.4	2.5	9.0	1.3	0.2	3.7	1.5	2.6	2.5	0.8	0.1	1.2	2.5
Developing regions													
I. Communicable, maternal and perinatal	30.7	49.5	16.2	8.1	5.1	23.2	29.4	52.2	46.4	9.7	5.5	34.5	28.9
A. Infectious & parasitic	11.2	47.1	13.3	6.5	3.1	16.3	10.3	49.5	24.5	6.9	3.3	20.1	18.2
B. Respiratory infections	3.2	2.4	2.9	1.6	2.0	2.6	3.2	2.7	2.2	2.1	2.1	2.5	2.6
C. Maternal conditions	-	-	-	-	-	-	-	-	19.5	0.8	-	7.9	4.0
D. Perinatal conditions	16.3	-	-	-	-	4.3	16.0	-	-	-	-	4.0	4.1
II. Noncommunicable	57.1	31.7	53.6	83.9	90.6	59.1	57.8	32.6	46.6	86.0	89.5	56.4	57.7
A. Malignant neoplasms	0.4	2.1	2.4	9.6	5.5	3.1	0.8	0.8	1.9	9.6	4.2	2.5	2.8
B. Other neoplasm	-	-	-	-	-	-	-	-	-	-	-	-	-
C. Diabetes mellitus	-	-	0.3	1.3	0.4	0.3	-	-	0.2	1.8	0.5	0.3	0.3
D. Nutritional/endocrine	23.9	3.9	5.8	2.6	1.4	9.3	23.7	4.3	5.3	3.6	1.7	9.2	9.2
E. Neuropsychiatric	3.1	13.1	26.0	18.7	17.0	15.9	2.8	11.9	20.9	15.2	15.2	13.9	14.9
F. Sense organ	0.3	-	0.5	7.6	5.4	1.8	0.3	0.1	0.4	11.2	5.2	2.0	1.9
G. Cardiovascular diseases	1.5	1.7	4.3	16.8	35.0	8.3	1.0	2.6	3.3	16.7	36.7	7.9	8.1
H. Chronic respiratory diseases	4.6	5.8	3.8	4.5	12.5	5.4	4.8	5.2	2.9	5.8	10.7	4.9	5.2
I. Diseases of the digestive system	5.3	1.9	3.5	6.0	4.7	4.2	6.7	2.9	2.1	5.3	4.0	3.9	4.0
J. Diseases of the genito-urinary system	0.5	1.9	1.2	8.3	3.2	2.3	0.3	1.8	1.3	3.6	3.0	1.5	1.9
K. Skin disease	-	-	-	-	-	-	-	-	-	-	-	-	-
L. Diseases of the musculo-skeletal system	-	0.5	2.5	5.1	2.6	1.9	-	2.0	5.8	8.9	5.1	4.1	3.0
M. Congenital abnormalities	17.1	-	-	-	-	4.5	16.8	-	-	-	-	4.2	4.3
N. Oral health	0.4	0.8	3.3	3.3	2.8	2.1	0.4	0.9	2.5	4.3	3.1	2.0	2.0
III. Injuries	12.2	18.8	30.2	8.0	4.3	17.7	12.8	15.2	7.0	4.2	5.1	9.1	13.3
A. Unintentional	10.2	16.6	18.4	5.9	4.0	12.7	10.3	13.5	4.8	3.4	4.8	7.2	9.9
B. Intentional	2.0	2.2	11.8	2.1	0.3	5.1	2.4	1.7	2.2	0.9	0.2	1.8	3.4

[a] A dash represents less than 0.1%.

to treat a disease with a wider confidence interval as somewhat more important than the midpoint or expectation of the confidence interval. For all other conditions, the most reasonable approach, in the absence of other information, is to make decisions on the basis of the best estimate. In other words, we propose that for society as a whole the utility function of the magnitude of burden due to a particular disease is usually linear. Where wide confidence intervals appear to be concerned, investing resources in reducing the uncertainty around the estimates is also part of the optimal response.

One attempt to define the degree of uncertainty qualitatively for each estimate has already been initiated. Disease experts have been asked to grade estimates on a five-part quality-scoring scale. The reliability and validity of this quality-scoring system are still to be assessed. The results will ultimately be made available in the more detailed volume on the global burden of disease (8).

The total number of years lived with a disability is probably biased downwards because of omission of diseases and omission of idiopathic disabilities. More than 100 conditions were included in the study but many diseases have not been included. Disabilities from these missing diseases have been crudely estimated and included in the total. Deaths from residual categories of diseases not included in the GBD list have been estimated. Missing disabilities from these diseases causing mortality have been estimated by using the average relationship by Groups I, II and III between years lived with a disability and years of life lost due to premature mortality. But some conditions that lead only to disability and not to death may not have been covered by this procedure. Future work on expanding the number of conditions detailed in the GBD will eventually address most of this problem.

Perhaps of greater concern are the idiopathic disabilities where by definition there is no known cause. Take, for example, disabilities due to blindness. Blindness is included in the estimated burden through trachoma, onchocerciasis, glaucoma, cataract, congenital or perinatal factors, diabetes, neurological damage from malaria, and motor vehicle accidents and other trauma. Some idiopathic causes of blindness may not be included. (But for blindness the omissions are likely small.) In the future, cross-sectional datasets on the prevalence of certain impairments and disabilities could be used to assess the degree of omission of idiopathic outcomes.

While errors of omission may bias total YLD downwards, the problem of comorbidity biases the results upwards. The Global Burden of Disease estimates are built up from a disease perspective. Total

disability in each disability severity class is just the sum of all disability incidence in that class across the 100 causes. Disability, however, afflicts individuals. The fact that individuals can have more than one disability of the same or different Classes at the same time cannot be ignored. When someone suffering a Class I disability gets a further disability the effect is not simply additive. Presumably several Class I disabilities may combine to raise someone's total disability severity to a higher Class. However, the effect of three distinct Class I disabilities will not be to triple the disability severity weight for the individual as is currently implied in the aggregation method.

Comorbidity will occur at random but may be exacerbated if having a disability means that one's probability of getting others is higher. A simple numerical example will illustrate the comorbidity effect, even if the probabilities of becoming disabled are all independent. Imagine a population where there are ten disabling conditions, each with an annual incidence rate of 1 per 1000 which is constant across all age groups. There is no remission or case-fatality for these ten disabilities. In the age group 60+, the prevalence of each disability is expected to be 6.8%. However, the total prevalence of individuals with one or more Class I disability is not 68% but only 50.6%. Fig. 5 shows the expected percentage of the population with one, two, three, or four or more disabilities. The net overestimation of YLD due to comorbidity even in this simple example depends on whether having two, three or more Class I disabilities moves one into a higher disability class. If two Class I disabilities moved one into Class II, but three or four was still Class II, then the overestimate of YLD would not be large since most of the comorbid effect is captured by those with two Class I disabilities.

Fig. 5. **Comorbidity: hypothetical distribution of population by number of disabilities.**

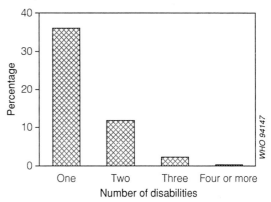

The magnitude of the overestimation of YLD due to comorbidity will be greater if the probabilities of getting different disabilities are dependent on each other. A diabetic has an increased risk of blindness, angina pectoris, amputation, neuropathy and renal failure. Household interview survey data suggest that there is considerable concentration of disability in an unlucky minority (18–20). At this stage of the measurement of disability, it is not feasible to take into account the interdependence of disability probabilities. Substantial further research is required to define a manageable method of accounting for these groups at high risk for disability.

Total YLD are not easily comparable estimates in the literature on the application of the ICIDH (International classification of impairments, disabilities and handicaps) to a population. In that work, disability is measured using a health expectancy: disability-free life expectancy. It would be desirable to use the wealth of data and expert estimates on the incidence and prevalence of disability by severity class and by age, sex and region to compute comparable health expectancy measures. For our DALY estimates to be directly comparable with the current publications (17), Class I, II and perhaps III disabilities would have to be ignored since their disability-free life expectancy ignores disability below some ill-defined threshold of moderate disability. Or one could define a hierarchy of health expectancies: disability-free life expectancy, life free of Class II or higher disability, life free of Class III or higher disability, and so on. Building a bridge between the sets of indicators will hopefully facilitate communication and sharing of information.

Traditionally, disability has been assessed in a cross-sectional fashion which defines the prevalence, by age and sex, of disabling conditions in a population. While this may be essential for determining the volume and nature of rehabilitation services, these data are of limited use for evaluating or monitoring primary or secondary prevention strategies. Cross-sectional surveys rarely provide insight into the causes of disability or indeed into the dynamics of the disabling process which often follows the occurrence of disease or injury. There is a clear need for monitoring systems which can identify new disabilities and then follow the evolution of these disabilities. Such systems will allow reliable retrospective assessment of the underlying cause of disabilities and will yield valuable prospective information on the nature, timing, and severity of subsequent complications and associated morbidities and the impact of interventions. If monitoring the burden of disease becomes a priority, then establishing cost-effective mechanisms to measure the burden of disability over a period of time will be critical.

Many countries in the Commonwealth of Independent States (CIS) already have in place monitoring systems for disability for determining eligibility for state benefits. These registries record all individuals with disabilities that interfere even partially with the capacity to work. Each disabled person is examined by a panel of physicians and social workers each year. For example, in Uzbekistan nearly half a million adults aged 18 to 60 years are registered with disabilities. Disabilities are classified according to severity and cause. Such detailed information on disabilities can be used both to validate the efforts to measure the National Burden of Disease in these countries and also to monitor trends in the burden of disability. By expanding such systems to the entire population, not just the age group 18 to 60, these systems in the CIS hold great promise for monitoring disability trends and causes. For other countries, a sample registration system for disability akin to the sample Registration Scheme for mortality in India or the Disease Surveillance Points system in China may provide a cost-effective alternative to complete registration of the disabled. Development of sample disability registration schemes should be a major theme for future research.

This study is a first attempt at quantifying a complex phenomenon in a way that can inform health policy debates. Six recommendations for future effort emerge. (1) Those conditions, which are estimated to cause many YLD and are the most uncertain, should be the focus of further epidemiological research. (2) Further work on the burden of disease should concentrate on improving the mapping from disease to impairment and then to disability. We hope that the publication of the results of the Global Burden of Disease study will install a new sensitivity to disability issues among some disease epidemiologists. (3) This sensitivity to disability issues should extend to better quantification of the cost-effectiveness of health interventions that prevent or treat disability. (4) Simple methods to adjust the results of the burden of disease exercises for comorbidity should be developed. (5) The number of conditions included in the Global Burden of Disease analysis should be expanded and the coverage of particular disabilities validated through cross-sectional work. (6) Methods for prospective monitoring of disability on a sample or general basis should be developed and applied.

Acknowledgements

We should like to acknowledge the financial and/or technical support of the Edna McConnel Clark Foundation, the Rockefeller Foundation, the World Bank and the World Health Organization. We would particularly like to thank

Richard Peto for his comments on earlier drafts of this article. Many others generously contributed time and technical advice to this undertaking (please see list of names in acknowledgements on page 31).

Résumé

La mesure quantitative de l'incapacité: données, méthodes, résultats

Une méthode destinée à remplacer les méthodes transversales d'évaluation de l'incapacité est exposée ici et ses résultats sont indiqués pour 1990. La méthode ne fournit pas d'estimation de la prévalence de l'incapacité, mais permet d'estimer le nombre de DALY (*disability-adjusted life years*: années de vie ajustées sur l'incapacité), supposées être vécues *ultérieurement*, d'après le profil estimé de l'incidence des maladies et des traumatismes survenus en 1990, puis en estimant la proportion de ces événements susceptibles de conduire à l'incapacité, la durée moyenne de ces incapacités et leur gravité comparée en termes de limitation de l'activité. Dans le présent article, ces DALY ont été désignées par YLD, de *years of life lived with disability*, ou années de vie vécues avec une incapacité, pour les distinguer de l'autre composante des DALY, à savoir celle qui résulte du décès prématuré. Les hypothèses, les méthodes et les modèles utilisés pour estimer les YLD sont indiqués en détail dans l'article. On y trouvera notamment la description du modèle de base de maladie utilisé dans cette étude (le Harvard incidence-prevalence model) montrant comment on peut obtenir les taux d'incidence, les durées, les taux de prévalence et de létalité de façon à garantir leur validité interne. Des exemples de résultats donnés par le modèle sont présentés, ainsi que la distribution de la gravité de l'incapacité concernant quelques maladies et traumatismes précis.

Dans la mesure où la base de données empirique utilisée pour estimer les paramètres nécessaires à l'estimation des YLD est extrêmement limitée, les estimations données dans cet article ont nécessairement des intervalles de confiance étendus. Elles indiquent néanmoins qu'à l'échelle mondiale, seul un quart environ de toutes les DALY de 1990 a pour origine une maladie transmissible ou une affection maternelle ou périnatale. Plus de 60% sont imputables aux maladies non transmissibles et environ 13% aux traumatismes. Par exemple, les maladies non transmissibles représentent plus de YLD en Inde que dans l'ensemble des pays industrialisés. Au fur et à mesure que les pays effectuent leur transition

sanitaire, la répartition des YLD se déplace vers les maladies non transmissibles, ce qui correspond au profil observé de la mortalité.

Concernant les classes d'âge, un quart du nombre de YLD dans le monde est imputable aux maladies et aux traumatismes chez le jeune enfant. Toutefois, elles représentent chez le jeune adulte (15–44 ans) une part significativement supérieure (35%). Cette tendance se retrouve dans toutes les régions, donnant à penser que la protection et la promotion de la santé chez le jeune adulte est une priorité mondiale. Le taux de YLD tend à être plus grand chez les hommes que chez les femmes, à l'exception de la classe d'âge apte à la procréation pour ces dernières.

Les causes spécifiques majeures de YLD varient d'une région à l'autre; deux causes cependant, les affections psychiatriques et les traumatismes, occupent le devant du tableau partout dans le monde. Cette conclusion ne ressort pas clairement de l'analyse des causes de décès et il est donc urgent de mettre en œuvre des systèmes ciblés de surveillance de l'incapacité pour développer les connaissances concernant les séquelles invalidantes des maladies et des traumatismes, et pour ainsi disposer d'une meilleure information lorsqu'il s'agit des programmes de prévention de l'incapacité.

References

1. **Murray CJL.** Quantifying the burden of disease: the technical basis for disability-adjusted life years. *Bulletin of the World Health Organization*, 1994, **72**: 429–445.
2. **Murray CJL, Lopez AD.** Global and regional cause-of-death patterns in 1990. *Bulletin of the World Health Organization*, 1994, **72**: 447–480.
3. **Murray CJL, Lopez AD, Jamison DT.** The global burden of disease in 1990: summary results, sensitivity analysis and future directions. *Bulletin of the World Health Organization*, 1994, **72**: 495–509.
4. **Omran AR.** The epidemiologic transition: a theory of the epidemiology of population change. *Milbank Memorial Fund quarterly*, 1971, **49**: 509–538.
5. **Bobadilla JL et al.** The epidemiological transition and health priorities. In: Jamison D, Mosley H, eds. *Disease control priorities in developing countries.* Oxford, Oxford University Press (for the World Bank), 1993.
6. **Murray CJL, Yang G, Qiao X.** Adult mortality: levels, patterns and trends. In: Feachem RG et al., eds. *The health of adults in the developing world.* Oxford, Oxford University Press (for the World Bank), 1992.
7. **World Bank.** *World development report 1993: Investing in health.* Oxford, Oxford University Press, 1993.

8. **Murray CJL, Lopez AD.** The global burden of disease and injury (text in preparation for the World Health Organization and the World Bank).
9. **Bebbington AC.** The expectation of life without disability in England and Wales: 1976–1988. *Population trends*, 1991, **66**: 26–29.
10. **Branch LG et al.** Active life expectancy for 10,000 Caucasian men and women in three communities. *Journal of gerontology*, 1991, **46**: M145–M150.
11. **Crimmins E, Saito Y, Ingegneri D.** Changes in life expectancy and disability-free life expectancy in the United States. *Population and development review*, 1989, **15**: 235–267.
12. **Mathers CD.** *Health expectancies in Australia 1981 and 1988.* Canberra, Australian Institute of Health, 1991.
13. **Robine JM, Colvez A.** Espérance de vie sans incapacité en France en 1981. *Population*, 1986, **41**: 1025–1042.
14. **Rogers RG, Rogers A, Belanger A.** Active life among the elderly in the United States: multistate life-table estimates and population projections. *Mil-*

bank Memorial Fund quarterly, 1989, **67**: 370–411.
15. **van Ginneken JK et al.** Results of two methods to determine health expectancy in the Netherlands in 1981–1985. *Social science and medicine*, 1991, **32**: 1129–1136.
16. **Wilkins R, Adams OB.** Health expectancy in Canada, late 1970s: demographic, regional and social dimensions. *American journal of public health*, 1983, **73**: 1073–1080.
17. **Réseau Espérance de Vie en Santé.** *Statistical world yearbook. Retrospective 1993 issue.* Montpellier, INSERM, 1993.
18. **Verbrugge LM, Lepkowski JM, Imanaka Y.** Comorbidity and its impact on disability. *Milbank Memorial Fund quarterly*, 1989, **67**: 450–484.
19. **Centers for Disease Control.** Comorbidity of chronic conditions and disability among older persons—United States, 1984. *Journal of the American Medical Association*, 1990, **263**: 209–210.
20. **Rice DP, Laplante MP.** Medical expenditure for disability and disabling comorbidity. *American journal of public health*, 1992, **82**: 739–741.

Annex

Years lived with a disability (YLDs, in thousands): Established Market Economies

Disease or injury (ICD 9 code)	Both sexes all ages	Males						Females					
		0–4	5–14	15–44	45–59	60+	All ages	0–4	5–14	15–44	45–59	60+	All ages
All Causes	44,765	1,503	790	7,642	4,934	7,800	22,669	1,378	619	7,922	3,530	8,647	22,096
I. Communicable, maternal & perinatal (001-139,320-322,460-465,466,480-487,614-616, 630-676,760-779)	4,223	357	79	485	108	112	1,140	339	74	2,410	113	146	3,083
A. Infectious & parasitic dis. (001-139,320-322,614-616)	2,143	37	39	236	32	36	380	33	36	1,623	30	40	1,763
A1. Tuberculosis (010-018,137)	47	–	1	16	7	6	31	–	–	8	4	4	16
A2. STDs excluding HIV (090-099,614-616)	1,553	–	–	15	–	–	16	–	–	1,531	4	1	1,537
a. Syphilis (090-097)	95	–	–	12	–	–	13	–	–	76	4	1	82
b. Chlamydia	8	–	–	3	–	–	3	–	–	5	–	–	5
c. Gonorrhoea (098)													
d. Pelvic inflammatory disease (614-616)	1,450	–	–	–	–	–	–	–	–	1,450	1	–	1,450
A3. HIV infection	165	–	–	126	7	2	135	–	–	28	1	1	30
A4. Diarrhoeal diseases (001,002,004,006-009)	210	9	13	58	15	9	104	8	12	57	15	13	106
a. Acute watery	175	7	11	49	12	8	87	7	10	47	13	11	88
b. Persistent	11	–	–	3	–	–	6	–	–	3	–	–	6
c. Dysentery	24	–	1	7	2	1	12	–	1	6	2	1	12
A5. Childhood cluster (032-33,037,045,050,055-56,138)	79	19	22	–	–	–	41	17	21	–	–	–	38
a. Pertussis (133)	70	16	19	–	–	–	36	16	18	–	–	–	34
b. Poliomyelitis (045,138)													
c. Diphtheria (032)	4	–	1	–	–	–	2	–	1	–	–	–	2
d. Measles (055)	5	1	2	–	–	–	3	1	1	–	–	–	2
e. Tetanus (037)													
A6. Meningitis (036,320-322)	11	4	–	–	–	–	6	4	–	–	–	–	5
A7. Hepatitis (070)	17	–	–	4	3	4	10	–	–	2	1	–	7
A8. Malaria (084)													
A9. Tropical cluster (085,086,120,125)													
a. African trypanosomiasis (086.3,086.4,086.5)													
b. Chagas disease (086.0,086.1,086.2)													
c. Schistosomiasis (120)													
d. Leishmaniasis (085)													
e. Lymphatic filariasis (125.0, 125.1)													
f. Onchocerciasis (125.3)													
A10. Leprosy (030)													
A11. Trachoma (076)													
A12. Intestinal helminths (126-129)													
a. Ascaris (127.0)													
b. Trichuris (127.3)													
c. Hookworm (126)													
B. Respiratory infections (381-382,460-466,480-487)	1,206	145	40	248	76	76	585	138	38	261	78	106	621
B1. Acute lower respiratory inf. (460-465)	495	1	13	129	46	50	239	1	13	125	47	70	256
B2. Acute upper respiratory inf. (466,480-487)	432	1	27	119	30	26	203	1	25	135	31	36	229
B3. Otitis media (381-382)	278	143	–	–	–	–	143	136	–	–	–	–	136

Years lived with a disability (YLDs, in thousands): Established Market Economies

Disease or injury (ICD 9 code)	Both sexes all ages	Males 0-4	Males 5-14	Males 15-44	Males 45-59	Males 60+	Males All ages	Females 0-4	Females 5-14	Females 15-44	Females 45-59	Females 60+	Females All ages
C. Maternal conditions (630-676)	531	–	–	–	–	–	–	–	–	525	5	–	531
C1. Haemorrhage (666,667)	89	–	–	–	–	–	–	–	–	88	–	–	89
C2. Sepsis (670)	198	–	–	–	–	–	–	–	–	196	2	–	198
C3. Eclampsia (642.4-642.6)	3	–	–	–	–	–	–	–	–	3	–	–	3
C4. Hypertension (642 minus 642.4-642.6)	–	–	–	–	–	–	–	–	–	–	–	–	–
C5. Obstructed labour (660)	229	–	–	–	–	–	–	–	–	227	2	–	229
C6. Abortion (630-639)	10	–	–	–	–	–	–	–	–	10	–	–	10
D. Perinatal causes (760-779)	343	175	–	–	–	–	175	169	–	–	–	–	169
II. Noncommunicable (140-628,680-759) (minus 320-322,460-465,466,480-487, 614-616)	37,185	1,021	576	5,883	4,613	7,328	19,420	944	469	5,106	3,334	7,911	17,765
A. Malignant neoplasms (140-208)	5,320	20	41	407	926	1,552	2,946	16	35	379	738	1,207	2,375
A1. Mouth and oropharynx (140-149)	120	–	–	11	42	34	87	–	–	5	13	15	33
A2. Oesophagus (150)	36	–	–	1	11	15	27	–	–	–	3	6	10
A3. Stomach (151)	216	–	–	9	44	75	129	–	–	9	24	56	88
A4. Colorectal (152,153,154)	689	–	–	22	110	216	349	–	–	20	94	226	341
A5. Liver (155)	32	–	–	1	9	10	20	–	–	–	4	7	12
A6. Pancreas (157)	45	–	–	1	8	15	24	–	–	–	5	15	21
A7. Lung (162)	360	–	–	9	90	153	252	–	–	6	39	63	108
A8. Melanoma and other skin (172-173)	56	–	–	9	9	6	24	–	–	14	10	8	32
A9. Breast (174)	364	–	–	–	–	–	–	–	–	75	151	138	364
A10. Cervix (180)	63	–	–	–	–	–	–	–	–	27	22	14	63
A11. Corpus uteri (179,181-182)	67	–	–	–	–	–	–	–	–	5	31	30	67
A12. Ovary (183)	58	–	–	–	–	–	–	–	–	11	24	22	58
A13. Prostate (185)	288	–	–	–	37	250	288	–	–	–	–	–	–
A14. Bladder (188)	210	–	–	9	49	103	161	–	–	3	13	33	48
A15. Lymphoma (200-202)	202	2	2	33	35	41	111	–	–	22	26	42	91
A16. Leukemia (204-208)	57	2	2	7	8	14	32	–	–	5	6	12	25
B. Other neoplasm (210-239)	–	–	–	–	–	–	–	–	–	–	–	–	–
C. Diabetes mellitus (250)	536	–	–	73	114	58	244	–	–	75	131	85	291
D. Nutritional/endocrine (240-285, minus 250)	1,093	137	55	89	85	98	464	129	49	248	83	120	629
D1. Protein-energy malnutrition (260-263)	221	113	–	–	–	–	113	108	–	–	–	–	108
D2. Iodine deficiency (243)	–	–	–	–	–	–	–	–	–	–	–	–	–
D3. Vitamin A deficiency (264)	–	–	–	–	–	–	–	–	–	–	–	–	–
D4. Anaemias (280-285)	514	3	39	50	51	32	175	3	37	203	52	45	340
E. Neuro-psychiatric (290-359, minus 320-322)	12,533	71	263	3,514	1,423	1,664	6,936	54	201	2,379	893	2,071	5,597
E1. Major affective disorder	2,108	–	–	528	109	44	680	–	–	1,073	231	123	1,428
E2. Bipolar affective disorder (296)	112	–	–	45	8	3	55	–	–	45	8	4	57
E3. Psychoses (295, 291-294,297-299)	560	–	–	300	–	–	300	–	–	260	–	–	260
E4. Epilepsy (345)	566	40	139	106	30	16	331	27	94	74	23	16	235
E5. Alcohol dependence (303)	2,602	–	–	1,259	708	308	2,275	–	–	179	102	45	327
E6. Alzheimer & other dementias (330,331,333-336,290)	3,570	–	–	–	332	1,149	1,482	–	–	–	368	1,721	2,089
E7. Parkinson disease (332)	255	–	–	–	46	63	109	–	–	–	51	95	146
E8. Multiple sclerosis (340)	145	–	–	71	1	–	72	–	–	71	1	–	73
E9. Drug dependence (304)	1,481	–	55	885	132	33	1,105	–	14	306	48	8	376
E10. Post-traumatic stress disorder	720	5	46	190	24	6	271	8	75	314	39	13	449

Years lived with a disability (YLDs, in thousands): Established Market Economies

Disease or injury (ICD 9 code)	Both sexes all ages	Males 0-4	Males 5-14	Males 15-44	Males 45-59	Males 60+	Males All ages	Females 0-4	Females 5-14	Females 15-44	Females 45-59	Females 60+	Females All ages
F. Sense organ (360-389)	80	2	-	-	12	13	27	2	-	-	23	28	53
F1. Glaucoma-related blindness (365)	47	-	-	-	8	3	11	-	-	-	19	17	36
F2. Cataract-related blindness (366)	28	-	-	-	3	10	13	-	-	4	-	10	15
G. Cardiovascular diseases (390-459)	7,073	32	14	454	787	2,366	3,653	25	11	217	338	2,829	3,420
G1. Rheumatic heart disease (390-398)	1,931	-	-	77	223	736	1,036	-	-	16	61	819	895
G2. Ischaemic heart disease (*)	1,638	-	2	61	99	549	713	-	2	43	60	819	925
G3. Cerebrovascular disease (430-438)	45	2	2	5	5	14	25	2	2	2	2	16	20
G4. Inflammatory cardiac disease (+)	1,910	34	105	304	153	469	1,064	25	85	280	130	326	847
H. Chronic respiratory dis. (460-519, minus 460-466,480-487)	1,630	-	-	-	-	-	967	-	-	-	-	-	663
H1. Chronic obstructive lung dis. (490-492,495-496)	954	15	-	-	76	356	468	12	-	-	38	351	486
H2. Asthma (493)	508	19	100	246	306	32	325	13	6	-	-	58	182
I. Diseases of the digestive system (520-579)	888	5	13	-	57	-	549	3	1	63	38	-	340
I1. Peptic ulcer disease (531-533)	288	-	-	71	131	118	173	-	-	26	46	76	115
I2. Cirrhosis of the liver (571)	467	5	1	40	131	332	320	3	1	28	38	269	147
J. Genito-urinary (580-629)	476	3	-	-	35	166	233	3	-	28	24	199	243
J1. Nephritis/nephrosis (580-589)	240	2	-	29	124	116	41	2	-	16	-	-	199
J2. Benign prostatic hypertrophy (600)	-	-	-	-	-	-	27	-	-	-	-	-	-
K. Skin disease (680-709)	1,385	-	-	-	-	-	1,385	-	-	-	-	-	-
L. Musculo-skeletal system (710-739)	3,705	-	77	507	496	304	1,384	-	68	1,141	657	454	2,321
L1. Rheumatoid arthritis (714)	1,324	-	-	79	83	65	228	-	-	718	239	109	1,096
L2. Osteoarthritis (715)	2,229	-	76	416	403	217	1,102	1	37	391	399	300	1,127
M. Congenital abnormalities (740-759)	1,372	698	13	216	138	107	698	674	12	215	153	160	674
N. Oral health (520-529)	1,017	2	13	216	138	107	476	2	12	215	153	160	541
N1. Dental caries (521.0)	73	2	-	16	3	3	37	2	-	15	3	4	37
N2. Periodontal disease (523)	53	-	-	24	2	2	27	-	-	23	2	2	26
N3. Edentulism (520)	891	-	-	176	134	103	413	-	-	176	148	154	478
III. Injuries (E800-999)	3,358	126	135	1,274	213	361	2,109	95	75	407	82	590	1,249
A. Unintentional (E800-949)	2,354	99	112	630	162	350	1,352	69	58	228	64	582	1,001
A1. Road traffic accidents (E810-819, 826-829)	421	6	41	181	16	4	248	4	20	125	20	4	173
A2. Poisoning (E850-869)	10	-	-	6	-	-	7	-	-	2	-	-	3
A3. Falls (E850-869)	1,108	14	15	143	66	280	519	9	6	26	18	529	589
A4. Fires (E890-899)	339	42	27	97	24	20	210	32	23	41	12	21	129
A5. Drowning (E910)	-	-	-	-	-	-	-	-	-	-	-	-	-
A6. Occupational (#)	16	-	-	9	4	1	14	-	-	1	1	-	2
B. Intentional (E950-969,990-999)	1,004	27	23	644	51	11	757	26	17	178	18	8	247
B1. Self-inflicted (E950-959)	-	-	-	-	-	-	-	-	-	-	-	-	-
B2. Homicide and violence (E960-969)	1,004	27	23	644	51	11	757	26	17	178	18	8	247
B3. War (E990-999)	-	-	-	-	-	-	-	-	-	-	-	-	-
Population (in millions)	797.8	26.4	53.3	184.1	66.1	60.5	390.5	25.1	50.7	179.2	67.8	84.6	407.3

Notes

A dash (-) symbol indicates less than 1,000 YLDs.

* ICD 9 codes for ischaemic heart disease are as follows: 410-414, 440.9, plus: at ages 45-59: 50% of 427.1, 427.4, 427.5, and 33% of 428; at ages 60+: 80% of 427.1, 427.4, 427.5 and 50% of 428.

+ ICD 9 codes for inflammatory cardiac diseases are as follows: 420, 421, 422, 425 plus: at ages 0-44: 50% of 428; at ages 45-59: 25% of 428; at ages 60+: 20% of 428.

There are no established ICD 9 codes specific for occupational injuries. Estimates have been based on reported occupational injuries and deaths tabulated by the International Labour Organisation.

Years lived with a disability (YLDs, in thousands): Formerly Socialist Economies of Europe

Disease or injury (ICD 9 code)	Both sexes all ages	Males 0-4	Males 5-14	Males 15-44	Males 45-59	Males 60+	Males All ages	Females 0-4	Females 5-14	Females 15-44	Females 45-59	Females 60+	Females All ages
All Causes	23,324	902	472	4,405	3,032	2,971	11,782	813	371	4,052	2,203	4,102	11,542
I. Communicable, maternal & perinatal (001-139, 320-322,460-465,466,480-487,614-616, 630-676,760-779)	1,856	196	41	153	44	34	468	185	38	1,059	50	56	1,389
A. Infectious & parasitic dis. (001-139,320-322,614-616)	717	30	20	50	13	8	120	24	18	532	12	10	597
A1. Tuberculosis (010-018,137)	20			7	3	2	12			3	2	2	7
A2. STDs excluding HIV (090-099,614-616)	510			8			8			500	1		502
a. Syphilis (090-097)	32			6			7			23	1		25
b. Chlamydia	3			1			1			2			2
c. Gonorrhoea (098)													
d. Pelvic inflammatory disease (614-616)	475									475	1		475
A3. HIV infection	10			8			8			1			2
A4. Diarrhoeal diseases (001,002,004,006-009)	94	6	7	24	6	3	46	5	6	24	7	6	48
a. Acute watery	78	5	6	20	5	3	38	5	5	20	6	5	40
b. Persistent	5			1			2			1			3
c. Dysentery	10			3			5			3			5
A5. Childhood cluster (032-33,037,045,050,055-56,138)	39	9	11				20	8	10				19
a. Pertussis (133)	35	8	10				18	8	9				17
b. Poliomyelitis (045,138)	2						1						1
c. Diphtheria (032)	2						1						1
d. Measles (055)													
e. Tetanus (037)													
A6. Meningitis (036,320-322)	4			2			2			2			2
A7. Hepatitis (070)	6						3						3
A8. Malaria (084)													
A9. Tropical cluster (085,086,120,125)													
a. African trypanosomiasis (086.3,086.4,086.5)													
b. Chagas disease (086.0,086.1,086.2)													
c. Schistosomiasis (120)													
d. Leishmaniasis (085)													
e. Lymphatic filariasis (125.0, 125.1)													
f. Onchocerciasis (125.3)													
A10. Leprosy (030)													
A11. Trachoma (076)													
A12. Intestinal helminths (126-129)													
a. Ascaris (127.0)													
b. Trichuris (127.3)													
c. Hookworm (126)													
B. Respiratory infections (381-382,460-466,480-487)	538	76	21	103	31	26	256	72	20	109	34	46	281
B1. Acute lower respiratory inf. (460-465)	207		7	53	19	17	97		7	52	21	30	110
B2. Acute upper respiratory inf. (466,480-487)	185		14	49	12	9	85		13	57	14	15	100
B3. Otitis media (381-382)	145	74					74	71					71
C. Maternal conditions (630-676)	422									418	4		422
C1. Haemorrhage (666,667)	44									44			44
C2. Sepsis (670)	151									149	2		151
C3. Eclampsia (642.4-642.6)	2									2			2
C4. Hypertension (642 minus 642.4-642.6)													
C5. Obstructed labour (660)	203									201	2		203
C6. Abortion (630-639)	15									15			15
D. Perinatal causes (760-779)	180	91					91	89					89

Years lived with a disability (YLDs, in thousands): Formerly Socialist Economies of Europe

Disease or injury (ICD 9 code)	Both sexes all ages	Males						Females					
		0-4	5-14	15-44	45-59	60+	All ages	0-4	5-14	15-44	45-59	60+	All ages
II. Noncommunicable (140-628,680-759) (minus 320-322,460-465,466,480-487, 614-616)	19,138	591	309	3,180	2,757	2,814	9,651	543	278	2,729	2,076	3,861	9,487
A. Malignant neoplasms (140-208)	2,116	19	30	234	480	396	1,158	15	24	176	348	394	958
A1. Mouth and oropharynx (140-149)	45	-	-	5	19	11	34	-	-	1	4	5	10
A2. Oesophagus (150)	14	-	-	-	5	5	10	-	-	-	2	3	4
A3. Stomach (151)	107	-	-	5	27	29	61	-	-	4	15	27	46
A4. Colorectal (152,153,154)	128	-	-	5	25	32	62	-	-	6	23	38	66
A5. Liver (155)	12	-	-	-	3	3	6	-	-	-	3	3	6
A6. Pancreas (157)	13	-	-	-	3	3	7	-	-	-	2	4	6
A7. Lung (162)	106	-	-	5	45	36	86	-	-	1	7	11	20
A8. Melanoma and other skin (172-173)	8	-	-	1	1	-	3	-	-	1	2	1	5
A9. Breast (174)	65							-	-	15	31	19	65
A10. Cervix (180)	31							-	-	9	13	9	31
A11. Corpus uteri (179,181-182)	18							-	-	1	10	6	18
A12. Ovary (183)	17							-	-	3	8	6	17
A13. Prostate (185)	29	-	-	-	5	23	29						
A14. Bladder (188)	35	-	-	1	11	16	28	-	-	-	2	4	6
A15. Lymphoma (200-202)	32	-	-	6	7	4	17	-	-	5	5	4	14
A16. Leukemia (204-208)	16	-	-	2	3	2	8	-	-	2	2	2	7
B. Other neoplasm (210-239)	1												
C. Diabetes mellitus (250)	143	-	-	18	30	13	61	-	-	20	38	25	82
D. Nutritional/endocrine (240-285, minus 250)	488	82	72	49	14	8	224	76	69	88	17	14	264
D1. Protein-energy malnutrition (260-263)	114	58	-	-	-	-	58	56	-	-	-	-	56
D2. Iodine deficiency (243)	1												
D3. Vitamin A deficiency (264)	-												
D4. Anaemias (280-285)	278	5	68	35	7	4	118	5	65	76	8	6	160
E. Neuro-psychiatric (290-359, minus 320-322)	5,748	48	122	1,624	749	647	3,190	38	105	1,111	434	870	2,559
E1. Major affective disorder	1,140	-	-	280	55	19	353	-	-	589	131	67	787
E2. Bipolar affective disorder (296)	63	-	-	25	4	-	30	-	-	26	5	2	33
E3. Psychoses (295, 291-294,297-299)	226	-	-	119	-	-	119	-	-	107	-	-	107
E4. Epilepsy (345)	260	20	70	43	12	5	150	14	49	31	10	7	110
E5. Alcohol dependence (303)	1,780	-	-	861	484	211	1,557	-	-	122	70	31	224
E6. Alzheimer & other dementias (330,331,333-336,290)	1,355	-	-	-	126	370	496	-	-	-	156	703	859
E7. Parkinson disease (332)	131	-	-	-	23	27	51	-	-	-	29	52	81
E8. Multiple sclerosis (340)	59	-	-	28	-	-	29	-	-	29	-	-	30
E9. Drug dependence (304)	237	-	9	143	21	5	178	-	2	48	7	1	59
E10. Post-traumatic stress disorder	314	-	24	79	10	2	117	-	39	131	17	5	197
F. Sense organ (360-389)	53	3	-	-	5	12	19	1	-	-	11	21	33
F1. Glaucoma-related blindness (365)	21	-	-	-	2	4	7	-	-	-	7	7	14
F2. Cataract-related blindness (366)	28	-	-	-	3	8	11	-	-	-	4	13	18
G. Cardiovascular diseases (390-459)	4,442	14	6	349	614	1,187	2,171	12	4	122	299	1,834	2,271
G1. Rheumatic heart disease (*)	1,439	-	-	111	228	363	703	-	-	16	67	654	736
G2. Ischaemic heart disease (390-398)	1,249	-	-	52	127	306	487	-	-	27	95	639	762
G3. Cerebrovascular disease (430-438)	22	-	-	3	7	3	13	-	-	-	-	9	9
G4. Inflammatory cardiac disease (+)													
H. Chronic respiratory dis. (460-519, minus 460-466,480-487)	965	15	54	144	139	208	561	12	45	122	66	159	405
H1. Chronic obstructive lung dis. (490-492,495-496)	255	-	-	2	39	123	163	-	-	-	11	81	92
H2. Asthma (493)	417	8	52	101	30	11	201	6	44	103	39	24	216

Years lived with a disability (YLDs, in thousands): Formerly Socialist Economies of Europe

Disease or injury (ICD 9 code)	Both sexes all ages	Males 0-4	5-14	15-44	45-59	60 +	All ages	Females 0-4	5-14	15-44	45-59	60 +	All ages
I. Diseases of the digestive system (520-579)	1,025	34	7	205	223	152	621	22	5	91	123	163	405
I1. Peptic ulcer disease (531-533)	120	-	1	42	23	5	71	-	-	26	17	5	49
I2. Cirrhosis of the liver (571)	122	-	-	22	37	26	86	-	-	7	13	16	37
J. Genito-urinary (580-629)	474	3	4	67	118	98	290	2	3	52	58	70	185
J1. Nephritis/nephrosis (580-589)	193	-	2	46	31	25	105	-	2	31	25	28	87
J2. Benign prostatic hypertrophy (600)	106	-	-	-	62	43	106	-	-	-	-	-	-
K. Skin disease (680-709)	-	-	-	-	-	-	-	-	-	-	-	-	-
L. Musculo-skeletal system (710-739)	1,353	-	2	134	116	11	263	-	2	578	353	155	1,089
L1. Rheumatoid arthritis (714)	567	-	-	55	100	4	159	-	-	320	60	28	407
L2. Osteoarthritis (715)	721	-	-	68	10	3	81	-	-	242	280	118	640
M. Congenital abnormalities (740-759)	718	363	-	-	-	-	363	355	-	-	-	-	355
N. Oral health (520-529)	1,606	10	13	357	266	82	728	10	19	368	328	154	878
N1. Dental caries (521.0)	146	10	13	27	11	6	68	10	19	27	13	11	79
N2. Periodontal disease (523)	36	-	-	15	2	-	18	-	-	15	2	2	18
N3. Edentulism (520)	1,424	-	-	315	253	75	642	-	-	326	314	142	781
III. Injuries (E800-999)	2,330	114	122	1,072	232	123	1,663	85	55	264	77	185	667
A. Unintentional (E800-949)	1,643	108	113	633	176	114	1,144	78	47	146	51	175	499
A1. Road traffic accidents (E810-819, 826-829)	177	3	21	72	6	1	103	2	10	51	8	2	74
A2. Poisoning (E850-869)	32	3	3	14	3	-	24	2	2	3	-	-	8
A3. Falls (E850-869)	531	18	27	157	51	75	328	12	10	24	12	145	203
A4. Fires (E890-899)	239	26	14	89	28	9	166	22	9	21	9	12	73
A5. Drowning (E910)	-	-	-	-	-	-	-	-	-	-	-	-	-
A6. Occupational (#)	25	-	-	15	6	-	21	-	-	2	1	-	3
B. Intentional (E950-969,990-999)	687	7	9	438	56	9	519	7	8	117	26	10	168
B1. Self-inflicted (E950-959)	687	7	9	438	56	9	519	7	8	117	26	10	168
B2. Homicide and violence (E960-969)	-	-	-	-	-	-	-	-	-	-	-	-	-
B3. War (E990-999)	-	-	-	-	-	-	-	-	-	-	-	-	-
Population (in millions)	346.2	13.8	27.3	76.3	27.0	21.0	165.3	13.1	26.4	75.0	30.0	36.4	180.9

Notes

A dash (-) symbol indicates less than 1,000 YLDs.

* ICD 9 codes for ischaemic heart disease are as follows: 410-414, 440.9, plus: at ages 45-59: 50% of 427.1, 427.4, 427.5, and 33% of 428; at ages 60+: 80% of 427.1, 427.4, 427.5 and 50% of 428.

+ ICD 9 codes for inflammatory cardiac diseases are as follows: 420, 421, 422, 425 plus: at ages 0-44: 50% of 428; at ages 45-59: 25% of 428; at ages 60+: 20% of 428.

* There are no established ICD 9 codes specific for occupational injuries.

Estimates have been based on reported occupational injuries and deaths tabulated by the International Labour Organisation.

Years lived with a disability (YLDs, in thousands): India

Disease or injury (ICD 9 code)	Both sexes all ages	Males						Females					
		0-4	5-14	15-44	45-59	60+	All ages	0-4	5-14	15-44	45-59	60+	All ages
All Causes	92,070	13,881	6,517	12,690	6,272	5,256	44,616	14,613	5,719	17,835	4,599	4,689	47,455
I. Communicable, maternal & perinatal (001-139,320-322,460-465,466,480-487,614-616, 630-676,760-779)	24,788	3,941	2,480	2,246	580	310	9,557	3,776	2,241	8,453	453	307	15,231
A. Infectious & parasitic dis. (001-139,320-322,614-616)	13,157	928	2,292	1,760	471	186	5,637	898	2,065	4,067	304	187	7,520
A1. Tuberculosis (010-018,137)	1,984	26	181	697	184	100	1,189	25	187	478	71	34	795
A2. STDs excluding HIV (090-099,614-616)	2,989	-	-	103	5	-	110	4	4	2,862	12	1	2,879
a. Syphilis (090-097)	85	-	-	48	3	-	51	-	-	31	2	-	34
b. Chlamydia	317	-	-	51	2	-	54	3	3	249	10	1	263
c. Gonorrhoea (098)	16	-	-	4	-	-	4	-	-	11	-	-	12
d. Pelvic inflammatory disease (614-616)	2,570	-	-	-	-	-	-	-	-	2,570	-	-	2,570
A3. HIV infection	189	-	-	115	4	-	120	-	-	67	-	-	69
A4. Diarrhoeal diseases (001,002,004,006-009)	823	35	158	200	22	10	426	33	148	183	22	10	396
a. Acute watery	637	24	123	158	18	7	330	23	115	144	17	7	307
b. Persistent	10	3	-	-	-	-	5	3	-	-	-	-	5
c. Dysentery	176	7	34	42	5	3	91	7	31	39	5	3	85
A5. Childhood cluster (032-33,037,045,050,055-56,138)	1,738	364	657	-	-	-	1,022	258	456	2	-	-	716
a. Pertussis (133)	199	47	55	-	-	-	102	44	52	-	-	-	97
b. Poliomyelitis (045,138)	1,484	306	587	-	-	-	893	204	387	-	-	-	591
c. Diphtheria (032)	35	8	9	-	-	-	17	6	10	2	-	-	18
d. Measles (055)	19	4	6	-	-	-	10	4	6	-	-	-	10
e. Tetanus (037)	1	-	-	-	-	-	-	-	-	-	-	-	-
A6. Meningitis (036,320-322)	61	29	1	-	1	1	31	28	1	-	-	-	30
A7. Hepatitis (070)	17	-	3	4	-	-	9	-	3	4	-	-	8
A8. Malaria (084)	165	5	20	49	8	4	86	4	18	45	8	4	79
A9. Tropical cluster (085,086,120,125)	1,023	13	139	310	150	19	632	9	93	126	135	28	391
a. African trypanosomiasis (086.3,086.4,086.5)	-	-	-	-	-	-	-	-	-	-	-	-	-
b. Chagas disease (086.0,086.1,086.2)	-	-	-	-	-	-	-	-	-	-	-	-	-
c. Schistosomiasis (120)	-	-	-	-	-	-	-	-	-	-	-	-	-
d. Leishmaniasis (085)	581	13	139	192	2	3	349	9	93	126	3	2	232
e. Lymphatic filariasis (125.0, 125.1)	442	-	-	118	149	17	284	-	-	-	131	27	158
f. Onchocerciasis (125.3)	-	-	-	-	-	-	-	-	-	-	-	-	-
A10. Leprosy (030)	521	33	209	14	3	-	259	31	216	13	1	-	262
A11. Trachoma (076)	309	-	-	49	33	30	112	-	-	89	15	93	197
A12. Intestinal helminths (126-129)	1,907	5	826	134	9	8	983	5	779	123	9	8	924
a. Ascaris (127.0)	1,101	5	562	-	-	-	567	5	529	-	-	-	534
b. Trichuris (127.3)	457	-	235	-	-	-	235	-	222	-	-	-	222
c. Hookworm (126)	349	-	30	134	9	8	181	-	28	123	9	8	168
B. Respiratory infections (381-382,460-466,480-487)	2,435	355	188	486	109	124	1,263	337	176	428	110	121	1,172
B1. Acute lower respiratory inf. (460-465)	1,275	26	120	313	87	112	658	25	113	286	84	108	616
B2. Acute upper respiratory inf. (466,480-487)	530	5	68	173	22	13	281	5	64	142	25	12	249
B3. Otitis media (381-382)	630	323	-	-	-	-	323	307	-	-	-	-	307
C. Maternal conditions (630-676)	3,998	-	-	-	-	-	-	-	-	3,958	40	-	3,998
C1. Haemorrhage (666,667)	217	-	-	-	-	-	-	-	-	215	2	-	217
C2. Sepsis (670)	1,986	-	-	-	-	-	-	-	-	1,967	20	-	1,986
C3. Eclampsia (642.4-642.6)	11	-	-	-	-	-	-	-	-	11	-	-	11
C4. Hypertension (642 minus 642.4-642.6)	-	-	-	-	-	-	-	-	-	-	-	-	-
C5. Obstructed labour (660)	1,558	-	-	-	-	-	-	-	-	1,543	15	-	1,558
C6. Abortion (630-639)	181	-	-	-	-	-	-	-	-	179	2	-	181
D. Perinatal causes (760-779)	5,199	2,657	-	-	-	-	2,657	2,542	-	-	-	-	2,542

C.J.L. Murray & A.D. Lopez

Years lived with a disability (YLDs, in thousands): India

Disease or injury (ICD 9 code)	Both sexes all ages	Males 0-4	Males 5-14	Males 15-44	Males 45-59	Males 60+	Males All ages	Females 0-4	Females 5-14	Females 15-44	Females 45-59	Females 60+	Females All ages
II. Noncommunicable (140-628,680-759) (minus 320-322, 460-465,466,480-487, 614-616)	57,225	8,467	2,448	8,482	5,336	4,806	29,538	9,176	2,175	8,121	3,954	4,261	27,687
A. Malignant neoplasms (140-208)	3,163	41	132	437	912	369	1,892	155	25	362	581	148	1,271
A1. Mouth and oropharynx (140-149)	560	–	–	78	201	120	400	–	–	39	89	31	161
A2. Oesophagus (150)	63	–	–	4	18	15	37	–	–	5	16	6	27
A3. Stomach (151)	65	–	–	9	21	14	45	–	–	5	11	5	20
A4. Colorectal (152,153,154)	75	–	–	16	16	13	45	–	–	7	14	9	30
A5. Liver (155)	8	–	–	–	3	2	6	–	–	–	2	–	3
A6. Pancreas (157)	6	–	–	–	2	2	4	–	–	–	1	1	2
A7. Lung (162)	43	–	–	4	18	13	35	–	–	–	4	3	7
A8. Melanoma and other skin (172-173)	2	–	–	–	–	1	1	–	–	–	1	–	1
A9. Breast (174)	61	–	–	–	–	–	–	–	–	18	33	10	61
A10. Cervix (180)	125	–	–	–	–	–	–	–	–	48	64	12	125
A11. Corpus uteri (179,181-182)	6	–	–	–	–	–	–	–	–	1	4	2	6
A12. Ovary (183)	13	–	–	–	–	–	–	–	–	6	5	2	13
A13. Prostate (185)	23	–	–	–	6	17	23	–	–	–	–	–	–
A14. Bladder (188)	4	–	–	1	–	–	1	–	–	–	1	–	3
A15. Lymphoma (200-202)	47	–	4	13	9	5	32	–	2	6	5	3	15
A16. Leukemia (204-208)	29	–	4	9	3	2	18	–	2	5	2	–	11
B. Other neoplasm (210-239)	325	–	–	45	89	30	164	–	–	42	90	29	161
C. Diabetes mellitus (250)	13,432	–	–	1,552	253	119	6,946	–	–	1,330	288	137	6,486
D. Nutritional/endocrine (240-285, minus 250)	3,723	4,520	502	502	3	–	1,909	4,315	416	1,330	–	–	1,814
D1. Protein-energy malnutrition (260-263)	1,284	1,909	18	18	195	–	659	1,814	17	22	3	–	625
D2. Iodine deficiency (243)	3,639	614	–	477	3	–	1,864	583	–	–	–	–	1,774
D3. Vitamin A deficiency (264)	3,420	1,864	477	–	–	–	1,623	1,774	446	1,042	188	83	1,797
D4. Anaemias (280-285)	13,771	439	1,037	3,824	1,045	865	7,210	517	861	3,858	643	683	6,561
E. Neuro-psychiatric (290-359, minus 320-322)	3,089	–	–	916	118	33	1,066	–	–	1,733	228	62	2,023
E1. Major affective disorder (296)	204	–	–	93	10	2	105	–	–	87	10	2	99
E2. Bipolar affective disorder (296)	1,996	–	–	904	36	14	904	–	–	1,092	25	9	1,092
E3. Psychoses (295, 291-294,297-299)	1,438	147	–	202	484	211	868	98	307	130	70	31	570
E4. Epilepsy (345)	1,780	–	–	861	215	524	1,557	–	–	122	217	519	224
E5. Alcohol dependence (303)	1,476	–	–	–	25	24	740	–	–	–	25	24	737
E6. Alzheimer & other dementias (330,331,333-336,290)	98	–	–	–	–	14	49	–	–	–	–	9	49
E7. Parkinson disease (332)	145	–	–	74	47	12	75	–	5	69	16	3	70
E8. Multiple sclerosis (340)	522	–	19	314	17	3	392	–	141	106	26	4	130
E9. Drug dependence (304)	838	–	88	207	623	422	327	–	9	321	570	378	511
E10. Post-traumatic stress disorder	–	–	5	115	165	48	–	–	–	93	118	49	–
F. Sense organ (360-389)	2,297	136	–	91	458	374	1,201	134	182	90	452	329	1,096
F1. Glaucoma-related blindness (365)	398	4	120	638	1,094	2,039	231	4	69	505	747	2,062	166
F2. Cataract-related blindness (366)	1,811	–	73	79	4	–	932	–	–	82	4	–	880
G. Cardiovascular diseases (390-459)	7,656	9	11	160	451	792	4,026	10	21	46	187	686	3,630
G1. Rheumatic heart disease (390-398)	320	6	6	96	166	506	160	10	16	121	192	622	920
G2. Ischaemic heart disease (*)	2,324	–	–	68	81	114	1,404	–	–	40	50	100	967
G3. Cerebrovascular disease (430-438)	1,755	624	313	384	189	291	788	837	229	397	182	175	216
G4. Inflammatory cardiac disease (+)	493	–	–	–	–	–	277	–	–	–	–	–	1,820
H. Chronic respiratory dis. (460-519, minus 460-466,480-487)	3,621	–	–	–	–	–	1,801	–	–	–	–	–	162
H1. Chronic obstructive lung dis. (490-492,495-496)	420	3	3	6	58	188	258	3	2	5	56	95	455
H2. Asthma (493)	962	32	180	228	52	15	506	25	144	210	57	19	962

Years lived with a disability (YLDs, in thousands): India

Disease or injury (ICD 9 code)	Both sexes all ages	Males						Females					
		0-4	5-14	15-44	45-59	60+	All ages	0-4	5-14	15-44	45-59	60+	All ages
I. Diseases of the digestive system (520-579)	4,821	792	133	651	435	275	2,287	1,385	228	450	279	193	2,534
I1. Peptic ulcer disease (531-533)	408	-	8	178	77	13	277	-	4	83	38	7	131
I2. Cirrhosis of the liver (571)	639	2	4	155	194	97	451	3	8	67	73	38	188
J. Genito-urinary (580-629)	1,900	83	150	137	431	189	990	58	154	256	228	215	911
J1. Nephritis/nephrosis (580-589)	843	16	131	96	93	90	426	11	138	126	74	69	417
J2. Benign prostatic hypertrophy (600)	329	-	-	-	295	34	329	-	-	-	-	-	-
K. Skin disease (680-709)		-	-	-	-	-	-	-	-	-	-	-	-
L. Musculo-skeletal system (710-739)	933	4	21	163	74	46	308	14	33	335	161	81	625
L1. Rheumatoid arthritis (714)	198	-	-	85	9	3	96	-	-	78	18	6	102
L2. Osteoarthritis (715)	432	-	-	57	52	14	122	-	-	166	116	28	310
M. Congenital abnormalities (740-759)	3,466	1,771	-	-	-	-	1,771	1,694	-	-	-	-	1,694
N. Oral health (520-529)	1,813	20	34	535	187	157	934	19	32	489	185	155	879
N1. Dental caries (521.0)	324	20	34	69	25	19	167	19	32	63	24	18	157
N2. Periodontal disease (523)	1,104	-	-	466	75	33	574	-	-	426	73	32	530
N3. Edentulism (520)	384	-	-	-	87	106	192	-	-	-	87	105	192
III. Injuries (E800-999)	10,058	1,474	1,588	1,962	357	141	5,521	1,661	1,303	1,261	191	120	4,536
A. Unintentional (E800-949)	9,346	1,435	1,554	1,546	326	135	4,996	1,652	1,299	1,112	176	112	4,351
A1. Road traffic accidents (E810-819, 826-829)	278	8	29	166	11	2	216	4	11	41	4	1	61
A2. Poisoning (E850-869)	7	1	2	-	-	-	4	-	2	-	-	-	2
A3. Falls (E850-869)	4,289	808	738	653	189	69	2,457	1,014	523	139	85	71	1,832
A4. Fires (E890-899)	954	314	78	28	10	7	437	180	227	102	3	4	517
A5. Drowning (E910)		-	-	-	-	-	-	-	-	-	-	-	-
A6. Occupational (#)	41	-	-	19	5	-	24	-	-	15	2	-	17
B. Intentional (E950-969,990-999)	711	39	33	416	31	6	526	9	4	149	15	9	186
B1. Self-inflicted (E950-959)		-	-	-	-	-	-	-	-	-	-	-	-
B2. Homicide and violence (E960-969)	609	30	27	367	26	5	456	-	-	132	13	9	153
B3. War (E990-999)	102	9	6	49	5	-	69	9	4	17	2	-	32
Population (in millions)	849.5	59.8	101.8	200.5	47.6	29.8	439.4	56.7	95.3	183.2	46.0	28.9	410.1

Notes

A dash (-) symbol indicates less than 1,000 YLDs.

* ICD 9 codes for ischaemic heart disease are as follows: 410-414, 440.9, plus: at ages 45-59: 50% of 427.1, 427.4, 427.5, and 33% of 428; at ages 60+: 80% of 427.1, 427.4, 427.5 and 50% of 428.

+ ICD 9 codes for inflammatory cardiac diseases are as follows: 420, 421, 422, 425 plus: at ages 0-44: 50% of 428; at ages 45-59: 25% of 428; at ages 60+: 20% of 428.

There are no established ICD 9 codes specific for occupational injuries.

Estimates have been based on reported occupational injuries and deaths tabulated by the International Labour Organisation.

Years lived with a disability (YLDs, in thousands): China

Disease or injury (ICD 9 code)	Both sexes all ages	Males 0-4	5-14	15-44	45-59	60+	All ages	Females 0-4	5-14	15-44	45-59	60+	All ages
All Causes	85,791	6,980	5,650	13,901	6,367	8,364	41,263	7,335	5,082	18,479	5,063	8,569	44,529
I. Communicable, maternal & perinatal (001-139,320-322,460-465,466,480-487,614-616, 630-676,760-779)	19,259	1,032	3,625	2,040	481	332	7,510	1,004	3,340	6,597	462	346	11,750
A. Infectious & parasitic dis. (001-139,320-322,614-616)	14,629	216	3,519	1,629	392	220	5,976	215	3,241	4,603	366	228	8,653
A1. Tuberculosis (010-018,137)	1,531	15	94	579	153	90	931	14	96	403	54	33	601
A2. STDs excluding HIV (090-099,614-616)	3,374	–	–	63	2	–	66	–	3	3,293	10	2	3,307
a. Syphilis (090-097)	358	–	–	52	2	–	55	–	2	290	10	1	303
b. Chlamydia	26	–	–	10	–	–	11	–	–	14	–	–	15
c. Gonorrhoea (098)	2,989	–	–	–	–	–	–	–	–	2,989	–	–	2,989
d. Pelvic inflammatory disease (614-616)	–	–	–	–	–	–	–	–	–	–	–	–	–
A3. HIV infection	3	–	–	2	–	–	3	–	–	–	–	–	–
A4. Diarrhoeal diseases (001,002,004,006-009)	2,089	36	151	715	120	60	1,081	35	141	663	106	63	1,008
a. Acute watery	1,626	25	117	563	94	42	842	24	109	522	84	44	784
b. Persistent	10	4	2	–	–	–	5	3	1	–	–	–	5
c. Dysentery	453	8	32	151	25	18	234	7	30	140	22	19	219
A5. Childhood cluster (032-33,037,045,050,055-56,138)	336	73	112	–	–	–	184	61	90	–	–	–	151
a. Pertussis (133)	125	29	35	–	–	–	64	28	33	–	–	–	61
b. Poliomyelitis (045,138)	198	41	74	–	–	–	114	31	53	–	–	–	84
c. Diphtheria (032)	2	–	–	–	–	–	–	–	–	–	–	–	–
d. Measles (055)	10	2	3	–	–	–	5	2	3	–	–	–	5
e. Tetanus (037)	5	3	–	–	–	–	3	2	–	–	–	–	2
A6. Meningitis (036,320-322)	65	31	1	–	–	–	33	30	1	–	–	–	32
A7. Hepatitis (070)	61	–	–	20	14	8	42	–	–	7	3	8	18
A8. Malaria (084)	6	–	–	–	–	–	3	–	–	–	–	–	3
A9. Tropical cluster (085,086,120,125)	493	16	177	64	39	7	304	10	105	38	28	8	189
a. African trypanosomiasis (086.3,086.4,086.5)	–	–	–	–	–	–	–	–	–	–	–	–	–
b. Chagas disease (086.0,086.1,086.2)	–	–	–	–	–	–	–	–	–	–	–	–	–
c. Schistosomiasis (120)	412	16	177	64	–	–	258	10	105	38	–	–	153
d. Leishmaniasis (085)	–	–	–	–	–	–	–	–	–	–	–	–	–
e. Lymphatic filariasis (125.0, 125.1)	81	–	–	–	38	7	46	–	–	–	28	8	36
f. Onchocerciasis (125.3)	–	–	–	–	–	–	–	–	–	–	–	–	–
A10. Leprosy (030)	4	–	–	–	2	–	2	–	–	–	2	–	2
A11. Trachoma (076)	472	–	–	39	36	40	115	–	–	110	149	98	357
A12. Intestinal helminths (126-129)	6,015	16	3,005	72	2	5	3,103	16	2,820	67	2	5	2,912
a. Ascaris (127.0)	3,701	16	1,895	–	–	–	1,911	16	1,774	–	–	–	1,789
b. Trichuris (127.3)	2,143	–	1,103	–	–	–	1,103	–	1,040	–	–	–	1,040
c. Hookworm (126)	172	–	7	72	5	5	89	–	7	67	4	5	83
B. Respiratory infections (381-382,460-466,480-487)	2,066	343	106	410	89	112	1,060	329	99	381	79	118	1,006
B1. Acute lower respiratory inf. (460-465)	931	14	60	245	62	97	478	14	56	227	55	102	453
B2. Acute upper respiratory inf. (466,480-487)	496	3	46	165	28	16	257	3	42	153	25	16	239
B3. Otitis media (381-382)	639	326	–	–	–	–	326	313	–	–	–	–	313
C. Maternal conditions (630-676)	1,631	–	–	–	–	–	–	–	–	1,613	17	–	1,631
C1. Haemorrhage (666,667)	217	–	–	–	–	–	–	–	–	214	2	–	217
C2. Sepsis (670)	580	–	–	–	–	–	–	–	–	574	6	–	580
C3. Eclampsia (642.4-642.6)	11	–	–	–	–	–	–	–	–	11	–	–	11
C4. Hypertension (642 minus 642.4-642.6)	–	–	–	–	–	–	–	–	–	–	–	–	–
C5. Obstructed labour (660)	769	–	–	–	–	–	–	–	–	761	8	–	769
C6. Abortion (630-639)	6	–	–	–	–	–	–	–	–	6	–	–	6
D. Perinatal causes (760-779)	933	473	–	–	–	–	473	460	–	–	–	–	460

Years lived with a disability (YLDs, in thousands): China

	Both sexes	Males						Females					
Disease or injury (ICD 9 code)	all ages	0-4	5-14	15-44	45-59	60+	All ages	0-4	5-14	15-44	45-59	60+	All ages
II. Noncommunicable (140-628,680-759) (minus 320-322,460-465,466,480-487, 614-616)	56,393	4,547	1,468	8,433	5,501	7,615	27,565	4,570	1,298	10,967	4,358	7,636	28,828
A. Malignant neoplasms (140-208)	2,792	46	106	492	488	370	1,500	81	73	396	407	335	1,292
A1. Mouth and oropharynx (140-149)	88	-	-	12	27	14	54	-	-	11	15	8	34
A2. Oesophagus (150)	110	-	-	5	31	35	70	-	-	3	19	17	39
A3. Stomach (151)	241	-	-	18	73	76	168	-	-	11	29	34	74
A4. Colorectal (152,153,154)	126	-	-	15	26	23	63	-	-	16	20	27	63
A5. Liver (155)	77	-	-	14	25	13	52	-	-	8	10	7	25
A6. Pancreas (157)	29	-	-	3	8	5	15	-	-	1	5	7	14
A7. Lung (162)	138	-	-	10	36	44	90	-	-	6	17	24	48
A8. Melanoma and other skin (172-173)	3	-	-	-	-	-	2	-	-	-	-	-	2
A9. Breast (174)	66							-	-	27	24	14	66
A10. Cervix (180)	69							-	-	13	32	23	69
A11. Corpus uteri (179,181-182)	16							-	-	2	10	4	16
A12. Ovary (183)	26							-	-	10	10	5	26
A13. Prostate (185)	4	-	-	-	1	3	4						
A14. Bladder (188)	44	-	-	6	14	12	32	-	-	1	4	7	12
A15. Lymphoma (200-202)	61	-	1	19	14	5	39	-	-	7	8	6	21
A16. Leukemia (204-208)	58	-	3	22	6	3	35	2	2	13	5	2	23
B. Other neoplasm (210-239)	165	-	-	22	44	16	82	-	-	21	42	19	82
C. Diabetes mellitus (250)	4,836	1,254	209	490	164	82	2,198	1,232	200	973	143	90	2,638
D. Nutritional/endocrine (240-285, minus 250)	695	352	-	-	-	-	352	343	-	-	-	-	343
D1. Protein-energy malnutrition (260-263)	944	388	26	55	6	1	476	384	24	53	6	2	469
D2. Iodine deficiency (243)	946	480	-	-	-	-	480	466	-	-	-	-	466
D3. Vitamin A deficiency (264)	946	-	-	-	-	-	466	-	-	-	-	-	480
D4. Anaemias (280-285)	2,083	28	170	416	148	70	832	27	158	862	131	73	1,252
E. Neuro-psychiatric (290-359, minus 320-322)	14,370	188	493	4,152	1,156	1,187	7,177	144	392	4,590	860	1,207	7,193
E1. Major affective disorder	4,843	-	-	1,414	182	53	1,648	-	-	2,747	334	114	3,195
E2. Bipolar affective disorder (296)	319	-	-	144	15	4	163	-	-	137	14	4	156
E3. Psychoses (295, 291-294,297-299)	1,515	-	-	829	-	-	829	-	-	685	-	-	685
E4. Epilepsy (345)	1,311	125	354	246	45	18	789	86	233	161	29	13	522
E5. Alcohol dependence (303)	1,780	-	-	861	484	211	1,557	-	-	122	70	31	224
E6. Alzheimer & other dementias (330,331,333-336,290)	2,445	-	-	-	333	837	1,170	-	-	-	318	957	1,275
E7. Parkinson disease (332)	159	-	-	-	39	39	78	-	-	-	37	44	81
E8. Multiple sclerosis (340)	228	-	-	116	1	-	117	-	-	110	1	-	111
E9. Drug dependence (304)	190	-	7	114	17	4	143	-	-	38	6	1	47
E10. Post-traumatic stress disorder	1,138	12	84	316	26	5	443	19	133	498	37	1	695
F. Sense organ (360-389)	1,433	36	-	41	339	226	642	28	9	81	467	207	792
F1. Glaucoma-related blindness (365)	473	-	-	-	94	46	140	-	-	32	232	69	333
F2. Cataract-related blindness (366)	756	10	-	25	213	151	399	-	-	-	209	112	357
G. Cardiovascular diseases (390-459)	9,078	175	68	693	1,159	2,645	4,740	104	44	734	900	2,556	4,338
G1. Rheumatic heart disease (390-398)	89	6	18	23	-	-	41	3	17	29	2	-	47
G2. Ischaemic heart disease (*)	976	-	6	130	132	282	556	-	2	62	60	293	420
G3. Cerebrovascular disease (430-438)	3,744	14	19	248	498	1,228	2,007	11	8	189	372	1,157	1,737
G4. Inflammatory cardiac disease (+)	81	-	-	8	11	23	44	-	-	8	7	20	37
H. Chronic respiratory dis. (460-519, minus 460-466,480-487)	8,546	375	429	1,010	575	2,093	4,482	484	342	867	436	1,934	4,064
H1. Chronic obstructive lung dis. (490-492,495-496)	3,758	2	-	32	284	1,718	2,036	2	-	33	188	1,500	1,723
H2. Asthma (493)	3,028	90	414	843	177	53	1,579	74	333	790	180	73	1,450

Years lived with a disability (YLDs, in thousands): China

Disease or injury (ICD 9 code)	Both sexes all ages	Males 0-4	Males 5-14	Males 15-44	Males 45-59	Males 60+	Males All ages	Females 0-4	Females 5-14	Females 15-44	Females 45-59	Females 60+	Females All ages
I. Diseases of the digestive system (520-579)	3,313	466	94	516	348	332	1,755	556	103	330	253	316	1,558
I1. Peptic ulcer disease (531-533)	238	-	3	100	44	8	155	-	1	54	23	5	83
I2. Cirrhosis of the liver (571)	808	3	4	200	185	159	552	1	4	61	85	105	256
J. Genito-urinary (580-629)	1,766	20	41	360	574	213	1,208	21	27	278	100	132	558
J1. Nephritis/nephrosis (580-589)	1,102	14	41	345	102	126	629	21	27	255	75	96	474
J2. Benign prostatic hypertrophy (600)	503	-	-	-	450	53	503	-	-	-	-	-	-
K. Skin disease (680-709)	-	-	-	-	-	-	-	-	-	-	-	-	-
L. Musculo-skeletal system (710-739)	5,027	-	16	402	506	282	1,206	8	95	2,458	609	650	3,821
L1. Rheumatoid arthritis (714)	754	-	-	124	83	23	230	-	86	264	126	49	524
L2. Osteoarthritis (715)	3,962	-	-	251	407	190	848	-	-	2,112	456	546	3,114
M. Congenital abnormalities (740-759)	3,750	1,912	-	-	-	-	1,912	1,838	-	-	-	-	1,838
N. Oral health (520-529)	1,297	75	13	254	147	163	653	72	12	236	139	185	644
N1. Dental caries (521.0)	231	75	13	17	9	4	118	72	12	16	8	4	113
N2. Periodontal disease (523)	512	-	-	237	19	9	265	-	-	220	17	9	247
N3. Edentulism (520)	554	-	-	-	119	150	269	-	-	-	114	171	285
III. Injuries (E800-999)	10,139	1,401	557	3,429	384	417	6,188	1,761	444	915	244	587	3,951
A. Unintentional (E800-949)	8,201	1,155	500	2,675	339	404	5,073	1,304	365	676	214	569	3,128
A1. Road traffic accidents (E810-819, 826-829)	1,394	27	94	899	55	12	1,087	13	37	230	19	9	307
A2. Poisoning (E850-869)	43	9	6	7	1	-	24	3	9	7	-	-	20
A3. Falls (E850-869)	3,371	420	184	764	158	284	1,808	640	156	164	125	479	1,563
A4. Fires (E890-899)	930	194	55	221	27	48	546	137	82	87	27	51	384
A5. Drowning (E910)	46	-	-	-	-	-	46	-	-	-	-	-	-
A6. Occupational (#)	37	-	-	30	7	-	37	-	-	-	-	-	-
B. Intentional (E950-969,990-999)	1,938	246	57	753	45	13	1,115	457	79	240	30	17	823
B1. Self-inflicted (E950-959)	-	-	-	-	-	-	-	-	-	-	-	-	-
B2. Homicide and violence (E960-969)	1,938	246	57	753	45	13	1,115	457	79	240	30	17	823
B3. War (E990-999)	-	-	-	-	-	-	-	-	-	-	-	-	-
Population (in millions)	1,133.7	60.2	97.0	306.3	72.7	49.0	585.2	57.9	90.4	284.1	64.4	51.7	548.5

Notes

A dash (-) symbol indicates less than 1,000 YLDs.

* ICD 9 codes for ischaemic heart disease are as follows: 410-414, 440.9, plus: at ages 45-59: 50% of 427.1, 427.4, 427.5, and 33% of 428; at ages 60+: 80% of 427.1, 427.4, 427.5 and 50% of 428.

+ ICD 9 codes for inflammatory cardiac diseases are as follows: 420, 421, 422, 425 plus: at ages 0-44: 50% of 428; at ages 45-59: 25% of 428; at ages 60+: 20% of 428.

There are no established ICD 9 codes specific for occupational injuries. Estimates have been based on reported occupational injuries and deaths tabulated by the International Labour Organisation.

Years lived with a disability (YLDs, in thousands): Other Asia and Islands

Disease or injury (ICD 9 code)	Both sexes all ages	Males						Females					
		0-4	5-14	15-44	45-59	60+	All ages	0-4	5-14	15-44	45-59	60+	All ages
All Causes	63,421	6,856	6,551	11,235	4,100	3,304	32,046	6,316	5,342	12,570	3,612	3,535	31,375
I. Communicable, maternal & perinatal (001-139,320-322,460-465,466,480-487,614-616, 630-676,760-779)	18,281	1,735	3,545	1,644	337	199	7,461	1,598	3,355	5,308	334	225	10,820
A. Infectious & parasitic dis. (001-139,320-322,614-616)	11,890	415	3,389	1,260	259	115	5,439	323	3,206	2,564	226	131	6,451
A1. Tuberculosis (010-018,137)	1,665	20	156	582	137	71	966	19	163	433	57	28	700
A2. STDs excluding HIV (090-099,614-616)	1,309	-	-	53	2	-	56	-	3	1,241	7	-	1,253
a. Syphilis (090-097)	2	-	-	-	1	-	1	-	-	-	-	-	-
b. Chlamydia (098)	271	-	-	41	1	-	43	-	-	217	7	-	228
c. Gonorrhoea (098)	28	-	-	11	-	-	11	-	-	16	-	-	17
d. Pelvic inflammatory disease (614-616)	1,008	-	-	-	-	-	-	-	-	1,008	-	-	1,008
A3. HIV infection	94	-	-	57	-	-	60	-	-	34	-	-	34
A4. Diarrhoeal diseases (001,002,004,006-009)	479	26	88	106	16	7	242	25	84	105	16	8	237
a. Acute watery	370	18	68	84	12	5	187	17	65	83	13	5	183
b. Persistent	7	3	-	-	-	-	3	2	-	-	-	-	3
c. Dysentery	103	5	19	23	3	2	52	5	18	22	3	2	51
A5. Childhood cluster (032-33,037,045,050,055-56,138)	522	107	190	-	-	-	297	82	142	-	-	-	225
a. Pertussis (133)	152	37	44	-	-	-	81	32	38	-	-	-	70
b. Poliomyelitis (045,138)	338	63	137	-	-	-	200	44	94	-	-	-	138
c. Diphtheria (032)	16	3	4	-	-	-	8	3	5	-	-	-	8
d. Measles (055)	16	3	5	-	-	-	8	3	5	-	-	-	8
e. Tetanus (037)													
A6. Meningitis (036,320-322)	43	20	3	-	-	-	22	20	3	-	-	-	21
A7. Hepatitis (070)	19	-	-	5	-	-	10	-	-	5	-	-	10
A8. Malaria (084)	352	16	41	100	15	6	177	15	39	99	15	7	175
A9. Tropical cluster (085,086,120,125)	238	4	56	77	37	1	176	2	28	6	21	5	62
a. African trypanosomiasis (086.3,086.4,086.5)													
b. Chagas disease (086.0,086.1,086.2)													
c. Schistosomiasis (120)	99	4	51	11	-	-	66	2	25	6	-	-	32
d. Leishmaniasis (085)	28	-	5	18	-	-	24	-	3	-	-	-	4
e. Lymphatic filariasis (125.0, 125.1)	111	-	-	48	37	1	86	-	-	-	20	5	25
f. Onchocerciasis (125.3)													
A10. Leprosy (030)	161	8	61	11	1	-	81	8	59	12	1	-	80
A11. Trachoma (076)	931	-	-	177	37	21	235	-	-	523	98	74	695
A12. Intestinal helminths (126-129)	5,508	10	2,698	82	5	4	2,799	9	2,609	81	5	5	2,710
a. Ascaris (127.0)	3,048	10	1,540	-	-	-	1,550	9	1,490	-	-	-	1,499
b. Trichuris (127.3)	2,239	-	1,138	-	-	-	1,138	-	1,101	-	-	-	1,101
c. Hookworm (126)	221	-	20	82	5	4	111	-	19	81	5	5	110
B. Respiratory infections (381-382,460-466,480-487)	1,904	260	156	383	78	84	962	249	149	367	84	95	943
B1. Acute lower respiratory inf. (460-465)	1,007	19	99	244	63	76	502	19	95	243	64	85	505
B2. Acute upper respiratory inf. (466,480-487)	434	4	56	139	16	9	223	4	54	124	19	10	210
B3. Otitis media (381-382)	464	237	-	-	-	-	237	227	-	-	-	-	227
C. Maternal conditions (630-676)	2,401							-	-	2,378	24	-	2,401
C1. Haemorrhage (666,667)	162							-	-	161	2	-	162
C2. Sepsis (670)	1,189							-	-	1,178	12	-	1,189
C3. Eclampsia (642.4-642.6)	8							-	-	8	-	-	8
C4. Hypertension (642 minus 642.4-642.6)													
C5. Obstructed labour (660)	821							-	-	813	8	-	821
C6. Abortion (630-639)	166							-	-	165	2	-	166
D. Perinatal causes (760-779)	2,085	1,060	-	-	-	-	1,060	1,025	-	-	-	-	1,025

Years lived with a disability (YLDs, in thousands): Other Asia and Islands

Disease or injury (ICD 9 code)	Both sexes all ages	Males						Females					
		0-4	5-14	15-44	45-59	60+	All ages	0-4	5-14	15-44	45-59	60+	All ages
II. Noncommunicable (140-628,680-759) (minus 320-322,460-465,466,480-487, 614-616)	37,631	4,362	2,052	6,138	3,394	2,949	18,896	4,093	1,616	6,676	3,184	3,166	18,735
A. Malignant neoplasms (140-208)	1,781	25	149	208	369	169	920	42	31	301	358	129	861
A1. Mouth and oropharynx (140-149)	74	–	–	12	20	13	46	–	–	9	11	7	28
A2. Oesophagus (150)	12	–	–	–	4	3	8	–	–	2	2	1	4
A3. Stomach (151)	40	–	–	5	11	8	25	–	–	4	6	5	15
A4. Colorectal (152,153,154)	50	–	–	6	9	9	24	–	–	7	11	8	26
A5. Liver (155)	25	–	–	4	8	4	17	–	–	2	4	2	8
A6. Pancreas (157)	4	–	–	–	–	–	2	–	–	–	–	–	1
A7. Lung (162)	47	–	–	4	15	13	33	–	–	2	6	6	15
A8. Melanoma and other skin (172-173)	2	–	–	–	–	–	–	–	–	–	–	–	1
A9. Breast (174)	49	–	–	–	–	–	–	–	–	20	22	7	49
A10. Cervix (180)	66	–	–	–	–	–	–	–	–	29	31	7	66
A11. Corpus uteri (179,181-182)	5	–	–	–	–	–	–	–	–	1	3	1	5
A12. Ovary (183)	15	–	–	–	–	–	–	–	–	8	5	2	15
A13. Prostate (185)	6	–	–	–	1	5	6	–	–	–	–	–	–
A14. Bladder (188)	12	–	–	1	4	4	9	–	–	–	1	–	3
A15. Lymphoma (200-202)	29	–	1	7	5	3	17	–	2	6	4	2	12
A16. Leukemia (204-208)	22	–	2	6	2	–	11	–	2	6	2	–	10
*B. Other neoplasm (210-239)													
C. Diabetes mellitus (250)	247	–	–	35	65	17	117	–	–	36	74	20	129
D. Nutritional/endocrine (240-285, minus 250)	6,168	1,946	175	754	98	45	3,019	1,890	177	902	118	60	3,148
D1. Protein-energy malnutrition (260-263)	262	133	–	–	–	–	133	129	–	–	–	–	129
D2. Iodine deficiency (243)	1,205	560	18	24	2	–	605	556	17	24	2	–	600
D3. Vitamin A deficiency (264)	2,349	1,190	–	–	–	–	1,190	1,159	–	–	–	–	1,159
D4. Anaemias (280-285)	1,806	21	196	452	67	28	765	20	187	734	69	31	1,042
E. Neuro-psychiatric (290-359, minus 320-322)	10,023	253	936	2,766	725	597	5,278	199	657	2,806	512	571	4,745
E1. Major affective disorder	2,629	–	–	745	87	23	855	–	–	1,540	184	51	1,774
E2. Bipolar affective disorder (296)	171	–	–	76	7	2	85	–	–	77	8	2	87
E3. Psychoses (295, 291-294,297-299)	821	–	–	437	–	–	437	–	–	384	–	–	384
E4. Epilepsy (345)	1,168	109	385	162	26	9	691	74	260	115	20	7	477
E5. Alcohol dependence (303)	1,027	–	–	497	279	122	898	–	–	71	40	18	129
E6. Alzheimer & other dementias (330,331,333-336,290)	1,125	–	–	–	160	364	524	–	–	–	175	426	601
E7. Parkinson disease (332)	75	–	–	–	18	17	35	–	–	–	20	20	40
E8. Multiple sclerosis (340)	123	–	–	60	–	–	61	–	–	61	–	–	62
E9. Drug dependence (304)	854	–	32	514	76	19	642	14	8	173	26	5	212
E10. Post-traumatic stress disorder	697	8	73	166	12	2	262	21	118	280	20	3	436
F. Sense organ (360-389)	1,296	23	5	43	307	189	566	21	6	65	460	178	730
F1. Glaucoma-related blindness (365)	420	–	–	16	90	22	128	–	–	35	225	32	292
F2. Cataract-related blindness (366)	839	11	–	25	217	166	419	12	–	28	234	146	420
G. Cardiovascular diseases (390-459)	5,596	128	141	545	701	1,261	2,776	82	196	521	580	1,440	2,820
G1. Rheumatic heart disease (390-398)	178	1	39	48	–	–	91	1	38	45	2	–	87
G2. Ischaemic heart disease (*)	1,840	–	1	174	310	556	1,042	–	–	71	163	564	799
G3. Cerebrovascular disease (430-438)	1,060	6	13	57	106	275	457	3	22	88	135	354	602
G4. Inflammatory cardiac disease (+)	133	2	5	21	17	24	69	3	8	17	13	24	64
H. Chronic respiratory dis. (460-519, minus 460-466,480-487)	2,135	280	327	290	100	154	1,152	227	240	305	98	113	983
H1. Chronic obstructive lung dis. (490-492,495-496)	226	1	2	3	26	100	132	–	1	3	27	62	94
H2. Asthma (493)	1,041	49	219	228	40	10	546	44	191	211	38	11	495

Years lived with a disability (YLDs, in thousands): Other Asia and Islands

Disease or injury (ICD 9 code)	Both sexes all ages	Males						Females					
		0-4	5-14	15-44	45-59	60+	All ages	0-4	5-14	15-44	45-59	60+	All ages
I. Diseases of the digestive system (520-579)	2,251	356	132	310	230	163	1,191	346	155	271	158	130	1,059
I1. Peptic ulcer disease (531-533)	125	-	2	52	21	3	79	-	1	30	12	2	46
I2. Cirrhosis of the liver (571)	394	-	4	97	112	57	271	-	5	46	45	26	124
J. Genito-urinary (580-629)	1,188	38	145	77	297	114	671	16	106	151	124	121	517
J1. Nephritis/nephrosis (580-589)	588	8	127	57	51	59	302	4	94	82	50	55	285
J2. Benign prostatic hypertrophy (600)	247	-	-	-	225	21	247	-	-	-	-	-	-
K. Skin disease (680-709)	-	-	-	-	-	-	-	-	-	-	-	-	-
L. Musculo-skeletal system (710-739)	2,606	2	20	637	294	82	1,036	4	23	844	481	217	1,570
L1. Rheumatoid arthritis (714)	249	-	-	67	22	6	95	-	-	66	70	18	155
L2. Osteoarthritis (715)	2,172	-	-	561	265	59	886	-	-	721	394	171	1,286
M. Congenital abnormalities (740-759)	2,548	1,295	-	-	-	-	1,295	1,253	-	-	-	-	1,253
N. Oral health (520-529)	1,777	15	21	471	205	156	868	14	20	473	220	181	909
N1. Dental caries (521.0)	255	15	21	55	26	11	128	14	20	55	27	12	128
N2. Periodontal disease (523)	518	-	-	208	36	15	258	-	-	206	37	17	260
N3. Edentulism (520)	1,004	-	-	209	143	130	482	-	-	212	157	153	521
III. Injuries (E800-999)	7,509	759	954	3,454	368	155	5,690	625	371	586	94	144	1,820
A. Unintentional (E800-949)	5,273	662	830	1,961	276	142	3,871	523	307	361	74	137	1,402
A1. Road traffic accidents (E810-819, 826-829)	790	20	81	474	26	5	605	9	33	129	11	4	185
A2. Poisoning (E850-869)	11	2	3	3	-	-	8	1	2	-	-	-	3
A3. Falls (E850-869)	2,383	304	404	791	160	99	1,758	255	139	82	37	113	625
A4. Fires (E890-899)	489	127	70	93	14	6	310	87	52	30	5	5	179
A5. Drowning (E910)	-	-	-	-	-	-	-	-	-	-	-	-	-
A6. Occupational (#)	28	-	-	20	4	-	24	-	-	3	-	-	4
B. Intentional (E950-969,990-999)	2,237	97	124	1,493	92	12	1,819	102	64	225	20	7	418
B1. Self-inflicted (E950-959)	-	-	-	-	-	-	-	-	-	-	-	-	-
B2. Homicide and violence (E960-969)	2,103	86	116	1,429	86	12	1,729	90	58	201	18	7	374
B3. War (E990-999)	133	11	8	64	6	-	90	12	5	24	2	-	44
Population (in millions)	682.5	43.8	84.0	160.8	34.1	20.2	343.0	42.0	80.2	159.6	35.1	22.7	339.6

Notes

A dash (-) symbol indicates less than 1,000 YLDs.

* ICD 9 codes for ischaemic heart disease are as follows: 410-414, 440.9, plus: at ages 45-59: 50% of 427.1, 427.4, 427.5, and 33% of 428; at ages 60+: 80% of 427.1, 427.4, 427.5 and 50% of 428.

+ ICD 9 codes for inflammatory cardiac diseases are as follows: 420, 421, 422, 425 plus: at ages 0-44: 50% of 428; at ages 45-59: 25% of 428; at ages 60+: 20% of 428.

There are no established ICD 9 codes specific for occupational injuries.
Estimates have been based on reported occupational injuries and deaths tabulated by the International Labour Organisation.

Years lived with a disability (YLDs, in thousands): Sub-Saharan Africa

Disease or injury (ICD 9 code)	Both sexes all ages	Males						Females					
		0-4	5-14	15-44	45-59	60+	All ages	0-4	5-14	15-44	45-59	60+	All ages
All Causes	67,427	12,052	6,313	10,415	2,815	1,716	33,311	11,411	4,776	13,167	2,610	2,153	34,117
I. Communicable, maternal & perinatal (001-139,320-322,460-465,466,480-487,614-616, 630-676,760-779)	29,456	5,332	3,613	2,838	352	158	12,293	4,998	2,768	8,823	387	187	17,163
A. Infectious & parasitic dis. (001-139,320-322,614-616)	19,276	2,737	3,445	2,563	294	100	9,140	2,469	2,601	4,664	285	117	10,136
A1. Tuberculosis (010-018,137)	1,303	19	145	432	95	43	734	19	159	332	41	18	569
A2. STDs excluding HIV (090-099,614-616)	2,788	-	3	390	19	2	414	-	11	2,341	19	2	2,374
a. Syphilis (090-097)	556	-	2	292	16	2	313	-	1	225	14	2	243
b. Chlamydia	180	-	-	27	1	-	28	-	2	144	5	-	152
c. Gonorrhoea (098)	189	-	1	71	1	-	73	-	7	108	-	-	116
d. Pelvic inflammatory disease (614-616)	1,863	-	-	-	-	-	-	-	-	1,863	-	-	1,863
A3. HIV infection	1,073	24	-	488	12	1	526	24	5	508	10	7	548
A4. Diarrhoeal diseases (001,002,004,006-009)	662	41	164	104	14	6	329	40	163	107	16	5	333
a. Acute watery	509	28	128	82	11	4	253	28	127	84	12	5	256
b. Persistent	11	4	2	-	-	-	6	4	2	-	-	-	6
c. Dysentery	141	9	35	22	3	2	70	8	35	23	3	2	71
A5. Childhood cluster (032-33,037,045,050,055-56,138)	1,501	329	523	-	-	-	853	252	396	-	-	-	648
a. Pertussis (133)	276	67	79	-	-	-	146	60	71	-	-	-	130
b. Poliomyelitis (045,138)	1,187	254	434	-	-	-	688	185	314	-	-	-	499
c. Diphtheria (032)	10	2	3	-	-	-	5	2	3	-	-	-	5
d. Measles (055)	26	5	8	-	-	-	13	5	8	-	-	-	13
e. Tetanus (037)	1	-	-	-	-	-	-	-	-	-	-	-	-
A6. Meningitis (036,320-322)	109	23	16	15	-	-	54	23	16	16	-	-	54
A7. Hepatitis (070)	14	-	2	3	-	-	7	-	2	3	-	-	7
A8. Malaria (084)	4,708	1,576	350	391	29	10	2,356	1,561	347	400	32	13	2,353
A9. Tropical cluster (085,086,120,125)	3,627	151	1,607	486	88	21	2,354	80	850	248	77	19	1,273
a. African trypanosomiasis (086.3,086.4,086.5)	147	2	22	42	12	2	79	3	19	38	7	-	68
b. Chagas disease (086.0,086.1,086.2)	-	-	-	-	-	-	-	-	-	-	-	-	-
c. Schistosomiasis (120)	2,887	148	1,510	255	2	-	1,916	75	762	133	1	-	971
d. Leishmaniasis (085)	228	2	72	45	2	-	119	2	68	39	-	-	109
e. Lymphatic filariasis (125.0, 125.1)	184	-	-	90	40	3	132	-	-	37	45	7	51
f. Onchocerciasis (125.3)	182	-	3	55	34	16	108	-	2	37	23	11	74
A10. Leprosy (030)	209	8	91	7	-	-	107	8	85	7	-	-	102
A11. Trachoma (076)	901	-	-	168	29	14	210	-	-	558	79	53	690
A12. Intestinal helminths (126-129)	806	2	364	32	2	1	401	2	367	33	2	2	405
a. Ascaris (127.0)	419	2	207	-	-	-	209	2	209	-	-	-	211
b. Trichuris (127.3)	290	-	144	-	-	-	144	-	145	-	-	-	145
c. Hookworm (126)	97	-	13	32	2	1	48	-	13	33	2	-	49
B. Respiratory infections (381-382,460-466,480-487)	1,714	289	168	275	58	57	847	286	167	281	63	70	867
B1. Acute lower respiratory inf. (460-465)	909	28	109	208	49	52	445	27	109	213	53	63	464
B2. Acute upper respiratory inf. (466,480-487)	293	4	59	67	9	6	145	4	59	69	10	7	148
B3. Otitis media (381-382)	511	257	-	-	-	-	257	254	-	-	-	-	254
C. Maternal conditions (630-676)	3,916	-	-	-	-	-	-	-	-	3,878	38	-	3,916
C1. Haemorrhage (666,667)	207	-	-	-	-	-	-	-	-	205	2	-	207
C2. Sepsis (670)	1,938	-	-	-	-	-	-	-	-	1,919	19	-	1,938
C3. Eclampsia (642.4-642.6)	10	-	-	-	-	-	-	-	-	10	-	-	10
C4. Hypertension (642 minus 642.4-642.6)	-	-	-	-	-	-	-	-	-	-	-	-	-
C5. Obstructed labour (660)	1,489	-	-	-	-	-	-	-	-	1,474	15	-	1,489
C6. Abortion (630-639)	176	-	-	-	-	-	-	-	-	174	2	-	176
D. Perinatal causes (760-779)	4,550	2,306	-	-	-	-	2,306	2,244	-	-	-	-	2,244

Years lived with a disability (YLDs, in thousands): Sub-Saharan Africa

Disease or injury (ICD 9 code)	Both sexes all ages	Males 0-4	5-14	15-44	45-59	60+	All ages	Females 0-4	5-14	15-44	45-59	60+	All ages
II. Noncommunicable (140-628,680-759) (minus 320-322,460-465,466,480-487, 614-616)	28,595	5,375	1,700	3,870	2,151	1,515	14,612	5,095	1,410	3,527	2,113	1,839	13,983
A. Malignant neoplasms (140-208)	712	21	101	59	154	32	368	45	6	110	153	29	344
A1. Mouth and oropharynx (140-149)	28	–	–	5	8	4	17	–	–	3	2	3	10
A2. Oesophagus (150)	14	–	–	2	5	3	10	–	–	2	2	1	4
A3. Stomach (151)	22	–	–	3	6	3	12	–	–	2	5	3	10
A4. Colorectal (152,153,154)	16	–	–	2	3	2	8	–	–	2	3	3	8
A5. Liver (155)	22	–	–	6	6	2	14	–	–	3	3	1	8
A6. Pancreas (157)	3	–	–	–	–	–	1	–	–	–	–	–	2
A7. Lung (162)	9	–	–	1	3	2	6	–	–	–	1	–	2
A8. Melanoma and other skin (172-173)	7	–	–	–	2	–	3	–	–	–	2	2	4
A9. Breast (174)	24	–	–	–	–	–	–	–	–	8	12	5	24
A10. Cervix (180)	47	–	–	–	–	–	–	–	–	16	23	8	47
A11. Corpus uteri (179,181-182)	5	–	–	–	–	–	–	–	–	1	3	1	5
A12. Ovary (183)	8	–	–	–	–	–	–	–	–	3	4	1	8
A13. Prostate (185)	14	–	–	–	4	10	14	–	–	–	–	–	–
A14. Bladder (188)	12	–	–	1	4	3	8	–	–	1	2	–	4
A15. Lymphoma (200-202)	30	–	4	7	5	2	18	–	2	5	3	1	11
A16. Leukemia (204-208)	6	–	–	1	–	–	3	–	–	1	1	–	3
B. Other neoplasm (210-239)	6	–	–	–	–	–	3	–	–	–	–	–	3
C. Diabetes mellitus (250)	75	–	–	14	15	6	35	–	–	16	14	10	40
D. Nutritional/endocrine (240-285, minus 250)	5,717	2,377	43	445	37	15	2,918	2,397	53	246	75	29	2,800
D1. Protein-energy malnutrition (260-263)	1,243	620	–	–	–	–	620	623	–	–	–	–	623
D2. Iodine deficiency (243)	1,523	705	20	20	1	–	746	734	20	21	2	–	777
D3. Vitamin A deficiency (264)	1,991	990	–	–	–	–	990	1,001	–	–	–	–	1,001
D4. Anaemias (280-285)	433	9	80	76	17	6	188	9	79	130	19	8	245
E. Neuro-psychiatric (290-359, minus 320-322)	7,617	288	811	2,109	689	420	4,316	229	596	1,824	341	312	3,301
E1. Major affective disorder	1,647	–	–	464	50	11	525	–	–	986	109	27	1,122
E2. Bipolar affective disorder (296)	107	–	–	47	4	–	52	–	–	49	5	1	55
E3. Psychoses (295, 291-294,297-299)	518	–	–	272	–	–	272	–	–	246	–	–	246
E4. Epilepsy (345)	911	102	307	100	15	5	529	74	218	74	12	4	382
E5. Alcohol dependence (303)	1,643	–	–	795	447	195	1,437	–	–	113	65	28	206
E6. Alzheimer & other dementias (330,331,333-336,290)	602	–	–	–	91	181	272	–	–	–	104	226	330
E7. Parkinson disease (332)	42	–	–	–	11	8	19	–	–	–	12	10	22
E8. Multiple sclerosis (340)	77	–	–	37	–	–	38	–	–	39	–	–	40
E9. Drug dependence (304)	332	–	12	200	30	8	250	–	3	67	10	2	83
E10. Post-traumatic stress disorder	505	–	61	107	7	1	186	–	103	186	13	2	319
F. Sense organ (360-389)	1,345	36	5	44	296	193	574	29	6	54	409	274	771
F1. Glaucoma-related blindness (365)	171	–	–	–	3	1	4	–	–	1	89	78	168
F2. Cataract-related blindness (366)	1,130	18	–	43	293	193	547	16	–	53	319	195	583
G. Cardiovascular diseases (390-459)	3,107	86	61	292	398	598	1,435	47	96	251	420	857	1,671
G1. Rheumatic heart disease (390-398)	77	–	–	36	35	–	39	–	8	16	35	–	37
G2. Ischaemic heart disease (*)	340	–	–	17	129	88	187	–	–	12	35	106	153
G3. Cerebrovascular disease (430-438)	1,145	6	16	65	89	263	471	3	16	79	176	400	675
G4. Inflammatory cardiac disease (+)	236	4	6	40	35	39	124	3	11	24	29	46	113
H. Chronic respiratory dis. (460-519, minus 460-466,480-487)	2,532	416	364	274	89	83	1,225	308	296	289	312	102	1,307
H1. Chronic obstructive lung dis. (490-492,495-496)	144	2	3	3	20	50	78	1	1	2	28	33	66
H2. Asthma (493)	1,390	57	247	213	42	10	568	57	247	223	250	46	822

Years lived with a disability (YLDs, in thousands): Sub-Saharan Africa

Disease or injury (ICD 9 code)	Both sexes all ages	Males						Females					
		0-4	5-14	15-44	45-59	60+	All ages	0-4	5-14	15-44	45-59	60+	All ages
I. Diseases of the digestive system (520-579)	2,275	532	120	285	147	77	1,162	495	153	243	148	76	1,114
I1. Peptic ulcer disease (531-533)	61	-	1	21	8	1	32	-	1	19	8	1	29
I2. Cirrhosis of the liver (571)	315	1	3	101	74	26	207	1	5	46	40	15	108
J. Genito-urinary (580-629)	1,054	56	152	69	265	53	594	22	111	102	135	90	460
J1. Nephritis/nephrosis (580-589)	484	12	134	48	38	26	258	5	100	52	41	27	226
J2. Benign prostatic hypertrophy (600)	217	-	-	-	210	7	217	-	-	-	-	-	-
K. Skin disease (680-709)													
L. Musculo-skeletal system (710-739)	516	2	19	79	35	15	150	5	65	187	75	33	365
L1. Rheumatoid arthritis (714)	152	-	-	41	8	2	50	-	43	51	6	1	101
L2. Osteoarthritis (715)	223	-	-	30	22	5	57	-	-	99	54	12	166
M. Congenital abnormalities (740-759)	3,033	1,538	-	-	-	-	1,538	1,496	-	-	-	-	1,496
N. Oral health (520-529)	597	23	24	204	21	22	293	22	23	209	23	27	305
N1. Dental caries (521.0)	139	23	24	17	5	2	69	22	23	17	5	2	70
N2. Periodontal disease (523)	417	-	-	188	16	2	206	-	-	192	18	2	212
N3. Edentulism (520)	41	-	-	-	-	18	18	-	-	-	-	23	23
III. Injuries (E800-999)	9,376	1,345	999	3,707	312	43	6,406	1,317	598	818	111	127	2,971
A. Unintentional (E800-949)	5,322	990	740	1,643	176	35	3,584	934	417	218	53	117	1,738
A1. Road traffic accidents (E810-819, 826-829)	398	9	31	218	19	2	278	7	28	79	7	-	121
A2. Poisoning (E850-869)	10	2	2	2	-	-	6	2	2	-	-	-	4
A3. Falls (E850-869)	2,522	455	378	745	99	20	1,697	452	195	53	26	98	825
A4. Fires (E890-899)	607	190	66	88	8	1	353	155	73	18	3	4	254
A5. Drowning (E910)													
A6. Occupational (#)	18	-	-	14	2	-	16	-	-	2	-	-	2
B. Intentional (E950-969,990-999)	4,054	355	259	2,063	136	8	2,822	383	181	600	58	10	1,232
B1. Self-inflicted (E950-959)													
B2. Homicide and violence (E960-969)	1,421	90	76	947	38	3	1,153	112	57	86	9	4	268
B3. War (E990-999)	2,633	265	183	1,116	99	6	1,669	271	124	514	49	6	964
Population (in millions)	510.3	47.5	70.3	103.8	20.3	10.5	252.3	47.0	69.8	106.3	22.1	12.7	258.0

Notes

A dash (-) symbol indicates less than 1,000 YLDs.

* ICD 9 codes for ischaemic heart disease are as follows: 410-414, 440.9, plus: at ages 45-59: 50% of 427.1, 427.4, 427.5, and 33% of 428; at ages 60+: 80% of 427.1, 427.4, 427.5 and 50% of 428.

+ ICD 9 codes for inflammatory cardiac diseases are as follows: 420, 421, 422, 425 plus: at ages 0-44: 50% of 428; at ages 45-59: 25% of 428; at ages 60+: 20% of 428.

There are no established ICD 9 codes specific for occupational injuries.

Estimates have been based on reported occupational injuries and deaths tabulated by the International Labour Organisation.

Years lived with a disability (YLDs, in thousands): Latin America and the Caribbean

Disease or injury (ICD 9 code)	Both sexes all ages	Males 0-4	5-14	15-44	45-59	60+	All ages	Females 0-4	5-14	15-44	45-59	60+	All ages
All Causes	44,887	4,785	3,835	9,500	2,979	2,370	23,468	4,299	3,413	9,091	2,216	2,400	21,418
I. Communicable, maternal & perinatal (001-139,320-322,460-465,466,480-487,614-616, 630-676,760-779)	12,569	1,784	2,017	1,027	135	77	5,039	1,580	1,843	3,889	136	82	7,531
A. Infectious & parasitic dis. (001-139,320-322,614-616)	9,158	893	1,954	876	100	44	3,867	721	1,782	2,657	88	43	5,291
A1. Tuberculosis (010-018,137)	306	2	26	108	26	14	177	2	28	81	11	6	128
A2. STDs excluding HIV (090-099,614-616)	2,068	–	–	59	3	–	63	–	2	1,996	6	–	2,005
a. Syphilis (090-097)	46	–	–	25	2	–	27	–	–	18	1	–	19
b. Chlamydia	177	–	–	27	–	–	27	–	2	141	5	–	149
c. Gonorrhoea (098)	20	–	–	8	–	–	8	–	–	11	1	–	12
d. Pelvic inflammatory disease (614-616)	1,825	–	–	–	–	–	–	–	–	1,825	–	–	1,825
A3. HIV infection	237	–	–	175	6	–	182	–	–	51	2	2	55
A4. Diarrhoeal diseases (001,002,004,006-009)	616	140	44	103	16	7	310	116	63	103	13	12	307
a. Acute watery	477	110	31	82	12	5	240	100	33	81	10	13	237
b. Persistent	8	2	1	1	–	–	4	2	1	1	–	–	4
c. Dysentery	132	28	12	20	4	2	66	14	29	21	1	1	66
A5. Childhood cluster (032-33,037,045,050,055-56,138)	355	75	95	22	3	3	201	58	61	30	3	2	154
a. Pertussis (133)	124	60	5	2	–	–	67	54	2	1	–	–	57
b. Poliomyelitis (045,138)	216	13	85	26	2	1	127	2	56	28	2	1	89
c. Diphtheria (032)	4	1	1	–	–	–	2	1	1	–	–	–	2
d. Measles (055)	10	1	4	–	–	–	5	1	4	–	–	–	5
e. Tetanus (037)	–	–	–	–	–	–	–	–	–	–	–	–	–
A6. Meningitis (036,320-322)	27	12	1	1	–	–	14	11	1	1	–	–	14
A7. Hepatitis (070)	10	–	1	2	1	–	4	1	1	3	1	–	6
A8. Malaria (084)	97	2	11	29	4	2	48	2	11	29	5	2	49
A9. Tropical cluster (085,086,120,125)	2,571	653	457	297	30	7	1,444	523	344	231	24	5	1,127
a. African trypanosomiasis (086.3,086.4,086.5)	–	–	–	–	–	–	–	–	–	–	–	–	–
b. Chagas disease (086.0,086.1,086.2)	2,376	644	376	257	25	6	1,308	518	305	217	23	5	1,068
c. Schistosomiasis (120)	146	6	74	17	1	–	98	3	37	7	1	–	48
d. Leishmaniasis (085)	46	3	7	22	3	–	35	2	2	7	–	–	11
e. Lymphatic filariasis (125.0, 125.1)	3	–	–	3	–	–	3	–	–	–	–	–	–
f. Onchocerciasis (125.3)	–	–	–	–	–	–	–	–	–	–	–	–	–
A10. Leprosy (030)	59	3	4	20	2	1	30	3	5	18	2	1	29
A11. Trachoma (076)	110	–	5	28	4	1	38	–	12	52	5	3	72
A12. Intestinal helminths (126-129)	2,295	5	1,096	48	5	1	1,155	5	1,081	48	5	1	1,140
a. Ascaris (127.0)	1,299	5	649	–	–	–	654	5	640	–	–	–	645
b. Trichuris (127.3)	868	–	437	–	–	–	437	–	431	–	–	–	431
c. Hookworm (126)	128	–	10	48	5	1	64	–	10	48	5	1	64
B. Respiratory infections (381-382,460-466,480-487)	890	164	62	151	35	33	445	158	60	151	37	39	445
B1. Acute lower respiratory inf. (460-465)	357	7	32	83	25	28	176	6	32	83	26	33	181
B2. Acute upper respiratory inf. (466,480-487)	229	2	30	68	10	5	114	2	29	67	11	6	115
B3. Otitis media (381-382)	305	155	–	–	–	–	155	150	–	–	–	–	150
C. Maternal conditions (630-676)	1,092	–	–	–	–	–	–	–	10	1,082	–	–	1,092
C1. Haemorrhage (666,667)	109	–	–	–	–	–	–	–	1	107	1	–	109
C2. Sepsis (670)	336	–	–	–	–	–	–	–	1	332	3	–	336
C3. Eclampsia (642.4-642.6)	5	–	–	–	–	–	–	–	–	5	–	–	5
C4. Hypertension (642 minus 642.4-642.6)	–	–	–	–	–	–	–	–	–	–	–	–	–
C5. Obstructed labour (660)	500	–	–	–	–	–	–	–	5	495	–	–	500
C6. Abortion (630-639)	118	–	–	–	–	–	–	–	–	117	1	–	118
D. Perinatal causes (760-779)	1,428	727	–	–	–	–	727	701	–	–	–	–	701

Years lived with a disability (YLDs, in thousands): Latin America and the Caribbean

Disease or injury (ICD 9 code)	Both sexes all ages	Males						Females					
		0-4	5-14	15-44	45-59	60+	All ages	0-4	5-14	15-44	45-59	60+	All ages
II. *Noncommunicable* (140-322,460-465,466,480-487, 614-616)	24,159	2,610	1,070	4,144	2,509	2,149	12,481	2,412	1,077	4,048	1,949	2,193	11,678
A. Malignant neoplasms (140-208)	1,531	26	79	227	230	215	778	25	72	182	228	246	753
A1. Mouth and oropharynx (140-149)	31	-	-	4	12	8	24	-	-	1	3	3	7
A2. Oesophagus (150)	12	-	-	-	4	4	9	-	-	1	1	1	3
A3. Stomach (151)	55	-	-	4	14	17	36	-	-	3	7	9	19
A4. Colorectal (152,153,154)	51	-	-	4	9	11	25	-	-	4	10	12	26
A5. Liver (155)	4	-	-	-	1	-	2	-	-	-	-	-	2
A6. Pancreas (157)	6	-	-	-	1	2	3	-	-	1	1	1	2
A7. Lung (162)	38	-	-	3	12	13	28	-	-	1	4	5	10
A8. Melanoma and other skin (172-173)	6	-	-	-	1	-	3	-	-	1	1	-	3
A9. Breast (174)	60	-	-	-	-	-	-	-	-	19	27	14	60
A10. Cervix (180)	53	-	-	-	-	-	-	-	-	21	23	9	53
A11. Corpus uteri (179,181-182)	10	-	-	-	-	-	-	-	-	5	5	3	10
A12. Ovary (183)	9	-	-	-	-	-	-	-	-	3	4	2	9
A13. Prostate (185)	27	-	-	-	4	22	27	-	-	-	-	-	-
A14. Bladder (188)	17	-	-	-	5	8	13	-	-	1	1	2	4
A15. Lymphoma (200-202)	34	1	-	8	6	4	20	-	-	5	4	4	14
A16. Leukemia (204-208)	18	2	-	5	2	2	10	1	-	3	1	1	8
B. Other neoplasm (210-239)													
C. Diabetes mellitus (250)	227	-	-	39	53	16	108	-	-	40	59	20	119
D. Nutritional/endocrine (240-285, minus 250)	3,100	1,083	142	167	43	33	1,469	1,050	136	349	51	45	1,631
D1. Protein-energy malnutrition (260-263)	239	121	-	-	-	-	121	118	-	-	-	-	118
D2. Iodine deficiency (243)	496	232	7	10	-	-	249	229	7	10	1	-	247
D3. Vitamin A deficiency (264)	1,263	639	-	-	-	-	639	624	-	-	-	-	624
D4. Anaemias (280-285)	696	10	108	102	25	11	256	9	105	287	26	13	440
E. Neuro-psychiatric (290-359, minus 320-322)	7,223	149	348	2,322	709	518	4,045	120	282	1,927	401	449	3,178
E1. Major affective disorder	1,749	-	-	490	60	17	567	-	-	1,016	127	39	1,182
E2. Bipolar affective disorder (296)	114	-	-	50	5	1	56	-	-	51	6	2	58
E3. Psychoses (295, 291-294,297-299)	541	-	-	287	-	-	287	-	-	253	-	-	253
E4. Epilepsy (345)	593	58	188	83	13	5	347	40	131	60	11	4	246
E5. Alcohol dependence (303)	1,438	-	-	696	391	170	1,257	-	-	99	57	25	181
E6. Alzheimer & other dementias (330,331,333-336,290)	832	-	-	-	110	269	379	-	-	-	121	332	453
E7. Parkinson disease (332)	108	-	-	-	25	25	50	-	-	-	28	30	58
E8. Multiple sclerosis (340)	81	-	-	40	-	-	40	-	-	40	-	-	41
E9. Drug dependence (304)	806	-	30	486	72	18	606	-	8	163	25	5	200
E10. Post-traumatic stress disorder	450	6	45	108	8	1	168	9	75	182	13	3	282
F. Sense organ (360-389)	604	15	2	26	150	98	291	12	2	27	176	96	313
F1. Glaucoma-related blindness (365)	60	-	-	-	11	10	21	-	-	-	25	14	39
F2. Cataract-related blindness (366)	511	2	-	23	139	88	252	2	-	25	151	81	259
G. Cardiovascular diseases (390-459)	2,852	37	47	292	367	665	1,409	5	34	329	320	743	1,443
G1. Rheumatic heart disease (390-398)	159	-	34	45	2	-	82	-	34	40	2	-	77
G2. Ischaemic heart disease (*)	700	-	1	81	118	195	396	-	-	41	67	195	304
G3. Cerebrovascular disease (430-438)	784	2	7	93	102	169	373	2	6	104	101	199	411
G4. Inflammatory cardiac disease (+)	121	1	3	22	16	24	66	2	2	16	11	24	55
H. Chronic respiratory dis. (460-519, minus 460-466,480-487)	1,803	266	177	273	93	140	949	233	170	266	80	106	854
H1. Chronic obstructive lung dis. (490-492,495-496)	196	1	-	3	23	90	117	-	-	2	17	58	78
H2. Asthma (493)	875	30	157	197	40	12	436	29	153	200	43	14	440

Years lived with a disability (YLDs, in thousands): Latin America and the Caribbean

Disease or injury (ICD 9 code)	Both sexes all ages	Males 0-4	Males 5-14	Males 15-44	Males 45-59	Males 60+	Males All ages	Females 0-4	Females 5-14	Females 15-44	Females 45-59	Females 60+	Females All ages
I. Diseases of the digestive system (520-579)	1,378	96	50	316	203	145	810	69	40	204	124	131	568
I1. Peptic ulcer disease (531-533)	82	-	1	34	14	2	51	-	-	20	8	2	30
I2. Cirrhosis of the liver (571)	288	-	1	91	80	43	215	-	1	24	26	21	73
J. Genito-urinary (580-629)	761	28	23	77	241	88	457	21	23	129	55	76	304
J1. Nephritis/nephrosis (580-589)	380	11	17	63	35	57	182	8	18	77	38	56	198
J2. Benign prostatic hypertrophy (600)	206	-	-	-	196	10	206	-	-	-	-	-	-
K. Skin disease (680-709)													
L. Musculo-skeletal system (710-739)	2,057	3	86	268	337	152	846	2	195	457	369	187	1,211
L1. Rheumatoid arthritis (714)	710	-	-	76	137	39	253	-	107	238	87	25	458
L2. Osteoarthritis (715)	1,214	-	80	179	194	104	557	-	80	167	265	144	657
M. Congenital abnormalities (740-759)	1,745	888	-	-	-	-	888	857	-	-	-	-	857
N. Oral health (520-529)	870	18	114	137	82	76	426	17	111	137	87	92	444
N1. Dental caries (521.0)	436	18	114	84	3	2	220	17	111	83	4	2	216
N2. Periodontal disease (523)	285	-	-	54	59	26	139	-	-	54	62	31	146
N3. Edentulism (520)	149	-	-	-	20	48	68	-	-	-	22	59	81
III. Injuries (E800-999)	8,158	392	748	4,329	335	144	5,948	307	493	1,154	131	125	2,210
A. Unintentional (E800-949)	6,002	351	674	2,683	213	126	4,046	272	463	986	114	121	1,956
A1. Road traffic accidents (E810-819, 826-829)	3,908	97	411	1,924	99	22	2,553	72	352	838	83	9	1,354
A2. Poisoning (E850-869)	3	-	-	-	-	-	2	-	-	-	-	-	1
A3. Falls (E850-869)	782	66	110	267	48	67	558	46	45	31	10	92	224
A4. Fires (E890-899)	309	69	31	66	10	6	182	64	24	29	5	5	127
A5. Drowning (E910)	21	-	-	14	3	-	17	-	-	2	-	-	3
A6. Occupational (#)	-	-	-	-	-	-	-	-	-	-	-	-	-
B. Intentional (E950-969,990-999)	2,156	41	75	1,646	122	19	1,902	35	30	167	16	5	254
B1. Self-inflicted (E950-959)													
B2. Homicide and violence (E960-969)	1,948	23	63	1,545	112	18	1,760	17	22	133	13	4	188
B3. War (E990-999)	207	18	12	101	10	-	142	18	8	34	4	-	65
Population (in millions)	444.3	28.7	52.1	104.3	22.2	14.2	221.6	27.7	50.7	104.1	23.4	16.8	222.7

Notes

A dash (-) symbol indicates less than 1,000 YLDs.

* ICD 9 codes for ischaemic heart disease are as follows: 410-414, 440.9, plus: at ages 45-59: 50% of 427.1, 427.4, 427.5, and 33% of 428; at ages 60+: 80% of 427.1, 427.4, 427.5 and 50% of 428.

+ ICD 9 codes for inflammatory cardiac diseases are as follows: 420, 421, 422, 425 plus: at ages 0-44: 50% of 428; at ages 45-59: 25% of 428; at ages 60+: 20% of 428.

There are no established ICD 9 codes specific for occupational injuries.

Estimates have been based on reported occupational injuries and deaths tabulated by the International Labour Organisation.

Years lived with a disability (YLDs, in thousands): Middle Eastern Crescent

Disease or injury (ICD 9 code)	Both sexes all ages	Males						Females					
		0-4	5-14	15-44	45-59	60 +	All ages	0-4	5-14	15-44	45-59	60 +	All ages
All Causes	45,808	6,944	3,852	6,949	2,609	2,141	22,495	6,532	3,221	9,313	2,015	2,232	23,313
I. Communicable, maternal & perinatal (001-139,320-322,460-465,466,480-487,614-616, 630-676,760-779)	11,168	1,966	903	711	150	99	3,828	1,913	825	4,276	189	138	7,340
A. Infectious & parasitic dis. (001-139,320-322,614-616)	4,664	562	813	518	106	45	2,045	561	740	1,124	116	78	2,618
A1. Tuberculosis (010-018,137)	418	4	42	149	33	17	245	4	44	105	13	7	173
A2. STDs excluding HIV (090-099,614-616)	657	–	–	28	–	–	30	–	1	624	2	–	627
a. Syphilis (090-097)	83	–	–	24	–	–	25	–	–	55	2	–	57
b. Chlamydia	10	–	–	4	–	–	4	–	–	5	–	–	6
c. Gonorrhoea (098)	564	–	–	–	–	–	–	–	–	564	–	–	564
d. Pelvic inflammatory disease (614-616)	26	–	–	–	–	–	–	–	–	4	–	–	4
A3. HIV infection (090-099,614-616)	394	29	80	77	11	5	202	28	76	72	11	6	193
A4. Diarrhoeal diseases (001,002,004,006-009)	303	20	62	60	9	3	155	19	59	57	9	4	148
a. Acute watery	7	3	–	–	–	–	4	3	–	–	–	–	4
b. Persistent	84	6	17	16	2	1	43	6	16	15	2	2	41
c. Dysentery	212	11	45	44	7	2	108	10	43	42	7	2	103
A5. Childhood cluster (032-33,037,045,050,055-56,138)	702	150	248	–	–	–	398	117	187	–	–	–	304
a. Pertussis (133)	134	31	37	–	–	–	68	30	36	–	–	–	66
b. Poliomyelitis (045,138)	550	115	206	–	–	–	321	83	146	–	–	–	229
c. Diphtheria (032)	5	1	1	–	–	–	2	1	1	–	–	–	2
d. Measles (055)	12	3	3	–	–	–	6	3	3	–	–	–	6
e. Tetanus (037)	38	18	–	–	–	–	19	18	–	–	–	–	19
A6. Meningitis (036,320-322)	10	2	2	1	–	–	5	2	2	1	–	–	5
A7. Hepatitis (070)	68	2	9	20	3	1	35	2	8	19	3	1	33
A8. Malaria (084)	275	14	98	38	11	1	162	9	64	24	11	6	114
A9. Tropical cluster (085,086,120,125)	276	–	–	–	–	–	161	–	–	–	–	–	115
a. African trypanosomiasis (086.3,086.4,086.5)	–	–	–	–	–	–	–	–	–	–	–	–	–
b. Chagas disease (086.0,086.1,086.2)	–	–	–	–	–	–	–	–	–	–	–	–	–
c. Schistosomiasis (120)	64	–	33	7	3	–	43	–	16	3	2	–	21
d. Leishmaniasis (085)	188	11	64	31	3	–	109	3	48	21	7	–	79
e. Lymphatic filariasis (125.0, 125.1)	24	–	–	–	–	–	9	–	–	–	–	–	15
f. Onchocerciasis (125.3)	–	–	–	–	–	–	–	–	–	–	–	–	–
A10. Leprosy (030)	32	–	14	–	–	–	16	–	13	–	3	–	16
A11. Trachoma (076)	576	–	–	161	39	18	218	–	–	235	69	54	358
A12. Intestinal helminths (126-129)	527	–	250	16	–	–	269	–	239	15	–	–	258
a. Ascaris (127.0)	483	–	245	2	–	–	247	–	235	2	–	–	237
b. Trichuris (127.3)	44	–	5	14	–	–	22	–	4	15	–	–	21
c. Hookworm (126)	–	–	–	–	–	–	–	–	–	–	–	–	–
B. Respiratory infections (381-382,460-466,480-487)	1,225	242	89	193	44	53	621	233	85	181	44	61	604
B1. Acute lower respiratory inf. (460-465)	713	–	77	173	41	51	361	–	73	163	41	58	353
B2. Acute upper respiratory inf. (466,480-487)	74	18	12	20	3	2	38	18	11	19	3	3	36
B3. Otitis media (381-382)	438	223	–	–	–	–	223	215	–	–	–	–	215
C. Maternal conditions (630-676)	3,000	–	–	–	–	–	–	–	–	2,970	30	–	3,000
C1. Haemorrhage (666,667)	169	–	–	–	–	–	–	–	–	167	2	–	169
C2. Sepsis (670)	1,507	–	–	–	–	–	–	–	–	1,492	15	–	1,507
C3. Eclampsia (642.4-642.6)	8	–	–	–	–	–	–	–	–	8	–	–	8
C4. Hypertension (642 minus 642.4-642.6)	1,211	–	–	–	–	–	–	–	–	1,199	12	–	1,211
C5. Obstructed labour (660)	77	–	–	–	–	–	–	–	–	76	–	–	77
C6. Abortion (630-639)	28	–	–	–	–	–	–	–	–	28	–	–	28
D. Perinatal causes (760-779)	2,280	1,162	–	–	–	–	1,162	1,118	–	–	–	–	1,118

Years lived with a disability (YLDs, in thousands): Middle Eastern Crescent

Disease or injury (ICD 9 code)	Both sexes all ages	Males 0-4	Males 5-14	Males 15-44	Males 45-59	Males 60+	Males All ages	Females 0-4	Females 5-14	Females 15-44	Females 45-59	Females 60+	Females All ages
II. Noncommunicable (140-628,680-759) (minus 320-322,460-465,466,480-487, 614-616)	26,574	4,068	1,630	3,582	2,202	1,941	13,423	3,840	1,415	4,150	1,743	2,003	13,151
A. Malignant neoplasms (140-208)	1,189	31	107	142	253	116	649	49	23	151	208	109	540
A1. Mouth and oropharynx (140-149)	49	–	–	8	15	9	32	–	–	4	7	5	16
A2. Oesophagus (150)	13	–	–	1	3	3	7	–	–	3	2	–	5
A3. Stomach (151)	29	–	–	3	8	6	18	–	–	2	4	4	11
A4. Colorectal (152,153,154)	34	–	–	4	7	6	17	–	–	4	7	6	17
A5. Liver (155)	5	–	–	–	1	1	3	–	–	1	1	–	2
A6. Pancreas (157)	4	–	–	–	1	1	2	–	–	1	1	–	2
A7. Lung (162)	38	–	–	4	16	11	31	–	–	1	3	3	7
A8. Melanoma and other skin (172-173)	3	–	–	–	–	–	2	–	–	–	–	–	2
A9. Breast (174)	50	–	–	–	–	–	–	–	–	18	21	11	50
A10. Cervix (180)	26	–	–	–	–	–	–	–	–	9	12	4	26
A11. Corpus uteri (179,181-182)	6	–	–	–	–	–	–	–	–	–	3	2	6
A12. Ovary (183)	9	–	–	–	–	–	–	–	–	4	4	2	9
A13. Prostate (185)	6	–	–	–	2	4	6	–	–	–	–	–	–
A14. Bladder (188)	22	–	–	–	7	10	17	–	–	–	2	3	5
A15. Lymphoma (200-202)	31	–	2	9	5	4	20	–	–	5	3	3	11
A16. Leukemia (204-208)	14	–	1	4	2	1	8	–	–	2	1	2	5
B. Other neoplasm (210-239)													
C. Diabetes mellitus (250)	259	–	–	50	67	14	131	–	–	45	68	16	129
D. Nutritional/endocrine (240-285, minus 250)	3,555	1,116	203	332	55	24	1,730	1,073	192	471	58	30	1,824
D1. Protein-energy malnutrition (260-263)	394	200	–	–	–	–	200	194	–	–	–	–	194
D2. Iodine deficiency (243)	1,279	607	16	19	2	–	645	598	15	19	2	–	634
D3. Vitamin A deficiency (264)	423	214	–	–	–	–	214	209	–	–	–	–	209
D4. Anaemias (280-285)	1,112	21	208	190	34	15	468	20	197	376	34	17	644
E. Neuro-psychiatric (290-359, minus 320-322)	6,469	262	657	1,629	375	354	3,277	215	489	1,808	308	372	3,192
E1. Major affective disorder	1,791	–	–	530	58	16	603	–	–	1,036	117	34	1,188
E2. Bipolar affective disorder (296)	118	–	–	54	5	1	60	–	–	52	5	1	58
E3. Psychoses (295, 291-294,297-299)	570	–	–	311	–	–	311	–	–	259	–	–	259
E4. Epilepsy (345)	906	101	301	115	17	6	541	69	201	77	13	5	366
E5. Alcohol dependence (303)	411	–	–	199	112	48	359	–	–	28	16	8	52
E6. Alzheimer & other dementias (330,331,333-336,290)	752	–	–	–	106	245	351	–	–	–	111	290	401
E7. Parkinson disease (332)	50	–	–	–	12	11	23	–	–	–	13	13	26
E8. Multiple sclerosis (340)	85	–	–	43	–	–	43	–	–	41	1	–	42
E9. Drug dependence (304)	332	–	12	200	30	8	250	–	3	67	10	3	83
E10. Post-traumatic stress disorder	499	8	57	117	8	2	192	13	91	188	13	2	308
F. Sense organ (360-389)	667	19	3	28	194	126	370	18	4	20	165	90	297
F1. Glaucoma-related blindness (365)	38	–	–	–	20	5	25	–	–	–	10	3	13
F2. Cataract-related blindness (366)	597	7	–	27	173	121	329	7	–	19	154	88	268
G. Cardiovascular diseases (390-459)	4,103	228	118	323	510	887	2,066	157	161	345	382	992	2,036
G1. Rheumatic heart disease (390-398)	120	1	28	31	1	2	63	–	27	27	1	2	57
G2. Ischaemic heart disease (*)	659	–	–	51	121	209	381	–	–	21	51	206	278
G3. Cerebrovascular disease (430-438)	968	10	12	43	106	266	437	6	19	66	108	332	531
G4. Inflammatory cardiac disease (+)	119	4	5	16	17	22	64	4	7	13	10	22	56
H. Chronic respiratory dis. (460-519, minus 460-466,480-487)	1,996	406	286	231	85	124	1,133	348	166	194	67	90	864
H1. Chronic obstructive lung dis. (490-492,495-496)	180	2	2	1	23	80	108	1	1	2	18	50	72
H2. Asthma (493)	828	56	208	191	31	8	494	34	127	137	27	9	334

Years lived with a disability (YLDs, in thousands): Middle Eastern Crescent

Disease or injury (ICD 9 code)	Both sexes all ages	Males						Females					
		0-4	5-14	15-44	45-59	60 +	All ages	0-4	5-14	15-44	45-59	60 +	All ages
I. Diseases of the digestive system (520-579)	2,038	493	95	174	156	107	1,025	543	117	163	104	86	1,013
I1. Peptic ulcer disease (531-533)	86	-	2	37	14	2	55	-	-	20	8	2	31
I2. Cirrhosis of the liver (571)	171	-	3	36	46	25	110	-	4	24	20	12	61
J. Genito-urinary (580-629)	958	48	96	71	279	88	582	25	79	109	83	80	376
J1. Nephritis/nephrosis (580-589)	374	9	79	32	31	38	189	5	66	50	29	35	185
J2. Benign prostatic hypertrophy (600)	217	-	-	-	204	13	217	-	-	-	-	-	-
K. Skin disease (680-709)	-	-	-	-	-	-	-	-	-	-	-	-	-
L. Musculo-skeletal system (710-739)	787	2	14	85	35	19	156	6	135	351	98	42	631
L1. Rheumatoid arthritis (714)	406	-	-	43	4	1	48	-	118	208	25	7	358
L2. Osteoarthritis (715)	256	-	-	37	26	7	70	-	-	108	61	16	186
M. Congenital abnormalities (740-759)	2,787	1,420	-	-	-	-	1,420	1,367	-	-	-	-	1,367
N. Oral health (520-529)	1,755	42	49	517	193	78	880	41	47	494	202	92	875
N1. Dental caries (521,0)	335	42	49	52	17	10	170	41	47	49	17	11	165
N2. Periodontal disease (523)	303	-	-	147	6	3	155	-	-	138	6	3	147
N3. Edentulism (520)	1,117	-	-	318	170	66	554	-	-	306	179	78	563
III. Injuries (E800-999)	8,065	911	1,319	2,656	257	101	5,244	780	981	888	83	90	2,821
A. Unintentional (E800-949)	5,497	683	1,140	1,388	151	91	3,453	541	874	501	45	83	2,044
A1. Road traffic accidents (E810-819, 826-829)	2,847	123	680	834	42	14	1,692	66	692	379	13	4	1,154
A2. Poisoning (E850-869)	12	3	3	2	-	-	8	2	2	-	-	-	4
A3. Falls (E850-869)	1,142	209	202	242	60	54	767	188	74	33	16	66	375
A4. Fires (E890-899)	400	131	53	43	8	4	238	97	42	18	3	3	162
A5. Drowning (E910)	-	-	-	-	-	-	-	-	-	-	-	-	-
A6. Occupational (#)	14	-	-	9	2	-	11	-	-	2	-	-	2
B. Intentional (E950-969,990-999)	2,568	228	179	1,268	106	9	1,790	239	107	387	37	8	778
B1. Self-inflicted (E950-959)	-	-	-	-	-	-	-	-	-	-	-	-	-
B2. Homicide and violence (E960-969)	872	66	65	486	36	5	660	75	35	90	8	3	212
B3. War (E990-999)	1,696	162	114	781	70	4	1,130	164	72	296	29	4	566
Population (in millions)	503.1	41.2	65.3	113.9	22.3	13.7	256.4	39.7	62.0	107.2	22.3	15.5	246.7

Notes

A dash (-) symbol indicates less than 1,000 YLDs.

* ICD 9 codes for ischaemic heart disease are as follows: 410-414, 440.9, plus: at ages 45-59: 50% of 427.1, 427.4, 427.5, and 33% of 428; at ages 60+: 80% of 427.1, 427.4, 427.5 and 50% of 428.

+ ICD 9 codes for inflammatory cardiac diseases are as follows: 420, 421, 422, 425 plus: at ages 0-44: 50% of 428; at ages 45-59: 25% of 428; at ages 60+: 20% of 428.

There are no established ICD 9 codes specific for occupational injuries.

Estimates have been based on reported occupational injuries and deaths tabulated by the International Labour Organisation.

Years lived with a disability (YLDs, in thousands): World

Disease or injury (ICD 9 code)	Both sexes all ages	Males 0-4	Males 5-14	Males 15-44	Males 45-59	Males 60+	Males All ages	Females 0-4	Females 5-14	Females 15-44	Females 45-59	Females 60+	Females All ages
All Causes	467,493	53,903	33,979	76,736	33,109	33,922	231,649	52,697	28,543	92,430	25,847	36,327	235,844
I. Communicable, maternal & perinatal (001-139,320-322,460-465,466,480-487,614-616, 630-676,760-779)	121,601	16,342	16,302	11,142	2,188	1,321	47,295	15,393	14,484	40,816	2,124	1,489	74,306
A. Infectious & parasitic dis. (001-139,320-322,614-616)	75,635	5,819	15,472	8,893	1,667	754	32,605	5,244	13,690	21,834	1,427	834	43,029
A1. Tuberculosis (010-018,137)	7,274	88	647	2,569	638	343	4,285	84	679	1,842	252	132	2,989
A2. STDs excluding HIV (090-099,614-616)	15,248	–	6	719	32	3	762	1	25	14,388	62	9	14,486
a. Syphilis (090-097)	690	–	2	367	21	2	393	–	1	275	18	2	297
b. Chlamydia	1,512	–	3	240	8	–	252	–	14	1,195	44	7	1,260
c. Gonorrhoea (098)	301	–	2	113	2	–	117	–	10	173	–	–	184
d. Pelvic inflammatory disease (614-616)	12,744	–	–	–	–	–	–	–	–	12,744	–	–	12,744
A3. HIV infection	1,797	26	2	992	33	3	1,056	26	6	693	15	1	741
A4. Diarrhoeal diseases (001,002,004,006-009)	5,367	203	822	1,388	219	108	2,740	196	788	1,314	208	121	2,627
a. Acute watery	4,175	142	641	1,097	174	77	2,132	137	614	1,039	165	87	2,043
b. Persistent	69	20	9	4	1	–	35	19	9	4	1	1	34
c. Dysentery	1,123	41	172	286	44	30	573	40	165	270	42	33	550
A5. Childhood cluster (032-33,037,045,050,055-56,138)	5,271	1,126	1,888	–	–	–	3,015	854	1,398	4	–	–	2,256
a. Pertussis (133)	1,115	267	315	–	–	–	582	244	289	–	–	–	533
b. Poliomyelitis (045,138)	3,974	821	1,522	–	–	–	2,343	575	1,055	–	–	–	1,631
c. Diphtheria (032)	78	17	20	–	–	–	37	13	24	4	–	–	41
d. Measles (055)	100	21	30	–	–	–	51	20	29	–	–	–	49
e. Tetanus (037)	4	–	–	–	–	–	2	–	–	–	–	–	2
A6. Meningitis (036,320-322)	358	139	21	18	–	–	180	138	21	18	–	–	178
A7. Hepatitis (070)	154	1	12	41	21	15	90	1	12	28	8	15	64
A8. Malaria (084)	5,397	1,600	430	591	60	24	2,705	1,584	424	594	63	27	2,692
A9. Tropical cluster (085,086,120,125)	8,229	851	2,535	1,272	356	57	5,072	631	1,483	675	295	73	3,157
a. African trypanosomiasis (086.3,086.4,086.5)	147	2	22	42	12	2	79	3	19	38	7	–	68
b. Chagas disease (086.0,086.1,086.2)	2,376	644	376	257	25	6	1,308	518	305	217	23	6	1,068
c. Schistosomiasis (120)	3,607	177	1,846	354	3	–	2,381	91	944	189	–	–	1,226
d. Leishmaniasis (085)	1,073	29	289	309	6	4	637	20	214	193	6	3	436
e. Lymphatic filariasis (125.0, 125.1)	845	–	–	255	276	28	560	–	–	–	233	52	285
f. Onchocerciasis (125.3)	182	–	3	55	34	16	108	–	2	37	23	11	74
A10. Leprosy (030)	987	51	401	33	10	1	496	50	400	32	9	–	491
A11. Trachoma (076)	3,298	–	–	621	180	127	927	–	–	1,567	422	381	2,370
A12. Intestinal helminths (126-129)	17,059	40	8,239	384	25	22	8,710	38	7,896	366	25	23	8,349
a. Ascaris (127.0)	10,052	40	5,098	–	–	–	5,137	38	4,876	–	–	–	4,915
b. Trichuris (127.3)	5,996	–	3,057	–	–	–	3,057	–	2,939	–	–	–	2,939
c. Hookworm (126)	1,010	–	84	384	25	22	515	–	81	366	25	23	495
B. Respiratory infections (381-382,460-466,480-487)	11,978	1,872	830	2,249	521	567	6,039	1,802	794	2,159	529	655	5,939
B1. Acute lower respiratory inf. (460-465)	5,894	114	519	1,449	391	482	2,955	110	496	1,392	391	549	2,939
B2. Acute upper respiratory inf. (466,480-487)	2,673	20	311	800	130	85	1,346	19	298	766	137	105	1,326
B3. Otitis media (381-382)	3,411	1,738	–	–	–	–	1,738	1,673	–	–	–	–	1,673
C. Maternal conditions (630-676)	16,991	–	–	–	–	–	–	–	–	16,822	168	–	16,991
C1. Haemorrhage (666,667)	1,214	–	–	–	–	–	–	–	–	1,202	12	–	1,214
C2. Sepsis (670)	7,886	–	–	–	–	–	–	–	–	7,807	78	–	7,886
C3. Eclampsia (642.4-642.6)	59	–	–	–	–	–	–	–	–	58	–	–	59
C4. Hypertension (642 minus 642.4-642.6)	6,781	–	–	–	–	–	–	–	–	6,714	67	–	6,781
C5. Obstructed labour (660)	749	–	–	–	–	–	–	–	–	742	7	–	749
C6. Abortion (630-639)	–	–	–	–	–	–	–	–	–	–	–	–	–
D. Perinatal causes (760-779)	16,997	8,651	–	–	–	–	8,651	8,347	–	–	–	–	8,347

Years lived with a disability (YLDs, in thousands): World

Disease or injury (ICD 9 code)	Both sexes all ages	Males 0-4	5-14	15-44	45-59	60+	All ages	Females 0-4	5-14	15-44	45-59	60+	All ages
II. Noncommunicable (140-628,680-759) (minus 320-322,460-465,466,480-487, 614-616)	286,899	31,040	11,253	43,712	28,463	31,117	145,586	30,673	9,737	45,323	22,711	32,870	141,314
A. Malignant neoplasms (140-208)	18,604	230	745	2,205	3,812	3,218	10,210	428	290	2,058	3,021	2,598	8,394
A1. Mouth and oropharynx (140-149)	995	-	2	136	343	213	695	-	2	73	146	78	300
A2. Oesophagus (150)	274	-	-	15	80	82	177	-	-	11	49	36	97
A3. Stomach (151)	775	-	-	57	206	230	492	-	-	39	101	143	283
A4. Colorectal (152,153,154)	1,170	-	-	76	204	312	593	-	-	66	183	328	578
A5. Liver (155)	187	-	-	29	56	35	120	-	-	15	27	24	67
A6. Pancreas (157)	108	-	-	7	24	28	58	-	-	3	16	30	50
A7. Lung (162)	779	-	-	41	235	286	561	-	-	20	82	115	218
A8. Melanoma and other skin (172-173)	87	-	-	13	15	10	38	-	-	19	17	13	49
A9. Breast (174)	738							-	-	200	321	217	738
A10. Cervix (180)	480							-	-	174	221	85	480
A11. Corpus uteri (179,181-182)	133							-	-	14	69	49	133
A12. Ovary (183)	155							-	1	48	65	41	155
A13. Prostate (185)	397	-	-	3	61	334	397						
A14. Bladder (188)	355	-	-	23	93	153	270	-	-	7	26	52	86
A15. Lymphoma (200-202)	465	4	15	103	85	67	274	2	8	61	58	63	191
A16. Leukemia (204-208)	219	3	16	57	27	25	127	2	11	37	21	20	92
B. Other neoplasm (210-239)													
C. Diabetes mellitus (250)	1,976	-	-	291	483	169	943	-	-	289	523	221	1,033
D. Nutritional/endocrine (240-285, minus 250)	38,389	12,514	1,402	3,878	749	425	18,968	12,162	1,292	4,607	833	526	19,421
D1. Protein-energy malnutrition (260-263)	6,891	3,506	-	-	-	-	3,506	3,385	-	-	-	-	3,385
D2. Iodine deficiency (243)	6,734	3,105	104	152	15	4	3,380	3,085	100	149	16	4	3,353
D3. Vitamin A deficiency (264)	10,610	5,378	-	-	-	-	5,378	5,232	-	-	-	-	5,232
D4. Anaemias (280-285)	10,342	134	1,344	2,149	545	251	4,423	129	1,275	3,710	528	276	5,919
E. Neuro-psychiatric (290-359, minus 320-322)	77,755	1,698	4,667	21,939	6,871	6,254	41,429	1,514	3,583	20,303	4,391	6,535	36,326
E1. Major affective disorder (296)	18,996	-	-	5,366	717	216	6,299	-	-	10,720	1,460	517	12,697
E2. Bipolar affective disorder (296)	1,208	-	-	533	58	15	605	-	-	523	61	19	603
E3. Psychoses (295, 291-294,297-299)	6,746	-	-	3,461	-	-	3,461	-	-	3,286	-	-	3,286
E4. Epilepsy (345)	7,153	703	2,213	1,057	195	78	4,246	482	1,494	723	141	67	2,907
E5. Alcohol dependence (303)	12,461	-	-	6,030	3,389	1,477	10,896	-	-	857	491	218	1,565
E6. Alzheimer & other dementias (330,331,333-336,290)	12,158	-	-	-	1,473	3,939	5,413	-	-	-	1,570	5,175	6,745
E7. Parkinson disease (332)	918	-	-	-	200	215	415	-	-	-	215	289	504
E8. Multiple sclerosis (340)	942	-	-	470	6	-	475	-	-	461	6	-	467
E9. Drug dependence (304)	4,754	-	177	2,856	424	108	3,565	-	44	970	149	27	1,190
E10. Post-traumatic stress disorder	5,162	62	478	1,289	112	22	1,964	102	776	2,101	179	40	3,198
F. Sense organ (360-389)	7,775	168	20	298	1,926	1,279	3,691	156	37	340	2,280	1,271	4,084
F1. Glaucoma-related blindness (365)	1,627	-	-	35	393	139	567	-	-	67	725	268	1,061
F2. Cataract-related blindness (366)	5,701	60	-	234	1,499	1,110	2,903	58	-	238	1,526	975	2,799
G. Cardiovascular diseases (390-459)	43,907	836	575	3,587	5,631	11,648	22,277	565	740	3,023	3,988	13,313	21,630
G1. Rheumatic heart disease (390-398)	941	9	212	242	10	2	476	9	204	239	11	2	466
G2. Ischaemic heart disease (*)	10,209	9	10	819	1,644	3,222	5,704	5	5	283	690	3,522	4,505
G3. Cerebrovascular disease (430-438)	12,344	49	73	714	1,333	3,563	5,733	37	94	717	1,240	4,523	6,611
G4. Inflammatory cardiac disease (+)	1,249	19	26	184	185	267	681	21	45	121	123	258	569
H. Chronic respiratory dis. (460-519, minus 460-466,480-487)	23,510	2,416	2,055	2,909	1,424	3,563	12,367	2,474	1,572	2,721	1,371	3,006	11,143
H1. Chronic obstructive lung dis. (490-492,495-496)	5,687	11	11	52	500	2,645	3,218	9	7	49	360	2,043	2,469
H2. Asthma (493)	9,494	338	1,576	2,246	487	152	4,798	280	1,321	2,120	722	254	4,696

Years lived with a disability (YLDs, in thousands): World

Disease or injury (ICD 9 code)	Both sexes all ages	Males 0-4	Males 5-14	Males 15-44	Males 45-59	Males 60+	Males All ages	Females 0-4	Females 5-14	Females 15-44	Females 45-59	Females 60+	Females All ages
I. Diseases of the digestive system (520-579)	18,731	2,789	639	2,733	2,048	1,607	9,817	3,429	807	1,895	1,337	1,446	8,914
I1. Peptic ulcer disease (531-533)	1,408	1	20	564	258	50	893	-	11	314	152	37	515
I2. Cirrhosis of the liver (571)	3,206	9	19	772	860	551	2,212	7	27	302	350	308	994
J. Genito-urinary (580-629)	8,990	280	611	897	2,377	1,175	5,340	168	504	1,105	820	1,053	3,650
J1. Nephritis/nephrosis (580-589)	4,439	74	532	716	416	587	2,324	56	447	689	357	566	2,116
J2. Benign prostatic hypertrophy (600)	2,064	-	-	-	1,766	298	2,064	-	-	-	-	-	-
K. Skin disease (680-709)		-	-	-	-	-	-	-	-	-	-	-	-
L. Musculo-skeletal system (710-739)	16,985	14	255	2,276	1,894	912	5,351	41	618	6,352	2,804	1,820	11,634
L1. Rheumatoid arthritis (714)	4,361	-	-	569	446	143	1,159	-	384	1,943	631	244	3,202
L2. Osteoarthritis (715)	11,218	-	156	1,600	1,379	598	3,733	-	117	4,007	2,026	1,336	7,486
M. Congenital abnormalities (740-759)	19,421	9,886	-	-	-	-	9,886	9,535	-	-	-	-	9,535
N. Oral health (520-529)	10,733	205	281	2,691	1,240	841	5,257	197	276	2,620	1,336	1,046	5,476
N1. Dental caries (521.0)	1,940	205	281	336	99	56	977	197	276	325	100	65	963
N2. Periodontal disease (523)	3,228	-	-	1,338	215	89	1,642	-	-	1,274	216	97	1,587
N3. Edentulism (520)	5,564	-	-	1,017	926	695	2,639	-	-	1,021	1,021	884	2,926
III. Injuries (E800-999)	58,993	6,522	6,423	21,882	2,458	1,484	38,769	6,631	4,321	6,291	1,013	1,968	20,224
A. Unintentional (E800-949)	43,638	5,482	5,663	13,160	1,818	1,397	27,519	5,373	3,831	4,229	792	1,895	16,119
A1. Road traffic accidents (E810-819, 826-829)	10,212	293	1,386	4,767	274	64	6,783	177	1,182	1,871	165	33	3,429
A2. Poisoning (E850-869)	129	22	19	35	5	1	83	11	19	14	1	-	46
A3. Falls (E850-869)	16,128	2,294	2,058	3,761	831	949	9,893	2,616	1,147	551	329	1,592	6,235
A4. Fires (E890-899)	4,268	1,092	394	725	128	102	2,442	775	532	347	67	104	1,826
A5. Drowning (E910)		-	-	-	-	-	-	-	-	-	-	-	-
A6. Occupational (#)	208	-	-	130	33	2	165	-	-	34	9	-	43
B. Intentional (E950-969,990-999)	15,355	1,040	760	8,721	640	87	11,250	1,258	491	2,062	221	73	4,105
B1. Self-inflicted (E950-959)		-	-	-	-	-	-	-	-	-	-	-	-
B2. Homicide and violence (E960-969)	10,583	574	437	6,610	451	77	8,149	784	277	1,177	135	61	2,434
B3. War (E990-999)	4,771	466	324	2,111	190	10	3,101	474	214	885	86	12	1,671
Population (in millions)	5,267.4	321.3	551.2	1,249.9	312.4	218.9	2,653.7	309.3	525.5	1,198.6	311.1	269.2	2,613.7

Notes

A dash (-) symbol indicates less than 1,000 YLDs.

* ICD 9 codes for ischaemic heart disease are as follows: 410-414, 440.9, plus: at ages 45-59: 50% of 427.1, 427.4, 427.5, and 33% of 428; at ages 60+: 80% of 427.1, 427.4, 427.5 and 50% of 428.

+ ICD 9 codes for inflammatory cardiac diseases are as follows: 420, 421, 422, 425 plus: at ages 0-44: 50% of 428; at ages 45-59: 25% of 428; at ages 60+: 20% of 428.

There are no established ICD 9 codes specific for occupational injuries.

Estimates have been based on reported occupational injuries and deaths tabulated by the International Labour Organisation.

The global burden of disease in 1990: summary results, sensitivity analysis and future directions

C.J.L. Murray,[1] A.D. Lopez,[2] & D.T. Jamison[3]

A basic requirement for evaluating the cost-effectiveness of health interventions is a comprehensive assessment of the amount of ill health (premature death and disability) attributable to specific diseases and injuries. A new indicator, the number of disability-adjusted life years (DALYs), was developed to assess the burden of disease and injury in 1990 for over 100 causes by age, sex and region. The DALY concept provides an integrative, comprehensive methodology to capture the entire amount of ill health which will, on average, be incurred during one's lifetime because of new cases of disease and injury in 1990. It differs in many respects from previous attempts at global and regional health situation assessment which have typically been much less comprehensive in scope, less detailed, and limited to a handful of causes.

This paper summarizes the DALY estimates for 1990 by cause, age, sex and region. For the first time, those responsible for deciding priorities in the health sector have access to a disaggregated set of estimates which, in addition to facilitating cost-effectiveness analysis, can be used to monitor global and regional health progress for over a hundred conditions. The paper also shows how the estimates depend on particular values of the parameters involved in the calculation.

Introduction

Three perceived needs of the international public health information system motivated the design and implementation of the Global Burden of Disease (GBD) study reported here, which was undertaken collaboratively by WHO and the World Bank as background for the World Bank's *World development report 1993: investing in health* (*1*). The first is that if, ten years ago, one had summed the various estimates of mortality, by cause, for children and adults, they would have equalled several times the total deaths at each age. Through the efforts of the World Health Organization, stimulated in part by the World Bank's health sector priorities review, the estimates for deaths by cause under age 5 have been rationalized (*2*). Through a consultative process, the estimates for major causes of child mortality generated by WHO technical programmes now add up to the total mortality. For adults, however, a consistent set of estimates of mortality by cause did not exist prior to this study. Furthermore, claims about adult mortality by various disease advocates have not been scrutinized. The most detailed review of adult health, the World Bank's study on adult health in developing countries (*3*), indicated the weakness of measurements of adult mortality levels and causes. Providing a plausible, internally consistent, set of estimates of mortality by cause was an important goal for this exercise.

Second, most discussions of international public health priorities ignore issues of disability. For some, disability is considered only a problem for societies that have already undergone the epidemiological transition and where mortality rates are low. Considerable efforts have been made in recent years to measure disability, both by the United Nations and through national research projects (*4–13*). While these works are important advances in the measurement of disability, they have not much influenced the debate on health priorities—in large part because the burden of disability by cause or that part of it which is amenable to specific health interventions has not been measured. Estimating the amount of life lived with a disability and its relative significance vis-à-vis premature mortality by cause was thus a second major goal of the study.

Third, too often health planners or decision-makers are faced with a multitude of health problems and priorities for action. The disease or health problem with the most vocal or eloquent advocates often

[1] Assistant Professor of International Health Economics, Harvard Centre for Population and Development Studies, 9 Bow Street, Cambridge MA 02138, USA. Requests for reprints should be sent to this author.

[2] Scientist, Tobacco or Health Programme, World Health Organization, Geneva, Switzerland.

[3] Professor of Education, Professor of Public Health, and Director of the Center for Pacific Rim Studies, University of California at Los Angeles, USA.

Reprinted from *Bulletin of the World Health Organization*, 1994, **72** (3): 495–509.

garners the most attention. Some problems, however, do not have ready advocates and continue to be ignored. A major justification for the Global Burden of Disease study was to provide a process through which every disease or health problem would be evaluated in an objective fashion. The third goal was thus to provide a framework for objectively identifying epidemiological priorities, which together with information on the cost-effectiveness of interventions can help when decisions on the allocation of resources have to be made.

This paper is one of four in this issue of the *Bulletin of the World Health Organization* on the Global Burden of Disease study (*14–16*). Through the study, a new measure, the disability-adjusted life year (DALY), was developed and applied to estimating the burden of disease for more than 100 causes, for five age groups and the two sexes in eight regions of the world. The technical details of the strategy used to measure the time lived with a disability in a manner that can be meaningfully compared with the time lost because of premature mortality are provided in Murray (*14*). The methods, materials and results for the measurement of deaths by cause and disability by cause are provided elsewhere (*15, 16*). This article presents the main results, explores the sensitivity of the results to various assumptions, and proposes future directions for research.

Combined indicators of health or disease burden have a long history dating back to the mid-sixties. Only one attempt to measure the burden of disease in a comprehensive manner, however, was made before this study. The Ghana health assessment project team estimated the burden of disease due to mortality and morbidity in Ghana for 48 causes (*17*). In scope, their study is a landmark effort. The definition, measurement and weighting of disability were not, however, provided in detail or explained. Although its results were widely cited, the enormous effort undertaken in Ghana was not followed by applications of the same method in other countries or even subsequently in Ghana itself. The consequent lack of

interest in quantifying or monitoring the burden of disease may have been due to several factors including the extensive data requirements, the need for specific assumptions on the treatment of disability, and the lack of a direct channel into decision-making. With the expanding role of cost-effectiveness in planning the health sector, the need for a more comprehensive measurement of the burden of disease has become more apparent and urgent (*18*).

In 1987 the World Bank initiated a major analytical public health initiative, the Health Sector Priorities Review. This exercise, culminating in the publication of Disease Control Priorities for Developing Countries (*19*), has documented existing knowledge about the cost-effectiveness of health interventions in developing countries. With comparable information on the cost-effectiveness of nearly 50 interventions, interest in the allocative efficiency of the health sector has increased. The broadening analytical role for cost-effectiveness laid the foundation for the health policy message in the world development report for 1993 (*1*). In order to use cost-effectiveness to develop an essential package of health services, it is useful to know the burden of disease (*18*). The quantification reported here of the global and regional disease and injury burden to be addressed by the health services was thus a critical input to the World Development Report. The study has received financial and technical support from the World Bank, WHO, the Edna McConnell Clark Foundation, the Rockefeller Foundation, and the U.S. Centers for Disease Control and Prevention.

The assessment of disease burden reported here represents one major step in a larger programme of work that is further discussed in the concluding section of this paper. Fig. 1 illustrates that programme schematically; the burden of disease can be grouped in three separate ways for different age, sex and regional groupings of population. One group is by *risk-factor*—genetic, behavioural, environmental and physiological. The second is by *disease*. The third is by consequence—*premature mortality* at different

Fig. 1. **Three categories of the burden of disease.**

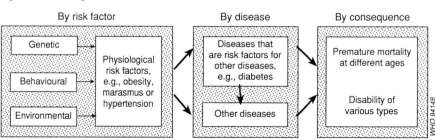

ages and different *types of disability* (e.g., sensory, cognitive functioning, sensor functioning, affective state, etc.). The analyses reported in this series of articles deal principally with the second group, by disease. Consequences are aggregated simply into premature mortality and disability; a fuller assessment of burden by consequence would provide highly relevant information to guide rehabilitation programmes. Likewise a decomposition of burden by risk factor would better guide primary prevention. This assessment of burden, by disease, is a precursor to the other groups while also providing a broad sense of disease burden to guide intervention.

Methods

Details of the methods, approaches and principles used to estimate causes of death by age, sex and region and the methods used for measuring disability incidence, duration, and severity have been described (*15, 16*). The study used a regional breakdown into two sets of regions: demographically developing countries—Sub-Saharan Africa (SSA), India (IND), China (CHI), Other Asia and Islands (OAI), Latin America and the Caribbean (LAC), and the Middle Eastern Crescent (MEC)—and two region with demographically mature populations, the Established Market Economies (EME) and the Formerly Socialist Economies of Europe (FSE).

The study began in January 1992 with the Version 1 results which were presented and discussed at an expert group meeting hosted by WHO in Geneva in December 1992. Version 2 results reflecting widespread technical review were produced in February 1993. Following a more intensive and critical appraisal of the assumptions about disability and the disabling sequelae of diseases and injuries by an independent group of experts, Version 3 results were prepared in April 1993 and are presented in the world development report (*1*). This paper provides Version 4 results incorporating further technical review and a relatively minor revision of specific disease estimates. In a short period of time (i.e., less than 18 months), more than 100 experts were recruited to assist in the study, estimates were generated and widely reviewed, and the final results calculated and interpreted. The exercise would not have succeeded without tremendous assistance from the technical experts, the support of the World Health Organization, and the active input of our Advisory Committee.[a]

[a] The Global Burden of Disease Advisory Committee met in Geneva at the World Health Organization on 9–11 December 1992. The committee consisted of Dr J.-P. Jardel (*Chairman*), Professor R. Feachem, Dr T. Godal, Mr D. Jamison, Dr J. Koplan, Dr A. Measham, Dr J.-M. Robine, and Professor P. Smith.

Results

Combining the contribution from both premature mortality and the years of life lived with a disability, where was the greatest burden of disease in 1990? As Fig. 2 shows, Sub-Saharan Africa and India were the two regions with the largest contribution (21.5% each) to the global total. The significant health gains recorded in China are reflected in the 15% contribution from this country, compared with a 21.5% share of the world's population. The two regions, EME and FSE, which have recorded most success in reducing Group I disease (communicable, maternal and perinatal causes), together account for only about 11% of the global burden of disease, but have about twice that share of the global population. Nearly 90% of the global burden of disease in 1990 therefore occurred because of disease and injury in the developing world. When population size is taken into account (see Fig. 3), the comparatively poor health profile of Sub-Saharan Africa is even more apparent. For every 1000 people living in the region about 580 DALYs were incurred in 1990, compared with just over 100 in EME. Much of the burden of disease (about 75%) in Sub-Saharan Africa is due to premature mortality, as it is (but to a lesser extent) in India, MEC and OAI. In the four remaining regions, where the overall level of the burden of disease is lowest, the contribution from disability and premature death is roughly the same. The rate of DALYs is similar in China and FSE (as is life expectancy), being about 50% higher than in the EME region. Most of the difference between regions is due to differences in premature mortality while disability rates are more equal across regions. It is worth noting, however, that crude disability DALY rates are higher in poor developing regions than in the Established Market Economies.

The sex ratio (male/female) of DALY rates is shown in Fig. 4 divided into the components due to

Fig. 2. **Total DALYs, by region, as a percentage of global DALYs.**

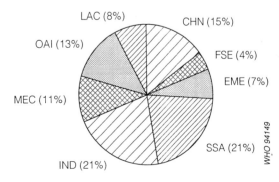

99

Fig. 3. **Total DALY rates, by region.**

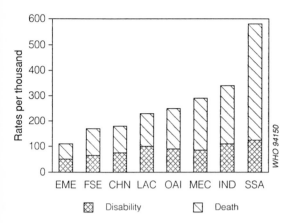

Fig. 4. **Male to female ratios of DALY rates for death and disability.**

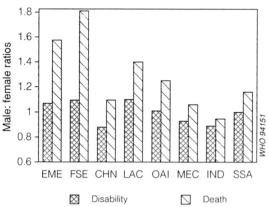

disability and premature death. DALYs due to years of life lived with a disability are indicated by YLD and the years of life lost due to premature mortality by YLL. It is immediately apparent that the rate of YLD is similar for both sexes in all regions, with male rates being 5–10% higher in EME, FSE, and LAC, and 5–15% lower in CHI, MEC and India, compared with the female rates. In OAI and SSA the disability rates, as measured by YLD, are identical for both males and females. This relative uniformity in disability levels for the sexes contrast sharply with the very marked variation across regions in the differential mortality of the sexes. In EME, and particularly in FSE, males rates of YLL are 60–80% higher than for females and are 40% higher in LAC. In FSE and LAC this excess male mortality, particularly in middle age, is due to higher death rates from chronic diseases, which in turn are significantly affected by smoking. As female smoking prevalence continues to rise and the male epidemic stabilizes we expect that the sex mortality ratio in these two regions will begin to decrease, as it has begun to do so in some countries (20). Much of the excess male mortality in LAC, as captured by the YLL rates, is due to extremely high male death rates from injuries. The burden of premature mortality is similar for males and females in MEC and China, and is estimated to be higher for females in India, which is consistent with other research showing excess female mortality during childhood and the reproductive years.[b]

More details on the relative contribution of each age group to the total DALYs estimated for each

region are given in Table 1. Overall, the burden of disease is greater among males in all regions except India (where it is shared equally between the sexes), with the male share of the total ranging from 51% in MEC and China to 57% in FSE. The age pattern of contributions varies markedly from one region to another, however. In EME, the region with the lowest DALY rate, the greatest contribution (21% each for both males and females) arises from diseases and injuries among the elderly. Only about 10% of the burden (half in males, half in females) is due to conditions affecting children below age 15. About 30% of all DALYs in both EME and FSE are attributable to the young adult ages (15–44 years), a pattern which is repeated across all regions. Even in Sub-Saharan Africa, one-quarter of the total burden of disease and injury arises from this age group, second in importance only to the massive contribution (53%) from diseases and injuries affecting young children.

The broad pattern of cause-specific contributions to total DALY rates during childhood (0–14 years), adulthood (15–59 years) and old age (60+) is given in Fig. 5 (females) and Fig. 6 (males). The pattern of regional variation is similar to what was observed for risks of death. At ages 0–14, much of the difference in DALY rates is due to differences in childhood risks of Group I diseases (communicable, maternal and perinatal), although even at these ages the contribution from Group II (noncommunicable disease) is significant, owing in large part to nutritional deficiencies and congenital abnormalities. Similarly, among women at least, almost all of the variation in DALY rates at ages 15–59 is due to differential rates of DALYs from Group I diseases across regions, being particularly high in Sub-Saharan Africa. A very different pattern emerges for men,

---

[b] **Dyson T.** *Excess female mortality in India: uncertain evidence on a narrowing differential.* Paper presented at the Workshop on Differential Female Health Care and Mortality, Dhaka, January 1987.

Table 1: Percentage distribution of total DALYs, by age and sex, for each region

Sex and age group (years)	Established Market Economies	Formerly Socialist Economies	China	Latin America and the Caribbean	Other Asia and Islands	Middle Eastern Crescent	India	Sub-Saharan Africa	All regions
Males:	56	58	51	56	54	51	50	52	52
0–4	4	5	12	18	21	26	23	29	20
5–14	1	2	4	6	8	6	5	7	6
15–44	17	20	16	20	14	10	11	12	14
45–59	12	16	9	6	6	4	6	3	6
60+	21	15	11	5	5	4	5	2	7
Females:	44	42	49	44	46	49	50	48	48
0–4	3	4	13	14	17	25	24	25	19
5–14	1	1	4	5	7	6	6	6	5
15–44	12	11	16	15	13	11	12	12	13
45–59	8	8	6	5	4	3	4	2	4
60+	21	18	10	5	5	4	5	2	7

however. Total DALY rates in FSE and LAC are significantly higher than in all other regions except India and SSA. In FSE, this reflects the prominence of noncommunicable diseases, as well as injuries, as major public health concerns among men. The higher rates in LAC, compared with China or MEC for example, arise from a high injury-attributable burden, as well as a significant residual burden of non-communicable disease even at these ages. DALY rates in Sub-Saharan Africa, half of which arise from Group I diseases, are also about twice as high as in most other regions of the developing world. There is thus a very major unfinished agenda in Africa in the conquest of infectious disease, which affects adults almost as much as young children. In the oldest age group (60+), the variation between developed and developing regions is still substantial, with women having twice as high DALY rates in SSA as in EME. Most of the difference is due to lower DALY rates of noncommunicable diseases in the developed regions. For men over 60, there are still higher rates in SSA as compared to EME but the excess is less pronounced than that for women.

Finally, a detailed summary of DALY numbers by age, sex and cause is given in the Annex (Tables 1, 2 and 3 for developed regions, developing regions and all regions, respectively, in 1990). The top half of each Table gives the absolute number of DALYs for the first level of cause disaggregation below the three large groups. The lower half of the Table gives the percentage of total DALYs within each age and sex group due to the next level of more specific causes. For each broad region, the list of specific causes has been chosen to include the top three causes in each age and sex group. Perhaps somewhat sur-

prisingly, the burden of disease from noncommunicable diseases is virtually the same as for communicable diseases for the world as a whole, although there are of course significant regional variations. Cardiovascular disease, neuropsychiatric disorders, cancers and nutritional/endocrine disorders are globally major health problems, as are injuries. These causes combined accounted for over 40% of the global burden of disease in 1990. At the same time, the major infectious diseases which have dominated public health for centuries remain as significant causes of the disease burden today and must continue to be a principal focus of public health attention. These include tuberculosis (3.4% of the global burden), diarrhoeal diseases (7.3%), the vaccine-preventable diseases (5.0%) and acute respiratory infections (8.4%). In the developing world, 50% of DALYs are attributable to Group I causes, the usual focus of international public health interest. Half the burden in the developing world is due to noncommunicable diseases and injuries. Important among the Group II causes are neoplasms (4.4%), nutritional/endocrine disorders (4.2%), neuropsychiatric illness (6%), cardiovascular disease (9%), chronic respiratory diseases (3.4%), digestive disorders (3.2%), and congenital abnormalities (3.1%). Among injuries, two-thirds of the burden is due to unintentional and one-third to intentional, with considerable regional diversity in the specific pattern of deaths from injury.

Sensitivity analysis

Quite apart from the numerous judgements required concerning the reliability, relevance and applicability of data and information about mortality and disabili-

Fig. 5. Total DALY rates for females within broad age ranges, by region, 1990.

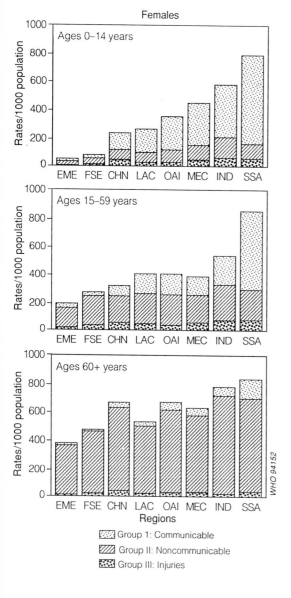

results to changing both discounting and age-weighting simultaneously has also been examined.

The discount rate (r) used in the calculation of DALYs has been varied from 0% to 10% in increments of 2.5%. To measure sensitivity of the results to the use of unequal age-weights, a new parameter must be introduced. The simple exponential age-weighting function in the original DALY formula

Fig. 6. Total DALY rates for males within broad age ranges, by region, 1990.

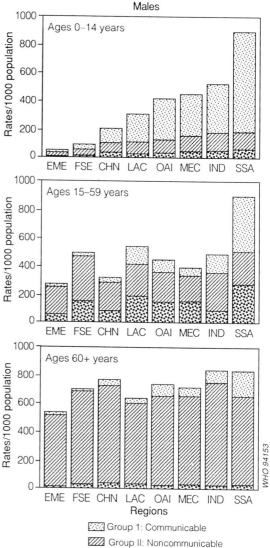

ty, the disability-adjusted life years incorporate some fundamental social values into its computation. We have tested the sensitivity of the results of the global burden of disease study to the most controversial of these assumptions, namely a positive discount rate and unequal valuation of the time lived at different ages. As described below, the sensitivity of the

(see ref. *14* for discussion) has been replaced with the following function:

$$KCxe^{-\beta x} + (1 - K)$$

where *K* is an age-weighting constant. When *K* equals one, then the age-weighting function is the same as in DALYs; whereas when *K* equals zero, then the age-weights are equal. Fig. 7 demonstrates the age-weighting for several values of *K* between zero and one.

The entire global burden of disease by cause, age, sex and region has been recalculated 25 times for each combination of discount rates at 0%, 2.5%, 5%, 7.5%, and 10% and *K* values of 0, 0.25, 0.5, 0.75 and 1. Of the 1.25 million figures generated, only a few can be discussed here. In the following discussion, the emphasis is on the qualitative impact of changing *r* and *K* on the final results.

Variations in *r* and *K* have little or no effect on the difference between sexes in total DALYs. At the global level, the proportion for males ranged from 51% to 52% and even within regions the largest variation was in FSE, only from 52% to 59%. While change in the discount rate has little effect on the male/female difference in total DALYs, it has a much greater effect on the distribution of total DALYs by the age of onset. For whatever value of *K*, increasing the discount rate will decrease the proportion of total burden in the age groups 0–4 and 5–14 years, and increase the share in the adult age group (45–59 years) and the elderly (60+ years). Fig. 8 illustrates the effects on ages 0–4 and 15–44 years; 15–44 is the transition age group where changing the discount rate has only a small effect on the share of total DALYs. Shifting from equal to unequal age-

Fig. 8. **Global burden of disease sensitivity results: proportion of total DALYs in age groups of 0–4 years and 15–59 years.**

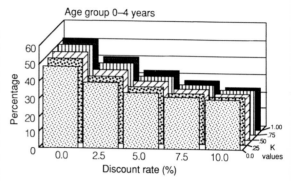

Age group 0–4 years

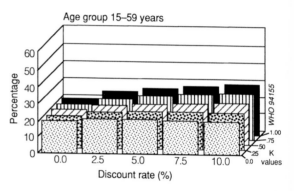

Age group 15–59 years

weights by increasing *K* from 0 to 1 has a much smaller and more complex effect on the age distribution of total DALYs. Up to a discount rate of 5%, unequal age-weights increase the burden at ages less than 45 years. For example, if we compare DALYs calculated with *r*=3% and *K*=1, the original formula, and a 'classical' version with a discount rate of zero and equal age-weights, the difference in age distribution of total DALYs is small since some of the effect of a 3% discount rate is counterbalanced by the unequal age weights. At high discount rates, raising *K* reinforces the effect of discounting on the age pattern.

Because the cause structure of burden is different at different age groups, changing the discount rate and age-weighting changes not only the overall age pattern of DALYs but also the relative importance of premature mortality and disability and different causes. Table 2 shows the proportion of burden due to disability which ranges from 25% to 45%, with the lowest proportion due to disability when the discount rate is zero and age-weights are equal, and the

Fig. 7. **Age-weight function at different values of *K*.**

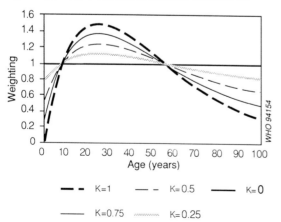

Table 2: **Years lived with a disability (YLD) as a percent of total DALYs at different K and r values (world total)**

r value (%)	% YLD at K value of:				
	0.00	0.25	0.50	0.75	1.00
0.0	25	26	26	27	29
2.5	33	33	33	33	33
5.0	37	38	38	38	38
7.5	41	41	41	41	41
10.0	45	44	44	44	45

highest when the discount rate is 10% and there is unequal age-weighting. As with the age pattern of total DALYs, changing the discount rate has a much larger effect than changing K. In fact, K has subtle qualitative effects depending on the level of the discount rate used.

Perhaps, the most important aspects of changing r and K to the study is the impact on DALYs by cause. Table 3 shows the proportion of the global burden due to Group I, Group II and Group III for different values of the discount rate and age-weighting patterns. Increasing the discount rate raises the importance of diseases affecting adults aged 15–59 and subsequently increases the share of Group II and decreases the share of Group I. Because Group III affects all age groups, changing the discount rate has a much less important effect on the share of total

Table 3: **The percent distribution of DALYs for the three cause groups at different K and r values (global total)**

r value (%)	% DALYs at K value of:				
	0.00	0.25	0.50	0.75	1.00
Group I					
0.0	51	51	52	53	53
2.5	43	44	45	46	47
5.0	39	39	40	41	42
7.5	36	37	37	38	39
10.0	35	35	36	36	37
Group II					
0.0	37	37	36	35	34
2.5	46	45	44	42	41
5.0	51	50	49	47	46
7.5	54	53	52	51	50
10.0	57	55	54	53	52
Group III					
0.0	12	12	12	12	13
2.5	11	11	12	12	12
5.0	10	11	11	12	12
7.5	10	10	11	11	12
10.0	9	9	10	11	11

DALYs due to causes in this group. Shifting from equal to unequal age-weights by going from $K=0$ to $K=1$ has nearly the opposite effect from increasing the discount rate on Groups I and II but little effect on Group III.

To test for the effect of changing r and K on the more detailed results by cause, the total DALYs due to each cause in each region and globally, calculated using different pairs of r and K, have each been regressed on the original results. The similarity of the cause-specific results with the GBD results can be measured using the r-squared from such regressions. In this case, the r-squared is a measure of how much of the variance in the burden of disease results, recalculated using a new set of assumptions, is captured in the original results. The Group I, II and III totals have been excluded because these spuriously raise the r-squared in the regressions. An r-squared of 1.0 would be a perfect match and an r-squared of 0.0 would mean there was no relationship between the two sets of estimates. Fig. 9 shows that at the global level, the r-squared ranges from 0.84 when $r=10\%$, $K=0$ to 0.99 when $r=2.5\%$, $K=1$. When r is non-zero, then increasing K makes the results closer to the original study whereas when the discount rate is zero, increasing K has the reverse effect.

The two extremes—a 'classical' approach when $r=0$ and $K=0$ and a 'development economist' approach where $r=10\%$ and $K=1$—can be compared. The GBD results are closer (r-squared of 0.98) to the 'classical' assumptions than to the 'development economist' assumptions (r-squared of 0.91). The results even for these two extremes are surprisingly similar. Nearly the entire effect of changing r or K is due to the effect on shifting the age pattern and thus the Group I versus Group II balance. The same regressions conducted on the results within each Group all give r-squared estimates between 0.97 and

Fig. 9. **Global burden of disease sensitivity results: r-squared from regressions of cause-specific DALYs compared with the study results.**

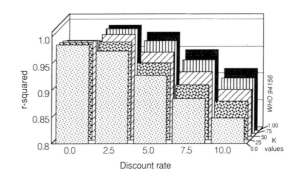

1.0 for Group I, 0.94 to 0.98 for Group II, and 0.99 to 1.0 for Group III.

This summary analysis of the sensitivity testing suggests several conclusions. First, discounting has a significant impact on the distribution of total DALYs by the age of onset. Second, unequal age-weighting has a much less pronounced effect than discounting and an effect that often runs counter to the effect of a time preference. Third, the overall impact of both discounting and age-weighting on the calculated burden due to specific causes is small. We conclude that the qualitative results of the burden of disease analysis are quite robust to the specific assumptions about time preference and age-weighting used. While we do not present in this paper a detailed analysis, we have also tested the results to changing the specific values of the disability class weights. At the aggregate level, these changes have little if any effect on the overall results as presented here.

Discussion

The sensitivity analysis has shown that the qualitative results of the Global Burden of Disease study are remarkably insensitive to the particular social preferences incorporated into the calculation of DALYs. The largest effect of changing the discount rate or age-weights is on the age distribution of DALYs. More importantly, the estimates for burden by cause do not change appreciably over a wide range of discount rates and age-weights. The most important choice is whether to use a zero or non-zero time preference. Specific values of a non-zero discount rate (between 0 and 10 percent) make much less difference and the same is true for equal or unequal age-weights. Further sensitivity analysis of changing the disability weights on high-prevalence, low-severity conditions will be useful. Nevertheless, we are reassured that specific value choices matter much less than the epidemiological details for any particular condition.

The global burden of disease results presented here are built upon more than 50 000 estimates of mortality, incidence, age of onset, duration and severity by cause, age, sex and region. The confidence intervals for some, such as deaths in EME, are likely narrow but for other estimates, such as the incidence of HIV infections in OAI, they are probably very wide. Nevertheless, we feel the results are interesting, informative and potentially useful. These estimates should be seen as a first tentative step in a process. Continued application of the process described in these papers will lead to improved estimates and more robust results. Where diseases appear to be significant contributors to the burden

and estimates are uncertain, we hope that the study will stimulate further work on local or regional epidemiology. The Tables of results must not be used as definitive and are not a substitute for future efforts to improve measurement.

How should these results and future versions of them be used to improve health policy decisions? Immediately, one can note the tremendous mismatch between international efforts on research and health policy analysis and the burden of disease by cause. Many of the major causes of burden in developing countries, as identified by this study, receive grossly disproportionate attention in international public health forums. For example, relatively few resources are devoted to controlling chronic respiratory, digestive, genitourinary or musculoskeletal diseases despite their contribution of 9% to the global burden. A review of the international health research system, with careful attention paid to the burden of disease and the current availability of cost-effective interventions, would be timely.

The burden of disease results in conjunction with information on the cost-effectiveness of health interventions should help in making international or regional resource allocation decisions. Already available information (1) on the burden of disease and the cost-effectiveness of interventions can identify "minimal packages" of public health and clinical interventions which, if implemented, would reduce the disease burden in low-income developing countries by about a quarter at a cost of $12 per person per year. Murray et al. have developed a computer model to define the optimal allocation of health resources, given the burden of disease, cost-effectiveness of health interventions, and the available human and physical resources in the health system (21). Regardless of the specific method, the burden of disease results are not the only input to a rational setting of priorities. They are, nevertheless, critical if the priorities are to be established objectively.

The results of the burden of disease exercise can be more useful at the national or subnational level. Combined with information on the global-effectiveness of health interventions, they can be used to assess objectively the allocative efficiency of the health sector and to propose the package of services that would maximize the DALYs gained, given a particular budget. The utility of this information for national health decision-makers has already been appreciated. Mexico and Mozambique began the first national burden of disease studies in early 1993. India (Andhra Pradesh), Colombia and Uzbekistan have recently initiated national or state burden of disease exercises as well. To this list must be added more than fifteen other countries that have expressed an interest in undertaking national burden of disease analyses, including two industrialized nations. These national burden of disease exercises not only generate useful results for the health policy debate, but also indicate substantial secondary benefits, as in Mexico and Mozambique. Through the process of review, collation and estimation for each disease, the strengths and weaknesses of existing information systems are identified, and a broad network of national experts on specific health problems is created.

A strong link between national burden of disease studies and maintenance of the global and regional burden of disease estimates has emerged. Efforts at country level unearth new data and shed light on the interpretation of known information. These advances enrich the regional estimates of disability and mortality by cause. National estimates in turn would be nearly impossible without the technical backup of existing regional epidemiological profiles for each disease. When no local data are available on incidence, duration or mortality, the epidemiological relationships between key parameters captured by disease experts can form the basis of a country estimate. In addition, the network of experts created by the study has been used to provide prompt answers to specific technical questions, such as the interaction between tuberculosis and HIV-2 infection in Mozambique.

Agenda for the future

Progress on the measurement of national, regional and global burdens of disease will require methodological advance on several topics which are briefly outlined below.

(1) The list of diseases included in burden of disease exercises needs to be improved and expanded. In particular, cardiovascular diseases and neuropsychiatric disorders are very heterogeneous groups with large shares in the total burden. More detailed disaggregations are required to clarify the debate on the application of specific interventions. In addition, diseases such as appendicitis, hernia and cysticercosis need to be added because they are locally important or alternatively consume a large share of health care resources.

(2) The measurement of the time lived with disabilities of different severities needs to be improved and validated. Methods to adjust the results for both independent and dependent comorbidity should be elaborated in the context of a full partitioning of the burden of disease by consequences as illustrated in Fig. 1. Prospective studies on the distribution of disabling sequelae due to particular diseases are also needed. Finally, the global or national burden of disease results should be validated through cross-sectional household surveys.

(3) Authors of conceptual frameworks about the nature and consequences of ill-health (e.g., 22–24) have repeatedly argued for the major role of individual behaviours and environmental factors in the causation of disease and injury. Assessing burden on the basis of medical diagnosis or disease nomenclature is thus only part of the information requirement of health planners. For a wide variety of conditions, certain behaviours or exposures have been repeatedly found to cause or contribute to disease or injury. Among the most important of these, at least in specific regions, are tobacco, alcohol abuse, poor diet, environmental degradation of various forms, malnutrition, sexual activity, certain occupations, and physical inactivity. Future work on extending the burden of disease approach to assess the contribution from these and other causes of disease and injury is urgently required to inform health policy-makers and assist in priority setting; this would involve a partitioning of the disease burden by risk factor (Fig. 1), an effort undertaken in the *World development report 1993* (*1*) for selected risk factors (nutritional, smoking and environmental). However, the analysis has not taken into account the fact that many diseases are themselves risk factors for other diseases in the sense that they increase the risk of related conditions. Diabetics, for example, have an increased risk of death and disability from cardiovascular diseases (*25*) and hepatitis B infection greatly increases the risk of dying from liver cancer (*26*). Estimates of the fractions of the burden of a specific disease that are more appropriately attributable to other conditions will also need to be developed if the approach is to reflect more reliably the impact of diseases in causing ill health.

(4) In the face of the HIV epidemic and present trends in many cancers and ischaemic heart disease and considering the known effects of changing population age-structure in many regions, projections of the burden of disease for the year 2000 or 2010 would be useful for health planners. Simple linear projections will not be adequate. Projection methods that incorporate known levels and trends of major risk factors such as smoking and trends in other diseases must be developed.

(5) If information on the burden of disease contributes useful baseline data for health policy-makers, the logical next step is to assess overall health sector performance with trends in the burden of disease. The information requirements for determining real trends in the burden of disease are much more exacting than for estimating the level of burden for an *ad hoc* study. Estimates of the level can be wrong by 5–10% without affecting the interpretation of results, but changes in the burden over a 5- or 10-year period may only be of this magnitude.

Monitoring systems that generate real estimates of mortality and disability by cause are required. Testing and application of successful sample monitoring systems for mortality and disability by cause are urgent priorities if monitoring the burden is to be a more reliable approach to assessing health priorities.

Acknowledgements

We should like to acknowledge the financial and or technical support of the Edna McConnel Clark Foundation, the Rockefeller Foundation, the World Bank and the World Health Organization. We would particularly like to thank Philip Musgrove for his comments on earlier drafts of this article. A large number of other individuals also generously contributed time and technical advice to this undertaking (see acknowledgements on page 31).

Résumé

Le poids de la morbidité dans le monde en 1990: récapitulation des résultats, analyse de la sensibilité et orientations futures

On trouvera décrit dans cet article le mécanisme utilisé pour regrouper les données existantes sur la mortalité et l'incapacité, assorti d'avis d'experts sur les séquelles incapacitantes des maladies et des traumatismes exprimées au moyen d'un indice récapitulatif unique appelé DALY (*Disability-adjusted life years*: années de vie ajustées sur l'incapacité). Les DALY mesurent, pour une année donnée et pour chaque cause, le nombre attendu d'années qui seront vécues avec une incapacité (où la gravité de l'incapacité est exprimée par les experts par un coefficient), ainsi que le nombre d'années de vie perdues par décès prématuré. Cet indice fournit donc une statistique globale et comparée du poids de la morbidité qui découle des cas incidents de maladie et de traumatisme survenus en 1990. On trouvera indiquée la valeur des DALY par âge (0–4, 5–14, 15–44, 45–59 et ≥60 ans), par sexe, et par région, selon les huit régions définies par la Banque mondiale.

Le calcul des DALY tient compte d'hypothèses supplémentaires concernant la préférence temporelle (actualisation) et la valeur des années de vie en fonction de l'âge (poids de l'âge). Les résultats obtenus en faisant varier ces paramètres à partir des valeurs choisies dans l'étude du poids de la morbidité dans le monde sont également indiqués. Cette analyse de la sensibilité montre que les résultats de l'étude sont remarquablement stables en dépit des variations des hypothèses concernant le poids de l'âge et le taux d'actualisation tant qu'il reste différent de zéro. La seule variation importante de l'estimation résulte de la fixation du taux d'actualisation soit à zéro, valeur utilisée traditionnellement en santé publique, soit à une autre valeur que zéro.

Près de 90% du nombre total des DALY estimées pour l'ensemble du monde en 1990 (1,36 milliard) concernent les pays en développement, dont 22% pour l'Inde et autant pour l'Afrique subsaharienne. Le taux de DALY est maximal en Afrique (580 pour 1000 habitants), l'Inde (340 pour 1000) venant ensuite. Les taux estimés les plus bas correspondent aux économies de marché bien établies (EMBE) (pays industrialisés, avec 110 pour 1000). Les variations régionales des taux de DALY sont pour la plus grande part dues aux différences de mortalité prématurée. Dans l'ensemble du monde, les hommes comptent un peu plus de DALY que les femmes (52% contre 48%), avec des variations régionales faibles. Toutefois, la contribution par âge des DALY varie considérablement d'une région à l'autre, les personnes âgées (60 ans et plus) représentant 42% des DALY dans les pays industrialisés (contre 9% dans la tranche d'âge 0–4 ans), tandis qu'à l'autre extrémité, en Afrique subsaharienne, 14% seulement des DALY sont attribuables à des maladies et des traumatismes chez les personnes âgées; près de 40% des DALY sont retrouvées dans la tranche d'âge 0–4 ans. Dans toutes les régions et pour les deux sexes, la morbidité et la mortalité chez le jeune adulte (15–44 ans) occupent une place importante de l'ensemble des DALY, représentant ordinairement 15 à 20% du poids total de la maladie.

L'article conclut en mentionnant une série de questions qui exigent un développement ultérieur pour renforcer la valeur de cette méthode utilisant le poids de la morbidité comme élément clé des systèmes d'information sanitaire. D'autres recherches sont nécessaires sur la dynamique des causes majeures entrant dans ce poids telles que les maladies cardio-vasculaires, les troubles neuro-psychiatriques et les traumatismes, au niveau de la population. Il est urgent de procéder à des études prospectives de la distribution et de la fréquence des séquelles incapacitantes de maladies et de traumatismes et d'établir des projections du poids de la maladie. Il est également important de disposer de méthodes d'évaluation du poids de la maladie et des traumatismes attribuables au mode de vie et à d'autres déterminants de la santé si l'on veut pouvoir utiliser réellement cette approche comme un outil nouveau, global et efficace, pour orienter les politiques et les stratégies sanitaires.

References

1. **World Bank.** *World development report 1993: Investing in health.* Oxford, Oxford University Press, 1993.
2. **Lopez AD.** Cause of death in industrial and developing countries: estimates for 1985–1990. In: Jamison DT et al., eds. *Disease control priorities in developing countries.* Oxford and New York, Oxford University Press (for the World Bank), 1993: 35–50.
3. **Feachem RG et al.** *The health of adults in the developing world.* Oxford, Oxford University Press (for the World Bank), 1992.
4. **Bebbington AC.** The expectation of life without disability in England and Wales: 1976–1988. *Population trends,* 1991, **66**: 26–29.
5. **Branch LG et al.** Active life expectancy for 10 000 Caucasian men and women in three communities. *Journal of gerontology,* 1991, **46**: M145–M150.
6. **Crimmins E, Saito Y, Ingegneri D.** Changes in life expectancy and disability-free life expectancy in the United States. *Population and development review,* 1989, **15**: 235–267.
7. **Mathers CD.** *Health expectancies in Australia 1981 and 1988.* Canberra, Australian Institute of Health, 1991.
8. **Robine JM, Colvez A.** Espérance de vie sans incapacité en France en 1981. *Population,* 1986, **41**: 1025–1042.
9. **Rogers RG, Rogers A, Belanger A.** Active life among the elderly in the United States: multistate life-table estimates and population projections. *Milbank Memorial Fund quarterly,* 1989, **67**: 370–411.
10. **van Ginneken JK et al.** Results of two methods to determine health expectancy in the Netherlands in 1981–1985. *Social science and medicine,* 1991, **32**: 1129–1136.
11. **Wilkins R, Adams OB.** Health expectancy in Canada, late 1970s: demographic, regional and social dimensions. *American journal of public health,* 1983, **73**: 1073–1080.
12. **Réseau Espérance de Vie en Santé.** *Statistical world yearbook. Retrospective 1993 issue.* Montpellier, INSERM, 1993.
13. **United Nations.** *Disability statistics compendium.* New York, 1990.
14. **Murray CJL.** Quantifying the burden of disease: the technical basis for disability-adjusted life years. *Bulletin of the World Health Organization,* 1994, **72**: 429–445.
15. **Murray CJL, Lopez AD.** Global and regional cause-of-death patterns in 1990. *Bulletin of the World Health Organization,* 1994, **72**: 447–480.
16. **Murray CJL, Lopez AD.** Quantifying disability: data, methods and results. *Bulletin of the World Health Organization,* 1994, **72**: 481–494
17. **Ghana Health Assessment Project Team.** A quantitative method for assessing the health impact of different diseases in less-developed countries. *International journal of epidemiology,* 1981, **10**: 73–80.
18. **Bobadilla JL et al.** Design, content and financing of an essential national package of health services. *Bulletin of the World Health Organization,* 1994, **72** (4) (in press).
19. **Jamison DH et al.** eds. *Disease control priorities in developing countries.* Oxford, Oxford University Press (for the World Bank), 1993.
20. **Lopez, AD.** Changes in tobacco consumption and lung cancer risk: evidence from national statistics. In: Parkin DM et al., eds. *Evaluating effectiveness of primary prevention of cancer.* Lyon, IARC, 1990: 57–76 (Scientific Publications No. 103).
21. **Murray CJL, Kreuser J, Whang W.** Cost-effectiveness analysis and policy choice: investing in health systems. *Bulletin of the World Health Organization,* 1994, **72**(4) (in press).
22. **Mosely WH, Chen L.** An analytical framework for the study of child survival in developing countries. *Population and development review,* 1984, **10**(suppl.): 25–45.
23. **Beaglehole R.** Conceptual frameworks for the investigation of mortality from major cardiovascular diseases. In: Lopez AD, Valkonen T, Caselli G, eds. *Adult mortality in developed countries.* Oxford, Oxford University Press (in press).
24. **Powles, J.** Socio-economic health determinants in working-age males. In: Diessendorf M, Bryan F, eds. *The impact of environment and lifestyle on human health.* Canberra, Society for Social Responsibility in Science. 1977: 31–51.
25. **King H, Zimmet P.** Trends in the prevalence and incidence of diabetes: non-insulin dependent diabetes mellitus. *World health statistics quarterly,* 1988, **41**(3–4): 190–196.
26. **Beasley RP et al.** Hepatocellular carcinoma and hepatitis B virus. A prospective study of 22 707 men in Taiwan. *Lancet,* 1981, **2**: 1129–1133.

Annex

Annex Table 1. **Total DALYs for major cause groups, by sex and age, 1990: Developed regions** [a,b]

	Males in age group (years):						Females in age group (years):						Both sexes
	0-4	5-14	15-44	45-59	60+	All ages	0-4	5-14	15-44	45-59	60+	All ages	All ages
All Causes	6,441	2,313	27,456	20,687	28,578	85,475	5,154	1,620	17,569	12,085	29,794	66,223	151,698
I. Communicable, maternal & perinatal	2,953	172	2,215	570	770	6,680	2,226	161	3,985	301	775	7,448	14,128
A. Infectious & parasitic	342	82	1,690	305	206	2,624	264	76	2,499	114	179	3,133	5,757
B. Respiratory infections	629	89	524	265	564	2,071	516	84	458	177	596	1,831	3,902
C. Maternal conditions	–	–	–	–	–	–	–	–	1,027	10	–	1,037	1,037
D. Perinatal conditions	1,983	1	–	–	–	1,985	1,446	1	–	–	–	1,447	3,432
II. Noncommunicable	2,836	1,284	14,681	17,916	26,638	63,355	2,474	1,061	11,113	11,082	27,753	53,483	116,838
A. Malignant neoplasms	115	229	2,257	5,423	7,026	15,050	91	172	2,096	3,806	5,470	11,635	26,684
B. Other neoplasm	11	14	57	54	67	204	10	11	47	46	68	182	386
C. Diabetes mellitus	–	1	190	283	316	792	1	3	161	284	498	947	1,739
D. Nutritional/endocrine	266	152	215	151	202	987	243	139	412	149	254	1,198	2,185
E. Neuro-psychiatric	196	451	5,675	2,427	2,600	11,349	153	356	3,725	1,459	3,268	8,961	20,311
F. Sense organ	6	–	2	18	26	52	5	–	9	35	49	90	142
G. Cardiovascular diseases	117	56	2,978	5,986	12,071	21,207	98	46	1,083	2,529	14,155	17,911	39,118
H. Chronic respiratory diseases	82	176	634	731	1,814	3,437	61	141	515	387	1,167	2,270	5,708
I. Diseases of the digestive system	109	27	1,092	1,367	1,243	3,837	72	22	472	628	1,156	2,350	6,187
J. Diseases of the genito-urinary system	22	12	234	414	703	1,385	15	11	172	204	609	1,010	2,395
K. Skin disease	2	–	10	7	14	34	2	–	9	7	26	44	78
L. Diseases of the musculo-skeletal system	3	82	665	631	348	1,729	2	75	1,770	1,050	692	3,590	5,319
M. Congenital abnormalities	1,892	57	98	16	9	2,072	1,709	53	69	16	11	1,858	3,930
N. Oral health	12	25	572	405	189	1,203	12	31	582	481	314	1,420	2,623
III. Injuries	652	856	10,561	2,201	1,170	15,440	454	398	2,471	702	1,266	5,292	20,732
A. Unintentional	594	769	6,673	1,476	933	10,445	399	346	1,494	435	1,125	3,799	14,244
B. Intentional	58	87	3,888	725	237	4,995	55	52	978	267	142	1,493	6,488
Top three causes in each age group (as percentage):													
STDs excluding HIV infection	0.01	0.01	0.09	–	–	0.04	0.01	0.07	11.59	0.06	0.01	3.09	1.37
Acute lower respiratory infections	6.07	2.10	1.29	1.07	1.84	1.81	5.70	2.78	1.51	1.09	1.82	1.93	1.86
Otitis media	3.62	0.04	0.97	–	–	0.27	4.25	0.05	0.56	–	–	0.33	0.30
Trachea/bronchus/lung	0.01	–	–	7.17	6.35	4.17	–	–	–	3.02	1.96	1.58	3.04
Breast	–	–	–	0.01	0.02	–	–	–	2.73	7.20	2.46	3.14	1.37
Protein-energy malnutrition	2.67	–	–	–	–	0.21	3.21	–	–	–	–	0.27	0.24
Major affective disorder	–	–	2.94	0.79	0.22	1.21	–	–	9.46	1.64	0.29	3.34	2.14
Epilepsy	1.04	9.64	0.92	0.32	0.11	0.75	0.89	9.39	0.93	0.38	0.10	0.66	0.71
Alcohol dependence	–	–	8.12	6.28	1.95	4.78	–	–	1.85	4.55	0.64	0.92	3.10
Alzheimer and other dementias	0.29	0.39	0.10	2.38	5.72	2.55	0.34	0.37	0.10	–	8.72	4.81	3.54
Ischaemic heart disease	0.03	0.05	4.42	15.44	20.15	11.90	0.02	0.03	1.09	7.25	20.41	10.80	11.42
Cerebrovascular disease	0.21	0.52	1.82	5.35	10.01	5.26	0.21	0.60	1.71	6.34	14.51	8.17	6.53
Asthma	0.38	6.92	1.46	0.74	0.33	0.98	0.37	8.11	2.24	1.33	0.46	1.27	1.11
Rheumatoid arthritis	–	–	0.49	0.90	0.27	0.47	–	1.85	5.92	2.55	0.55	2.33	1.28
Motor vehicle accidents	1.29	12.49	11.59	1.98	0.55	4.82	1.09	9.51	5.00	1.32	0.34	2.03	3.60
Homicide and violence	0.90	2.41	7.30	1.01	0.15	2.77	1.08	2.71	3.02	0.70	0.11	1.13	2.05

[a] DALYs are in thousands.
[b] A dash represents less than a thousand DALYs or less than 0.01%.

Annex Table 2. **Total DALYs for major cause groups, by sex and age, 1990: Developing regions** [a, b]

	Males in age group (years):						Females in age group (years):						Both sexes
	0-4	5-14	15-44	45-59	60+	All ages	0-4	5-14	15-44	45-59	60+	All ages	
All Causes	266,770	75,161	159,317	63,478	63,204	627,931	249,637	66,642	157,081	48,273	60,541	582,174	1,210,105
I. Communicable, maternal & perinatal	199,740	39,276	44,695	9,742	5,997	299,450	183,358	38,298	77,895	6,519	5,053	311,122	610,572
A. Infectious & parasitic	99,461	34,104	40,835	8,761	3,455	186,616	94,065	32,551	46,030	5,240	2,281	180,166	366,782
B. Respiratory infections	47,082	5,170	3,860	981	2,542	59,635	46,267	5,290	3,912	1,012	2,772	59,253	118,888
C. Maternal conditions	–	–	–	–	–	–	–	457	27,952	267	–	28,676	28,676
D. Perinatal conditions	53,197	1	–	–	–	53,199	43,026	–	–	–	–	43,027	96,226
II. Noncommunicable	52,351	20,292	59,460	47,834	54,724	234,660	52,059	18,631	59,875	39,169	53,209	222,943	457,604
A. Malignant neoplasms	727	2,545	6,873	10,353	9,152	29,651	1,294	723	7,024	8,341	6,297	23,679	53,330
B. Other neoplasm	94	167	236	145	88	729	151	1,189	297	108	89	1,835	2,564
C. Diabetes mellitus	10	6	701	1,036	927	2,680	11	19	680	1,372	1,466	3,548	6,228
D. Nutritional/endocrine	16,219	1,668	5,665	918	560	25,030	16,169	2,190	5,574	1,195	840	25,969	50,999
E. Neuro-psychiatric	2,773	6,904	19,167	5,488	4,456	38,787	2,673	5,078	18,464	3,398	4,058	33,671	72,458
F. Sense organ	269	40	325	1,946	1,291	3,871	249	74	373	2,277	1,256	4,228	8,098
G. Cardiovascular diseases	2,891	1,691	10,354	15,418	24,822	55,176	2,486	2,524	9,348	12,493	26,775	53,625	108,802
H. Chronic respiratory diseases	4,931	3,042	3,621	2,906	7,393	21,893	5,055	2,127	3,599	2,691	6,334	19,805	41,698
I. Diseases of the digestive system	5,630	1,372	6,335	4,679	3,044	21,049	6,934	1,734	4,226	2,877	2,325	18,095	39,145
J. Diseases of the genito-urinary system	672	1,503	1,797	2,727	1,507	8,207	419	1,254	2,266	1,557	1,512	7,008	15,215
K. Skin disease	116	57	44	23	56	296	119	26	209	17	98	468	764
L. Diseases of the musculo-skeletal system	25	273	1,724	1,336	751	4,110	79	661	4,994	1,928	1,399	9,061	13,171
M. Congenital abnormalities	17,797	765	503	17	10	19,092	16,232	770	774	55	6	17,837	36,929
N. Oral health	193	255	2,119	835	652	4,054	186	245	2,037	855	733	4,056	8,110
III. Injuries	14,679	15,593	55,162	5,902	2,584	93,821	14,220	9,714	19,312	2,585	2,278	48,109	141,930
A. Unintentional	12,440	13,609	32,653	4,153	1,923	64,777	11,621	8,406	10,027	1,664	1,824	22,541	93,318
B. Intentional	2,239	1,985	22,509	1,749	561	29,044	2,599	1,308	9,285	921	454	14,568	43,612
Top three causes in each age group (as percentage):													
Tuberculosis	0.46	4.12	8.27	9.48	4.02	4.15	0.53	5.69	6.92	5.72	1.87	3.42	3.80
STDs excluding HIV infection	0.51	0.03	1.47	0.17	0.01	0.61	0.49	0.06	8.76	0.26	0.02	2.61	1.57
HIV	0.50	0.07	9.25	0.65	0.03	2.64	0.49	0.34	6.55	0.32	–	2.05	2.35
Diarrhoeal diseases	15.77	6.08	1.68	0.65	0.36	7.95	16.28	7.11	1.71	0.88	0.38	8.37	8.15
Childhood cluster	10.66	8.09	0.10	0.09	0.04	5.54	10.70	8.60	0.11	0.13	0.05	5.62	5.58
Intestinal helminths	0.02	11.43	0.30	0.06	0.04	1.46	0.02	12.34	0.29	0.08	0.04	1.51	1.48
Acute lower respiratory infections	16.73	6.50	2.02	1.38	3.93	8.93	17.57	7.54	2.12	1.90	4.48	9.59	9.25
Ischaemic heart disease	0.03	0.07	1.51	7.71	11.67	2.36	0.01	0.04	0.64	4.83	11.48	1.78	2.08
Cerebrovascular disease	0.11	0.41	1.37	6.83	13.74	2.52	0.09	0.60	1.52	8.94	16.40	2.97	2.73
Chronic obstructive lung disease	0.14	0.18	0.25	2.77	9.57	1.39	0.12	0.14	0.25	2.91	8.03	1.21	1.30
Motor vehicle accidents	0.45	4.45	8.12	1.86	0.55	3.03	0.37	3.69	2.11	0.88	0.26	1.25	2.17

[a] DALYs are in thousands.
[b] A dash represents less than a thousand DALYs or less than 0.01%.

Annex Table 3. **Total DALYs for major cause groups, by sex and age, 1990: All regions**[a,b]

	Males in age group (years):						Females in age group (years):						Both sexes
	0-4	5-14	15-44	45-59	60+	All ages	0-4	5-14	15-44	45-59	60+	All ages	
All Causes	73,211	77,474	186,774	84,165	91,782	713,406	254,791	68,262	174,650	60,359	90,335	648,397	1,361,803
I. Communicable, maternal & perinatal	202,693	39,448	46,910	10,312	6,767	306,130	185,584	38,458	81,879	6,820	5,828	318,570	624,700
A. Infectious & parasitic	99,802	34,186	42,525	9,066	3,661	189,241	94,328	32,627	48,529	5,354	2,461	183,299	372,539
B. Respiratory infections	47,711	5,259	4,384	1,246	3,106	61,706	46,783	5,374	4,370	1,189	3,368	61,084	122,790
C. Maternal conditions							457	1	28,980	277	-	29,713	29,713
D. Perinatal conditions	55,180	2	-	-	-	55,183	44,472	1	-	-	-	44,474	99,658
II. Noncommunicable	55,187	21,576	74,141	65,750	81,362	298,016	54,533	19,692	70,988	50,252	80,962	276,426	574,442
A. Malignant neoplasms	843	2,774	9,130	15,777	16,178	44,701	1,385	895	9,119	12,148	11,767	35,314	80,015
B. Other neoplasm	105	181	293	199	155	933	161	1,200	345	153	157	2,017	2,950
C. Diabetes mellitus	11	7	891	1,319	1,243	3,473	12	22	841	1,656	1,964	4,495	7,968
D. Nutritional/endocrine	16,484	1,820	5,880	1,069	762	26,017	16,412	2,329	5,986	1,345	1,094	27,167	53,183
E. Neuro-psychiatric	2,969	7,355	24,842	7,915	7,056	50,137	2,826	5,434	22,189	4,857	7,326	42,632	92,768
F. Sense organ	276	40	327	1,963	1,316	3,923	253	74	374	2,311	1,305	4,318	8,240
G. Cardiovascular diseases	3,008	1,748	13,332	41,403	36,893	76,384	2,584	2,569	10,431	15,022	40,930	71,356	147,920
H. Chronic respiratory diseases	5,014	3,218	4,255	3,637	9,207	25,331	5,115	2,267	4,114	3,078	7,501	22,075	47,406
I. Diseases of the digestive system	5,739	1,399	7,417	6,046	4,286	24,887	7,006	1,756	4,697	3,505	3,481	20,445	45,332
J. Diseases of the genito-urinary system	694	1,515	2,032	3,141	2,210	9,562	434	1,265	2,437	1,761	2,122	8,018	17,610
K. Skin disease	119	58	54	30	69	330	121	26	218	23	124	512	842
L. Diseases of the musculo-skeletal system	28	355	2,389	1,968	1,099	5,839	81	736	6,763	2,979	2,092	12,651	18,490
M. Congenital abnormalities	19,689	822	601	32	19	21,164	17,941	823	843	72	17	19,695	40,859
N. Oral health	205	281	2,691	1,240	841	5,257	197	276	2,620	1,336	1,046	5,476	10,733
III. Injuries	15,331	16,450	65,273	8,103	3,654	109,261	14,674	10,112	21,783	3,287	3,545	53,401	162,662
A. Unintentional	13,034	14,377	39,326	5,629	2,856	75,222	12,020	8,752	11,521	2,099	2,949	37,340	112,562
B. Intentional	2,297	2,072	26,397	2,474	798	34,039	2,655	1,360	10,263	1,188	596	16,061	50,100
Top three causes in each age group (as percentage):													
Tuberculosis	0.45	4.00	7.15	7.31	2.86	3.71	0.52	5.56	6.24	4.62	1.29	3.08	3.41
STDs excluding HIV infection	0.49	0.03	1.27	0.13	0.01	0.54	0.48	0.06	9.05	0.22	0.02	2.66	1.55
HIV	0.50	0.07	8.55	0.62	0.03	2.51	0.50	0.34	6.07	0.28	-	1.89	2.22
Diarrhoeal diseases	15.43	5.93	1.48	0.52	0.27	7.03	15.98	6.97	1.59	0.74	0.28	7.55	7.28
Childhood cluster	10.42	7.89	0.08	0.07	0.03	4.88	10.49	8.44	0.10	0.11	0.03	5.05	4.96
Intestinal helminths	0.01	11.09	0.26	0.05	0.03	1.29	0.02	12.05	0.26	0.07	0.03	1.36	1.32
Acute lower respiratory infections	16.47	6.37	1.92	1.31	3.28	8.08	17.33	7.42	2.06	1.74	3.60	8.81	8.43
Major affective disorder	-	-	2.87	0.85	0.23	0.88	-	-	6.14	2.42	0.57	1.96	1.39
Ischaemic heart disease	0.03	0.07	1.94	9.61	14.31	3.50	0.01	0.04	0.68	5.31	14.43	2.70	3.12
Cerebrovascular disease	0.12	0.41	1.44	6.47	12.58	2.85	0.09	0.60	1.54	8.42	15.78	3.50	3.16
Chronic obstructive lung disease	0.14	0.18	0.23	2.49	7.99	1.46	0.12	0.14	0.24	2.56	6.17	1.22	1.35
Motor vehicle accidents	0.47	4.69	8.63	1.89	0.55	3.24	0.38	3.82	2.40	0.97	0.29	1.33	2.33

[a] DALYs are in thousands.
[b] A dash represents less than a thousand DALYs or less than 0.01%.

Annex Table 4. Disability-adjusted life years (DALYs, in thousands): Established Market Economies

Disease or injury (ICD 9 code)	Both sexes all ages	Males						Females					
		0-4	5-14	15-44	45-59	60+	All ages	0-4	5-14	15-44	45-59	60+	All ages
All Causes	93,919	3,475	1,295	16,127	11,584	19,719	52,200	2,865	944	11,431	7,183	19,296	41,719
I. Communicable, maternal & perinatal (001-139,320-322,460-465,466,480-487,614-616, 630-676,760-779)	9,108	1,500	100	1,674	324	627	4,226	1,168	95	2,768	204	648	4,882
A. Infectious & parasitic dis. (001-139,320-322,614-616)	4,101	128	50	1,333	160	150	1,821	104	48	1,905	77	146	2,280
A1. Tuberculosis (010-018,137)	152	–	2	34	30	40	106	–	–	14	10	20	46
A2. STDs excluding HIV (090-099,614-616)	1,564	–	–	17	1	–	20	–	–	1,535	5	2	1,544
a. Syphilis (090-097)	4	–	–	3	–	–	3	–	–	1	–	–	1
b. Chlamydia	99	–	–	13	–	–	14	–	–	78	5	–	85
c. Gonorrhoea (098)	8	–	–	3	–	–	3	–	–	5	–	–	5
d. Pelvic inflammatory disease (614-616)	1,453	–	–	–	–	–	–	–	–	1,451	–	–	1,453
A3. HIV infection	1,582	29	3	1,105	100	2	1,239	29	3	296	14	1	343
A4. Diarrhoeal diseases (001,002,004,006-009)	234	16	14	60	16	12	117	13	13	57	16	17	116
a. Acute watery	198	14	11	50	13	11	100	12	11	48	13	15	98
b. Persistent	12	1	–	3	–	–	6	–	–	3	–	–	6
c. Dysentery	24	1	–	7	2	1	12	–	–	6	2	2	12
A5. Childhood cluster (032-33,037,045,050,055-56,138)	87	21	23	–	–	–	45	19	22	–	–	–	42
a. Pertussis (133)	72	17	19	–	–	–	37	16	18	–	–	–	35
b. Poliomyelitis (045,138)	–	–	–	–	–	–	–	–	–	–	–	–	–
c. Diphtheria (032)	4	1	1	–	–	–	2	1	1	–	–	–	2
d. Measles (055)	10	3	2	–	–	–	5	3	2	–	–	–	5
e. Tetanus (037)	1	–	–	–	–	–	–	–	–	–	–	–	1
A6. Meningitis (036,320-322)	106	35	4	13	5	4	60	26	5	8	3	4	46
A7. Hepatitis (070)	65	1	1	18	11	9	40	1	1	10	5	8	25
A8. Malaria (084)	2	–	–	–	–	–	–	–	–	–	–	–	–
A9. Tropical cluster (085,086,120,125)	2	–	–	–	–	–	–	–	–	–	–	–	–
a. African trypanosomiasis (086.3,086.4,086.5)	–	–	–	–	–	–	–	–	–	–	–	–	–
b. Chagas disease (086.0,086.1,086.2)	–	–	–	–	–	–	–	–	–	–	–	–	–
c. Schistosomiasis (120)	–	–	–	–	–	–	–	–	–	–	–	–	–
d. Leishmaniasis (085)	1	–	–	–	–	–	–	–	–	–	–	–	–
e. Lymphatic filariasis (125.0, 125.1)	–	–	–	–	–	–	–	–	–	–	–	–	–
f. Onchocerciasis (125.3)	–	–	–	–	–	–	–	–	–	–	–	–	–
A10. Leprosy (030)	–	–	–	–	–	–	–	–	–	–	–	–	–
A11. Trachoma (076)	–	–	–	–	–	–	–	–	–	–	–	–	–
A12. Intestinal helminths (126-129)	–	–	–	–	–	–	–	–	–	–	–	–	–
a. Ascaris (127.0)	–	–	–	–	–	–	–	–	–	–	–	–	–
b. Trichuris (127.3)	–	–	–	–	–	–	–	–	–	–	–	–	–
c. Hookworm (126)	–	–	–	–	–	–	–	–	–	–	–	–	–
B. Respiratory infections (381-382,460-466,480-487)	2,416	216	50	341	164	477	1,247	185	46	315	122	501	1,170
B1. Acute lower respiratory inf. (460-465)	1,695	69	23	221	133	449	895	46	21	180	90	463	800
B2. Acute upper respiratory inf. (466,480-487)	439	2	27	120	31	28	207	1	26	136	31	38	232
B3. Otitis media (381-382)	283	146	–	–	–	–	146	137	–	–	–	–	137
C. Maternal conditions (630-676)	553	–	–	–	–	–	–	–	–	548	5	–	553
C1. Haemorrhage (666,667)	92	–	–	–	–	–	–	–	–	91	1	–	92
C2. Sepsis (670)	200	–	–	–	–	–	–	–	–	198	2	–	200
C3. Eclampsia (642.4-642.6)	7	–	–	–	–	–	–	–	–	7	–	–	7
C4. Hypertension (642 minus 642.4-642.6)	2	–	–	–	–	–	–	–	–	2	–	–	2
C5. Obstructed labour (660)	229	–	–	–	–	–	–	–	–	227	2	–	229
C6. Abortion (630-639)	13	–	–	–	–	–	–	–	–	13	–	–	13
D. Perinatal causes (760-779)	2,038	1,156	1	1	–	–	1,158	879	1	–	–	–	880

Annex Table 4. **Disability-adjusted life years (DALYs, in thousands): Established Market Economies**

Disease or injury (ICD 9 code)	Both sexes all ages	Males						Females					
		0-4	5-14	15-44	45-59	60+	All ages	0-4	5-14	15-44	45-59	60+	All ages
II. *Noncommunicable* (140-628,680-759) (minus 320-322,460-465,466,480-487, 614-616)	73,714	1,655	798	9,007	10,311	18,314	40,084	1,472	646	7,136	6,624	17,752	33,630
A. Malignant neoplasms (140-208)	18,019	54	122	1,370	3,247	5,229	10,022	45	96	1,367	2,514	3,976	7,997
A1. Mouth and oropharynx (140-149)	422	-	-	50	159	118	328	-	-	15	34	44	94
A2. Oesophagus (150)	353	-	-	23	124	137	284	-	-	4	21	44	69
A3. Stomach (151)	1,129	-	-	74	239	385	698	-	-	70	117	244	431
A4. Colorectal (152,153,154)	1,963	-	-	92	327	604	1,024	-	-	80	263	596	939
A5. Liver (155)	334	1	-	23	108	118	252	-	-	8	23	50	82
A6. Pancreas (157)	587	-	-	30	116	181	328	-	-	17	70	172	259
A7. Lung (162)	3,070	-	-	146	799	1,294	2,241	-	-	45	287	472	829
A8. Melanoma and other skin (172-173)	267	-	-	55	50	46	151	-	-	45	35	36	117
A9. Breast (174)	1,566	-	-	-	-	-	-	-	-	351	636	579	1,566
A10. Cervix (180)	235	-	-	-	-	-	-	-	-	97	78	60	235
A11. Corpus uteri (179,181-182)	227	-	-	-	-	-	-	-	-	24	81	122	227
A12. Ovary (183)	396	-	-	-	-	-	-	-	-	64	157	174	396
A13. Prostate (185)	667	-	-	4	80	583	667	-	-	-	-	-	-
A14. Bladder (188)	439	-	-	14	89	229	332	-	-	5	23	78	106
A15. Lymphoma (200-202)	833	3	10	146	137	182	478	1	5	82	92	175	355
A16. Leukemia (204-208)	612	11	35	125	68	110	350	10	24	84	54	90	262
B. Other neoplasm (210-239)	280	6	9	39	38	58	150	6	7	30	29	57	130
C. Diabetes mellitus (250)	1,331	-	-	140	218	260	619	-	2	116	208	385	712
D. Nutritional/endocrine (240-285, minus 250)	1,572	163	74	148	127	188	699	150	65	307	121	229	872
D1. Protein-energy malnutrition (260-263)	245	113	-	2	2	7	124	108	-	1	1	11	122
D2. Iodine deficiency (243)	-	-	-	-	-	-	-	-	-	-	-	-	-
D3. Vitamin A deficiency (264)	-	-	-	-	-	-	-	-	-	-	-	-	-
D4. Anaemias (280-285)	610	6	42	67	57	50	222	6	40	216	57	69	388
E. Neuro-psychiatric (290-359, minus 320-322)	14,038	117	298	3,891	1,599	1,926	7,832	90	228	2,529	986	2,374	6,207
E1. Major affective disorder	2,108	-	-	528	109	44	680	-	-	1,073	231	123	1,428
E2. Bipolar affective disorder (296)	115	-	-	45	8	3	56	-	-	45	9	5	59
E3. Psychoses (295, 291-294,297-299)	620	-	-	309	9	16	335	-	-	262	3	20	286
E4. Epilepsy (345)	695	43	144	160	44	23	413	30	98	102	30	22	281
E5. Alcohol dependence (303)	2,822	-	-	1,332	781	337	2,450	-	-	197	121	54	372
E6. Alzheimer & other dementias (330,331,333-336,290)	3,989	15	7	24	364	1,262	1,672	15	5	15	392	1,890	2,316
E7. Parkinson disease (332)	351	-	-	-	49	112	161	-	-	-	53	137	190
E8. Multiple sclerosis (340)	214	-	-	82	12	6	100	-	-	86	18	11	114
E9. Drug dependence (304)	1,576	-	55	962	133	34	1,183	-	14	322	48	9	393
E10. Post-traumatic stress disorder	720	-	46	190	24	6	271	-	75	314	39	13	449
F. Sense organ (360-389)	86	5	-	2	12	13	31	-	-	-	23	29	56
F1. Glaucoma-related blindness (365)	47	-	-	-	8	3	11	-	-	-	19	17	36
F2. Cataract-related blindness (366)	28	-	-	-	3	10	13	-	-	-	4	11	15
G. Cardiovascular diseases (390-459)	22,058	80	38	1,480	3,019	7,561	12,179	66	31	642	1,202	7,938	9,879
G1. Rheumatic heart disease (390-398)	138	-	-	12	15	22	49	-	-	13	24	51	89
G2. Ischaemic heart disease (*)	9,362	2	1	474	1,528	3,639	5,643	1	6	95	413	3,208	3,718
G3. Cerebrovascular disease (430-438)	4,974	10	8	248	447	1,601	2,314	8	5	178	292	2,176	2,660
G4. Inflammatory cardiac disease (+)	658	10	5	122	108	163	408	11	6	42	43	149	249
H. Chronic respiratory dis. (460-519, minus 460-466,480-487)	3,633	57	118	410	333	1,212	2,131	42	93	353	245	770	1,502
H1. Chronic obstructive lung dis. (490-492,495,496)	1,596	3	2	19	139	865	1,028	2	1	10	84	470	567
H2. Asthma (493)	1,138	16	106	278	95	65	561	13	86	274	109	95	577

Annex Table 4. Disability-adjusted life years (DALYs, in thousands): Established Market Economies

Disease or injury (ICD 9 code)	Both sexes all ages	Males 0-4	5-14	15-44	45-59	60+	All ages	Females 0-4	5-14	15-44	45-59	60+	All ages
I. Diseases of the digestive system (520-579)	3,880	40	14	634	826	876	2,390	27	11	291	362	798	1,490
I1. Peptic ulcer disease (531-533)	444	-	2	115	83	68	268	-	1	68	47	59	176
I2. Cirrhosis of the liver (571)	1,685	1	-	307	506	358	1,174	-	-	113	184	213	512
J. Genito-urinary (580-629)	1,470	15	3	85	227	520	849	10	3	59	81	467	621
J1. Nephritis/nephrosis (580-589)	874	12	2	62	78	292	446	8	2	36	54	327	427
J2. Benign prostatic hypertrophy (600)	252	-	-	-	124	128	252	-	-	-	-	-	-
K. Skin disease (680-709)	49	-	-	4	3	12	20	-	-	4	3	22	29
L. Musculo-skeletal system (710-739)	3,896	1	78	520	509	333	1,442	1	71	1,174	682	526	2,454
L1. Rheumatoid arthritis (714)	1,372	-	-	80	86	73	240	-	30	720	247	135	1,132
L2. Osteoarthritis (715)	2,239	-	76	416	403	217	1,112	-	37	391	399	300	1,127
M. Congenital abnormalities (740-759)	2,356	1,116	30	67	12	8	1,233	1,029	27	47	12	10	1,124
N. Oral health (520-529)	1,017	2	13	216	138	107	476	2	12	215	153	160	541
N1. Dental caries (521.0)	73	2	13	16	3	3	37	2	12	15	3	4	37
N2. Periodontal disease (523)	53	-	-	24	2	1	27	-	-	23	2	2	26
N3. Edentulism (520)	891	-	-	176	134	103	413	-	-	176	148	154	478
III. Injuries (E800-999)	11,096	319	397	5,446	950	778	7,890	225	203	1,527	354	897	3,207
A. Unintentional (E800-949)	7,375	274	344	3,237	594	635	5,084	182	170	911	208	819	2,291
A1. Road traffic accidents (E810-819, 826-829)	3,319	51	165	1,883	205	100	2,403	37	91	628	96	63	915
A2. Poisoning (E850-869)	272	3	3	169	22	7	204	2	2	48	10	6	68
A3. Falls (E850-869)	1,531	21	22	261	128	359	791	14	9	47	34	636	740
A4. Fires (E890-899)	517	63	41	149	38	31	323	48	34	63	19	30	194
A5. Drowning (E910)	270	34	36	116	20	12	217	18	8	16	5	6	53
A6. Occupational (#)	198	-	-	126	41	3	170	-	-	19	8	-	28
B. Intentional (E950-969,990-999)	3,722	45	53	2,209	356	143	2,806	43	33	616	146	78	916
B1. Self-inflicted (E950-959)	1,947	-	13	1,064	262	122	1,461	-	4	304	113	64	485
B2. Homicide and violence (E960-969)	1,774	45	39	1,144	93	21	1,343	43	29	312	33	14	431
B3. War (E990-999)	1	-	-	-	-	-	1	-	-	-	-	-	-
Population (in millions)	797.8	26.4	53.3	184.1	66.1	60.5	390.5	25.1	50.7	179.2	67.8	84.6	407.3

Notes

A dash (-) symbol indicates less than 1,000 DALYs.

* ICD 9 codes for ischaemic heart disease are as follows: 410-414, 440.9, plus: at ages 45-59: 50% of 427.1, 427.4, 427.5, and 33% of 428; at ages 60+: 80% of 427.1, 427.4, 427.5 and 50% of 428.

+ ICD 9 codes for inflammatory cardiac diseases are as follows: 420, 421, 422, 425 plus: at ages 0-44: 50% of 428; at ages 45-59: 25% of 428; at ages 60+: 20% of 428.

There are no established ICD 9 codes specific for occupational injuries.
  Estimates have been based on reported occupational injuries and deaths tabulated by the International Labour Organisation.

Annex Table 5. **Disability-adjusted life years (DALYs, in thousands): Formerly Socialist Economies of Europe**

Disease or injury (ICD 9 code)	Both sexes all ages	Males 0-4	5-14	15-44	45-59	60+	All ages	Females 0-4	5-14	15-44	45-59	60+	All ages
All Causes	57,779	2,966	1,018	11,330	9,102	8,859	33,275	2,289	676	6,138	4,903	10,498	24,504
I. Communicable, maternal & perinatal (001-139,320-322,460-465,466,480-487,614-616, 630-676,760-779)	5,020	1,453	72	541	246	143	2,454	1,059	66	1,217	97	128	2,566
A. Infectious & parasitic dis. (001-139,320-322,614-616)	1,656	213	32	357	145	56	803	160	28	594	37	33	853
A1. Tuberculosis (010-018,137)	361	2	–	156	109	40	308	1	1	22	14	14	53
A2. STDs excluding HIV (090-099,614-616)	514	–	–	9	–	–	10	–	2	502	2	–	504
a. Syphilis (090-097)	33	–	–	7	–	–	7	–	–	24	1	–	26
b. Chlamydia	3	–	–	1	–	–	1	–	–	2	–	–	2
c. Gonorrhoea (098)	476	–	–	–	–	–	–	–	–	476	–	–	476
d. Pelvic inflammatory disease (614-616)	20	–	–	–	–	–	–	–	–	18	2	–	20
A3. HIV infection	156	–	–	129	6	1	136	–	–	18	2	–	20
A4. Diarrhoeal diseases (001,002,004,006-009)	220	69	8	26	7	4	114	59	8	25	7	7	106
a. Acute watery	198	65	7	22	6	3	103	56	6	21	6	6	95
b. Persistent	10	3	–	1	–	–	5	2	–	1	–	–	5
c. Dysentery	12	1	–	3	–	–	6	1	–	3	–	–	6
A5. Childhood cluster (032-33,037,045,050,055-56,138)	47	11	12	1	–	–	25	10	11	1	–	–	22
a. Pertussis (133)	36	9	10	–	–	–	19	9	9	–	–	–	18
b. Poliomyelitis (045,138)	1	–	–	–	–	–	–	–	–	–	–	–	1
c. Diphtheria (032)	3	–	1	1	–	–	2	–	1	–	–	–	1
d. Measles (055)	5	2	1	–	–	–	3	2	–	–	–	–	2
e. Tetanus (037)	2	–	–	1	–	–	1	1	–	–	–	–	1
A6. Meningitis (036,320-322)	140	56	4	14	8	3	84	39	3	7	4	3	56
A7. Hepatitis (070)	41	7	2	7	3	3	22	6	1	8	2	2	19
A8. Malaria (084)	–	–	–	–	–	–	–	–	–	–	–	–	–
A9. Tropical cluster (085,086,120,125)	–	–	–	–	–	–	–	–	–	–	–	–	–
a. African trypanosomiasis (086.3,086.4,086.5)	–	–	–	–	–	–	–	–	–	–	–	–	–
b. Chagas disease (086.0,086.1,086.2)	–	–	–	–	–	–	–	–	–	–	–	–	–
c. Schistosomiasis (120)	–	–	–	–	–	–	–	–	–	–	–	–	–
d. Leishmaniasis (085)	–	–	–	–	–	–	–	–	–	–	–	–	–
e. Lymphatic filariasis (125.0, 125.1)	–	–	–	–	–	–	–	–	–	–	–	–	–
f. Onchocerciasis (125.3)	–	–	–	–	–	–	–	–	–	–	–	–	–
A10. Leprosy (030)	–	–	–	–	–	–	–	–	–	–	–	–	–
A11. Trachoma (076)	–	–	–	–	–	–	–	–	–	–	–	–	–
A12. Intestinal helminths (126-129)	–	–	–	–	–	–	–	–	–	–	–	–	–
a. Ascaris (127.0)	–	–	–	–	–	–	–	–	–	–	–	–	–
b. Trichuris (127.3)	–	–	–	–	–	–	–	–	–	–	–	–	–
c. Hookworm (126)	–	–	–	–	–	–	–	–	–	–	–	–	–
B. Respiratory infections (381-382,460-466,480-487)	1,486	413	40	184	101	87	824	331	38	143	56	94	662
B1. Acute lower respiratory inf. (460-465)	1,127	323	26	134	88	78	648	248	24	86	42	79	478
B2. Acute upper respiratory inf. (466,480-487)	190	2	14	50	13	9	88	2	13	57	14	16	102
B3. Otitis media (381-382)	169	88	–	–	–	–	88	81	–	–	–	–	81
C. Maternal conditions (630-676)	484	–	–	–	–	–	–	–	–	480	4	–	484
C1. Haemorrhage (666,667)	46	–	–	–	–	–	–	–	–	46	–	–	46
C2. Sepsis (670)	152	–	–	–	–	–	–	–	–	151	1	–	152
C3. Eclampsia (642.4-642.6)	3	–	–	–	–	–	–	–	–	3	–	–	3
C4. Hypertension (642 minus 642.4-642.6)	6	–	–	–	–	–	–	–	–	6	–	–	6
C5. Obstructed labour (660)	203	–	–	–	–	–	–	–	–	201	2	–	203
C6. Abortion (630-639)	44	–	–	–	–	–	–	–	–	43	–	–	44
D. Perinatal causes (760-779)	1,394	827	–	–	–	–	827	567	–	–	–	–	567

Annex Table 5. Disability-adjusted life years (DALYs, in thousands): Formerly Socialist Economies of Europe

Disease or injury (ICD 9 code)	Both sexes all ages	Males 0-4	Males 5-14	Males 15-44	Males 45-59	Males 60+	Males All ages	Females 0-4	Females 5-14	Females 15-44	Females 45-59	Females 60+	Females All ages
II. Noncommunicable (140-628,680-759) (minus 320-322,460-465,466,480-487, 614-616)	43,124	1,181	486	5,674	7,605	8,325	23,271	1,002	415	3,977	4,458	10,001	19,853
A. Malignant neoplasms (140-208)	8,665	62	107	886	2,177	1,797	5,028	46	76	729	1,292	1,494	3,637
A1. Mouth and oropharynx (140-149)	246			39	115	53	209			7	13	16	37
A2. Oesophagus (150)	156			12	69	46	127			2	9	18	29
A3. Stomach (151)	1,027			91	294	255	640			58	128	201	387
A4. Colorectal (152,153,154)	696			48	130	163	341			42	120	192	354
A5. Liver (155)	64			5	14	17	36			3	9	16	28
A6. Pancreas (157)	103			10	25	27	62			4	13	24	41
A7. Lung (162)	1,541			119	683	520	1,324			28	78	111	217
A8. Melanoma and other skin (172-173)	96			19	17	13	49			18	14	15	48
A9. Breast (174)	517									129	234	154	517
A10. Cervix (180)	202									64	74	64	202
A11. Corpus uteri (179,181-182)	57									8	24	25	57
A12. Ovary (183)	157									28	66	63	157
A13. Prostate (185)	114			3	24	86	114						
A14. Bladder (188)	238	3	2	16	71	87	179	2		6	19	32	60
A15. Lymphoma (200-202)	263	5	15	63	45	31	158	3	6	39	27	30	105
A16. Leukemia (204-208)	303	14	31	59	35	33	172	10	21	42	28	30	131
B. Other neoplasm (210-239)	106	5	5	18	16	9	54	4	4	17	16	11	52
C. Diabetes mellitus (250)	408			51	65	56	173		1	45	76	113	235
D. Nutritional/endocrine (240-285, minus 250)	613	103	79	68	24	14	288	93	75	104	28	25	325
D1. Protein-energy malnutrition (260-263)	117	59					59	57					57
D2. Iodine deficiency (243)	1												
D3. Vitamin A deficiency (264)													
D4. Anaemias (280-285)	306	7	70	40	10	6	132	6	67	81	10	10	174
E. Neuro-psychiatric (290-359, minus 320-322)	6,272	79	153	1,784	828	674	3,518	63	128	1,196	473	894	2,754
E1. Major affective disorder (296)	1,140			280	55	19	353			589	131	67	787
E2. Bipolar affective disorder (296)	69			25	4	1	31			26	5	7	38
E3. Psychoses (295, 291-294,297-299)	262			130	8	3	141			112	5	5	121
E4. Epilepsy (345)	382	24	79	93	23	8	226	16	55	60	16	9	156
E5. Alcohol dependence (303)	1,875			898	519	219	1,637			128	77	33	238
E6. Alzheimer & other dementias (330,331,333-336,290)	1,383	3	2	4	129	374	511	3	1	3	158	707	872
E7. Parkinson disease (332)	137				24	30	54				29	54	83
E8. Multiple sclerosis (340)	105			40	7	2	49			44	9	3	56
E9. Drug dependence (304)	238		9	144	21	5	179		2	48	7	1	59
E10. Post-traumatic stress disorder	314	3	24	79	10	2	117	4	39	131	17	5	197
F. Sense organ (360-389)	56	3			5	12	21	2			11	21	35
F1. Glaucoma-related blindness (365)	21				2	4	7				7	7	14
F2. Cataract-related blindness (366)	28				3	8	11				4	13	18
G. Cardiovascular diseases (390-459)	17,060	36	18	1,498	2,966	4,510	9,028	32	14	441	1,326	6,217	8,032
G1. Rheumatic heart disease (390-398)	343		2	66	67	23	158		2	43	89	51	185
G2. Ischaemic heart disease (*)	7,959			740	1,666	2,119	4,524			97	464	2,874	3,435
G3. Cerebrovascular disease (430-438)	4,928	4	4	252	659	1,260	2,179	3	3	122	474	2,147	2,749
G4. Inflammatory cardiac disease (+)	360	4	2	73	65	84	228	6	2	22	28	75	132
H. Chronic respiratory dis. (460-519, minus 460-466,480-487)	2,075	25	58	223	398	602	1,307	19	48	162	142	397	768
H1. Chronic obstructive lung dis. (490-492,495-496)	948	1		17	199	423	641			6	56	244	307
H2. Asthma (493)	540	8	54	123	58	29	273	7	45	119	52	44	267

Annex Table 5. **Disability-adjusted life years (DALYs, in thousands): Formerly Socialist Economies of Europe**

Disease or injury (ICD 9 code)	Both sexes all ages	Males						Females					
		0-4	5-14	15-44	45-59	60+	All ages	0-4	5-14	15-44	45-59	60+	All ages
I. Diseases of the digestive system (520-579)	2,307	70	13	457	541	367	1,448	45	11	180	265	358	859
I1. Peptic ulcer disease (531-533)	267	-	1	75	69	39	184	-	-	32	26	24	83
I2. Cirrhosis of the liver (571)	472	1	-	100	146	86	333	1	-	33	54	50	139
J. Genito-urinary (580-629)	925	7	9	150	187	183	536	5	7	112	122	143	389
J1. Nephritis/nephrosis (580-589)	439	3	6	108	73	54	244	3	5	70	57	59	194
J2. Benign prostatic hypertrophy (600)	134	-	-	-	64	69	134	-	-	-	-	-	-
K. Skin disease (680-709)	28	2	-	6	4	2	14	2	-	5	3	4	14
L. Musculo-skeletal system (710-739)	1,423	2	4	144	122	15	287	1	4	595	368	167	1,136
L1. Rheumatoid arthritis (714)	572	-	-	56	100	5	161	-	-	320	61	30	412
L2. Osteoarthritis (715)	721	-	-	68	10	3	81	-	-	242	280	118	640
M. Congenital abnormalities (740-759)	1,574	776	27	31	4	1	840	680	27	21	4	1	734
N. Oral health (520-529)	1,606	10	13	357	266	82	728	10	19	368	328	154	878
N1. Dental caries (521.0)	146	10	13	27	11	6	68	10	19	27	13	11	79
N2. Periodontal disease (523)	36	-	-	15	2	-	18	-	-	15	2	2	18
N3. Edentulism (520)	1,424	-	-	315	253	75	642	-	-	326	314	142	781
III. Injuries (E800-999)	9,635	333	460	5,115	1,251	392	7,550	229	195	945	347	370	2,085
A. Unintentional (E800-949)	6,869	320	425	3,436	882	298	5,361	216	176	583	227	306	1,508
A1. Road traffic accidents (E810-819, 826-829)	2,149	33	124	1,300	204	56	1,717	19	63	250	63	37	432
A2. Poisoning (E850-869)	849	32	16	403	186	32	670	22	12	75	50	19	179
A3. Falls (E850-869)	849	27	40	296	102	104	569	18	15	43	23	181	280
A4. Fires (E890-899)	374	40	21	140	46	15	262	33	14	33	14	19	112
A5. Drowning (E910)	569	32	89	302	51	11	485	13	30	28	8	5	84
A6. Occupational (#)	316	-	-	207	65	2	274	-	-	29	12	-	41
B. Intentional (E950-969,990-999)	2,766	13	35	1,679	369	94	2,189	12	19	362	121	63	577
B1. Self-inflicted (E950-959)	1,424	-	18	820	253	73	1,164	-	4	143	69	44	259
B2. Homicide and violence (E960-969)	1,342	13	16	859	117	20	1,025	12	15	219	52	20	318
B3. War (E990-999)	-	-	-	-	-	-	-	-	-	-	-	-	-
Population (in millions)	346.2	13.8	27.3	76.3	27.0	21.0	165.3	13.1	26.4	75.0	30.0	36.4	180.9

Notes

A dash (-) symbol indicates less than 1,000 DALYs.

* ICD 9 codes for ischaemic heart disease are as follows: 410-414, 440.9, plus: at ages 45-59: 50% of 427.1, 427.4, 427.5, and 33% of 428; at ages 60+: 80% of 427.1, 427.4, 427.5 and 50% of 428.

+ ICD 9 codes for inflammatory cardiac diseases are as follows: 420, 421, 422, 425 plus: at ages 0-44: 50% of 428; at ages 45-59: 25% of 428; at ages 60+: 20% of 428.

There are no established ICD 9 codes specific for occupational injuries.

Estimates have been based on reported occupational injuries and deaths tabulated by the International Labour Organisation.

Annex Table 6. Disability-adjusted life years (DALYs, in thousands): India

Disease or injury (ICD 9 code)	Both sexes all ages	Males 0-4	Males 5-14	Males 15-44	Males 45-59	Males 60+	Males All ages	Females 0-4	Females 5-14	Females 15-44	Females 45-59	Females 60+	Females All ages
All Causes	292,646	66,901	15,919	31,563	16,102	14,969	145,454	69,699	16,564	35,580	11,939	13,409	147,191
I. Communicable, maternal & perinatal (001-139,320-322,460-465,466,480-487,614-616, 630-676,760-779)	148,277	48,927	7,360	10,094	2,864	1,526	70,771	49,010	8,294	17,257	1,837	1,107	77,506
A. Infectious & parasitic dis. (001-139,320-322,614-616)	82,028	22,655	6,071	8,877	2,524	695	40,822	24,165	6,652	8,625	1,398	366	41,206
A1. Tuberculosis (010-018,137)	10,800	244	582	3,256	1,694	506	6,282	399	969	2,270	729	152	4,518
A2. STDs excluding HIV (090-099,614-616)	3,734	114	3	386	25	2	530	121	6	3,046	28	2	3,203
a. Syphilis (090-097)	808	114	3	327	23	1	468	121	2	198	19	1	340
b. Chlamydia	326	-	-	55	2	-	58	-	3	253	10	-	268
c. Gonorrhoea (098)	16	-	-	4	-	-	5	-	-	11	-	-	12
d. Pelvic inflammatory disease (614-616)	2,584	-	-	-	-	-	-	-	-	2,584	-	-	2,584
A3. HIV infection	4,066	12	9	2,567	112	7	2,707	14	15	1,314	14	1	1,358
A4. Diarrhoeal diseases (001,002,004,006-009)	28,037	11,586	1,129	804	102	21	13,643	12,268	1,305	688	113	20	14,394
a. Acute watery	15,390	5,913	856	638	76	16	7,498	6,260	988	545	84	15	7,892
b. Persistent	8,273	3,967	48	-	-	-	4,015	4,201	57	-	-	-	4,258
c. Dysentery	4,374	1,706	225	167	26	6	2,130	1,806	260	143	29	5	2,244
A5. Childhood cluster (032-33,037,045,050,055-56,138)	19,453	7,738	1,751	56	26	9	9,579	8,059	1,726	52	29	8	9,874
a. Pertussis (133)	2,950	1,189	236	-	-	-	1,425	1,255	270	-	-	-	1,525
b. Poliomyelitis (045,138)	1,835	362	725	-	-	-	1,087	246	502	-	-	-	748
c. Diphtheria (032)	108	20	28	-	-	-	48	17	38	-	-	-	60
d. Measles (055)	9,336	3,873	618	-	-	-	4,491	4,102	744	-	-	-	4,846
e. Tetanus (037)	5,224	2,293	145	56	26	9	2,528	2,440	172	47	29	8	2,696
A6. Meningitis (036,320-322)	2,006	589	370	178	40	13	1,191	516	168	116	12	5	815
A7. Hepatitis (070)	311	35	63	31	12	3	143	37	74	40	14	3	168
A8. Malaria (084)	951	59	151	219	39	8	476	62	175	187	43	8	475
A9. Tropical cluster (085,086,120,125)	2,425	90	447	725	166	30	1,459	67	355	280	234	30	966
a. African trypanosomiasis (086.3,086.4,086.5)	-	-	-	-	-	-	-	-	-	-	-	-	-
b. Chagas disease (086.0,086.1,086.2)	-	-	-	-	-	-	-	-	-	-	-	-	-
c. Schistosomiasis (120)	251	-	-	156	-	-	166	-	-	-	-	-	85
d. Leishmaniasis (085)	1,732	90	447	451	17	4	1,010	67	355	279	19	3	723
e. Lymphatic filariasis (125.0, 125.1)	442	-	-	118	149	17	284	-	-	-	131	27	158
f. Onchocerciasis (125.3)	-	-	-	-	-	-	-	-	-	-	-	-	-
A10. Leprosy (030)	521	33	209	14	3	-	259	31	216	13	1	-	262
A11. Trachoma (076)	309	-	-	49	33	30	112	-	-	89	15	93	197
A12. Intestinal helminths (126-129)	2,056	5	866	161	15	9	1,056	5	826	145	15	8	1,000
a. Ascaris (127.0)	1,166	5	589	2	-	-	597	5	562	2	-	-	569
b. Trichuris (127.3)	486	-	246	2	-	-	249	-	235	2	-	-	237
c. Hookworm (126)	404	-	31	157	14	9	211	-	29	142	14	8	194
B. Respiratory infections (381-382,460-466,480-487)	31,754	11,891	1,289	1,218	340	831	15,568	12,556	1,485	1,041	363	741	16,186
B1. Acute lower respiratory inf. (460-465)	30,133	11,351	1,217	1,042	308	816	14,734	12,020	1,420	896	338	726	15,399
B2. Acute upper respiratory inf. (466,480-487)	598	26	72	176	32	15	320	27	66	145	26	15	278
B3. Otitis media (381-382)	1,023	514	-	-	-	-	514	509	-	-	-	-	509
C. Maternal conditions (630-676)	7,824	-	-	-	-	-	-	-	156	7,592	76	-	7,824
C1. Haemorrhage (666,667)	1,365	-	-	-	-	-	-	-	47	1,305	13	-	1,365
C2. Sepsis (670)	2,752	-	-	-	-	-	-	-	31	2,693	27	-	2,752
C3. Eclampsia (642.4-642.6)	394	-	-	-	-	-	-	-	16	374	4	-	394
C4. Hypertension (642 minus 642.4-642.6)	191	-	-	-	-	-	-	-	8	182	2	-	191
C5. Obstructed labour (660)	1,941	-	-	-	-	-	-	-	16	1,906	19	-	1,941
C6. Abortion (630-639)	946	-	-	-	-	-	-	-	31	906	9	-	946
D. Perinatal causes (760-779)	26,671	14,381	-	-	-	-	14,381	12,290	-	-	-	-	12,290

Annex Table 6. **Disability-adjusted life years (DALYs, in thousands): India**

Disease or injury (ICD 9 code)	Both sexes all ages	Males						Females					
		0–4	5–14	15–44	45–59	60+	All ages	0–4	5–14	15–44	45–59	60+	All ages
II. Noncommunicable (140–628,680–759) (minus 320–322,460–465,466,480–487, 614–616)	117,642	15,202	4,700	14,701	12,226	13,080	59,908	17,525	5,002	13,567	9,589	12,051	57,734
A. Malignant neoplasms (140–208)	12,041	147	472	1,340	2,547	2,126	6,633	483	69	1,468	2,103	1,286	5,409
A1. Mouth and oropharynx (140–149)	1,908	3	9	226	385	658	1,280	13	2	131	202	280	627
A2. Oesophagus (150)	857			57	218	230	504			58	152	142	353
A3. Stomach (151)	713		1	86	202	181	471			52	103	87	242
A4. Colorectal (152,153,154)	445			71	65	117	253	2		48	47	95	192
A5. Liver (155)	220	1	4	22	76	52	156	4		14	23	22	64
A6. Pancreas (157)	124			11	32	35	78			8	18	19	46
A7. Lung (162)	561		1	65	207	200	474	2		13	32	39	86
A8. Melanoma and other skin (172–173)	18			2	4	3	10			2	4	2	8
A9. Breast (174)	609									217	260	131	609
A10. Cervix (180)	958									292	477	189	958
A11. Corpus uteri (179,181–182)	46									5	19	22	46
A12. Ovary (183)	206							4		93	62	47	206
A13. Prostate (185)	194				39	153	194						
A14. Bladder (188)	107			9	25	50	85	2		2	6	12	22
A15. Lymphoma (200–202)	447	23	75	98	42	70	308	25	5	34	23	53	140
A16. Leukemia (204–208)	557	41	133	87	22	41	325	121	18	55	14	24	233
B. Other neoplasm (210–239)	801	21	38	73	46	21	198	58	413	86	27	18	602
C. Diabetes mellitus (250)	1,868			218	312	308	840			188	397	442	1,028
D. Nutritional/endocrine (240–285, minus 250)	18,265	5,699	579	2,376	346	183	9,183	5,867	711	1,776	455	274	9,082
D1. Protein-energy malnutrition (260–263)	5,552	2,531	32	45	9	11	2,629	2,803	63	29	5	25	2,923
D2. Iodine deficiency (243)	1,398	641	25	34	8	4	713	613	31	34	4	3	685
D3. Vitamin A deficiency (264)	4,109	2,085					2,085	2,024					2,024
D4. Anaemias (280–285)	4,469	252	506	895	216	102	1,971	214	712	1,182	252	138	2,497
E. Neuro-psychiatric (290–359, minus 320–322)	17,837	823	1,730	4,511	1,331	1,032	9,426	1,085	1,450	4,350	726	799	8,411
E1. Major affective disorder	3,089			916	118	33	1,066			1,733	228	62	2,023
E2. Bipolar affective disorder (296)	208			94	11	3	107			87	10	3	101
E3. Psychoses (295, 291–294,297–299)	2,132		2	937	36	21	995		3	1,108	8	18	1,137
E4. Epilepsy (345)	2,280	190	628	394	90	29	1,331	155	434	303	40	17	949
E5. Alcohol dependence (303)	1,904			932	514	218	1,664			133	75	32	240
E6. Alzheimer & other dementias (330,331,333–336,290)	1,951	61	62	31	257	569	981	109	46	27	230	558	970
E7. Parkinson disease (332)	148				31	50	82				27	38	66
E8. Multiple sclerosis (340)	266		1	100	25	9	136		2	102	16	9	129
E9. Drug dependence (304)	647		24	394	49	12	479		8	140	16	3	168
E10. Post-traumatic stress disorder	838	12	88	207	17	3	327	19	141	321	26	4	511
F. Sense organ (360–389)	2,384	62	10	120	624	422	1,238	82	18	97	570	378	1,146
F1. Glaucoma-related blindness (365)	398			19	165	48	232				118	48	166
F2. Cataract-related blindness (366)	1,813	10		91	458	374	932	9		90	452	330	880
G. Cardiovascular diseases (390–459)	28,592	682	335	2,540	4,351	6,825	14,732	876	714	1,957	3,194	7,120	13,860
G1. Rheumatic heart disease (390–398)	1,874	14	86	190	152	160	602	24	110	285	395	459	1,272
G2. Ischaemic heart disease (*)	8,142	3	2	543	1,725	2,680	4,953	3	2	162	729	2,293	3,189
G3. Cerebrovascular disease (430–438)	6,248	58	47	352	663	1,632	2,752	69	93	462	784	2,088	3,496
G4. Inflammatory cardiac disease (+)	6,791	374	142	985	1,025	1,099	3,625	560	359	617	656	974	3,166
H. Chronic respiratory dis. (460–519, minus 460–466,480–487)	7,906	1,365	636	668	479	753	3,900	1,815	462	779	486	464	4,006
H1. Chronic obstructive lung dis. (490–492,495–496)	1,702	108	38	50	237	541	974	115	32	48	237	296	728
H2. Asthma (493)	1,719	77	337	316	84	36	850	81	266	366	112	44	869

Annex Table 6. **Disability-adjusted life years (DALYs, in thousands): India**

Disease or injury (ICD 9 code)	Both sexes all ages	Males 0-4	5-14	15-44	45-59	60+	All ages	Females 0-4	5-14	15-44	45-59	60+	All ages
I. Diseases of the digestive system (520-579)	11,240	1,619	281	1,657	1,298	751	5,607	2,822	496	1,096	742	478	5,634
I1. Peptic ulcer disease (531-533)	992	5	12	329	207	85	637	7	12	180	107	50	355
I2. Cirrhosis of the liver (571)	2,690	32	25	691	765	335	1,848	48	50	315	297	132	842
J. Genito-urinary (580-629)	3,932	195	375	307	606	401	1,884	139	393	568	484	464	2,048
J1. Nephritis/nephrosis (580-589)	2,101	61	337	226	222	196	1,041	43	361	307	177	172	1,060
J2. Benign prostatic hypertrophy (600)	371	-	-	-	296	74	371	-	-	-	-	-	-
K. Skin disease (680-709)	247	37	9	14	4	14	77	50	8	74	2	36	170
L. Musculo-skeletal system (710-739)	1,253	7	41	188	89	80	405	28	66	429	197	129	849
L1. Rheumatoid arthritis (714)	216	-	-	87	10	6	102	-	-	81	26	6	113
L2. Osteoarthritis (715)	432	-	-	57	52	14	122	-	-	166	116	28	310
M. Congenital abnormalities (740-759)	9,434	4,524	159	153	3	4	4,843	4,198	162	209	19	2	4,590
N. Oral health (520-529)	1,813	20	34	535	187	157	934	19	32	489	185	155	879
N1. Dental caries (521.0)	324	20	34	69	25	19	167	19	32	63	24	18	157
N2. Periodontal disease (523)	1,104	-	-	466	75	33	574	-	-	426	73	32	530
N3. Edentulism (520)	384	-	-	-	87	106	192	-	-	-	87	105	192
III. Injuries (E800-999)	26,727	2,773	3,859	6,768	1,013	363	14,775	3,164	3,268	4,756	513	251	11,952
A. Unintentional (E800-949)	23,134	2,696	3,679	5,038	892	336	12,640	3,138	3,113	3,560	456	228	10,494
A1. Road traffic accidents (E810-819, 826-829)	3,252	205	355	1,492	193	62	2,308	204	347	332	40	22	945
A2. Poisoning (E850-869)	288	50	34	104	19	4	211	27	31	17	-	-	77
A3. Falls (E850-869)	4,996	914	833	811	242	85	2,887	1,148	590	173	109	89	2,109
A4. Fires (E890-899)	1,557	508	125	47	18	13	710	292	365	178	6	7	847
A5. Drowning (E910)	1,729	182	380	292	31	11	897	217	302	273	31	10	832
A6. Occupational (#)	893	-	-	418	84	4	506	-	-	340	45	2	387
B. Intentional (E950-969,990-999)	3,593	77	180	1,730	121	27	2,136	26	155	1,196	57	23	1,457
B1. Self-inflicted (E950-959)	2,189	-	116	915	63	16	1,111	-	144	900	28	6	1,078
B2. Homicide and violence (E960-969)	1,105	52	47	661	51	10	821	-	-	243	25	16	285
B3. War (E990-999)	299	26	17	153	7	-	204	26	11	53	4	-	95
Population (in millions)	849.5	59.8	101.8	200.5	47.6	29.8	439.4	56.7	95.3	183.2	46.0	28.9	410.1

Notes

A dash (-) symbol indicates less than 1,000 DALYs.

* ICD 9 codes for ischaemic heart disease are as follows: 410-414, 440.9, plus: at ages 45-59: 50% of 427.1, 427.4, 427.5, and 33% of 428; at ages 60+: 80% of 427.1, 427.4, 427.5 and 50% of 428.

+ ICD 9 codes for inflammatory cardiac diseases are as follows: 420, 421, 422, 425 plus: at ages 0-44: 50% of 428; at ages 45-59: 25% of 428; at ages 60+: 20% of 428.

There are no established ICD 9 codes specific for occupational injuries.

Estimates have been based on reported occupational injuries and deaths tabulated by the International Labour Organisation.

Annex Table 7. Disability-adjusted life years (DALYs, in thousands): China

Disease or injury (ICD 9 code)	Both sexes all ages	Males						Females					
		0–4	5–14	15–44	45–59	60+	All ages	0–4	5–14	15–44	45–59	60+	All ages
All Causes	201,267	23,580	8,807	31,256	17,121	22,698	103,461	26,012	7,403	31,705	12,061	20,623	97,805
I. Communicable, maternal & perinatal (001–139,320–322,460–465,466,480–487,614–616, 630–676,760–779)	50,868	11,981	4,071	3,701	1,661	1,354	22,767	13,491	3,776	8,628	1,083	1,122	28,101
A. Infectious & parasitic dis. (001–139,320–322,614–616)	24,991	2,125	3,812	3,198	1,511	1,080	11,727	2,267	3,549	5,727	926	795	13,264
A1. Tuberculosis (010–018,137)	5,914	134	121	1,414	1,014	787	3,469	144	187	1,163	512	439	2,445
A2. STDs excluding HIV (090–099,614–616)	3,410	7	–	67	2	–	78	–	3	3,318	10	2	3,333
a. Syphilis (090–097)	12	7	–	–	–	–	8	–	–	5	–	–	5
b. Chlamydia (098)	367	–	–	56	2	–	58	–	2	294	10	2	308
c. Gonorrhoea (098)	27	–	–	11	–	–	11	–	–	15	–	–	15
d. Pelvic inflammatory disease (614–616)	3,004	–	–	–	–	–	–	–	–	3,004	–	–	3,004
A3. HIV infection	3	–	–	2	–	–	3	–	–	–	–	–	–
A4. Diarrhoeal diseases (001,002,004,006–009)	4,241	790	205	797	145	137	2,074	1,014	187	714	125	127	2,167
a. Acute watery	2,816	402	158	629	114	103	1,407	514	145	561	98	92	1,409
b. Persistent	628	268	4	–	–	–	272	346	4	3	–	3	357
c. Dysentery	797	121	43	30	10	33	395	154	39	151	26	32	402
A5. Childhood cluster (032–33,037,045,050,055–56,138)	1,743	691	200	168	25	4	930	616	163	23	7	4	813
a. Pertussis (133)	557	225	59	25	–	–	283	217	57	–	–	–	274
b. Poliomyelitis (045,138)	229	48	85	2	2	–	136	39	53	–	–	–	93
c. Diphtheria (032)	5	1	–	–	–	–	2	–	1	–	–	–	2
d. Measles (055)	299	133	19	–	–	–	152	129	19	–	–	–	147
e. Tetanus (037)	653	285	36	8	3	–	357	230	33	22	7	3	296
A6. Meningitis (036,320–322)	680	244	77	15	8	3	402	154	30	70	14	11	278
A7. Hepatitis (070)	661	64	7	58	119	36	446	53	19	75	24	45	216
A8. Malaria (084)	13	–	–	9	–	–	10	–	–	2	–	–	3
A9. Tropical cluster (085,086,120,125)	606	29	202	87	52	9	379	19	121	50	28	9	227
a. African trypanosomiasis (086.3,086.4,086.5)	–	–	–	–	–	–	–	–	–	–	–	–	–
b. Chagas disease (086.0,086.1,086.2)	–	–	–	–	–	–	–	–	–	–	–	–	–
c. Schistosomiasis (120)	429	16	177	67	13	2	275	10	105	38	–	–	154
d. Leishmaniasis (085)	–	–	–	–	–	–	–	–	–	–	–	–	–
e. Lymphatic filariasis (125.0, 125.1)	96	13	25	20	–	–	58	9	16	11	–	–	37
f. Onchocerciasis (125.3)	81	–	–	–	38	7	46	–	–	–	28	8	36
A10. Leprosy (030)	4	–	–	–	–	–	–	–	–	–	–	–	–
A11. Trachoma (076)	472	–	–	39	36	40	115	–	–	110	149	98	357
A12. Intestinal helminths (126–129)	6,313	16	3,116	109	9	6	3,257	16	2,925	100	9	6	3,056
a. Ascaris (127.0)	3,862	16	1,967	10	1	–	1,995	16	1,841	9	–	–	1,868
b. Trichuris (127.3)	2,253	–	1,142	15	2	–	1,160	–	1,077	14	1	–	1,093
c. Hookworm (126)	197	–	7	84	6	5	102	–	7	77	6	5	95
B. Respiratory infections (381–382,460–466,480–487)	12,904	4,816	258	503	150	274	6,001	5,784	228	450	114	327	6,903
B1. Acute lower respiratory inf. (460–465)	11,317	4,287	212	337	122	257	5,214	5,223	184	296	89	310	6,103
B2. Acute upper respiratory inf. (466,480–487)	550	25	46	166	28	16	281	30	43	154	25	18	269
B3. Otitis media (381–382)	1,037	505	–	–	–	–	505	532	–	–	–	–	532
C. Maternal conditions (630–676)	2,495	–	–	–	–	–	–	–	–	2,452	43	–	2,495
C1. Haemorrhage (666,667)	640	–	–	–	–	–	–	–	–	625	15	–	640
C2. Sepsis (670)	632	–	–	–	–	–	–	–	–	625	7	–	632
C3. Eclampsia (642.4–642.6)	71	–	–	–	–	–	–	–	–	69	2	–	71
C4. Hypertension (642 minus 642.4–642.6)	26	–	–	–	–	–	–	–	–	25	–	–	26
C5. Obstructed labour (660)	786	–	–	–	–	–	–	–	–	778	8	–	786
C6. Abortion (630–639)	93	–	–	–	–	–	–	–	–	90	3	–	93
D. Perinatal causes (760–779)	10,479	5,039	–	–	–	–	5,039	5,439	–	–	–	–	5,439

Annex Table 7. **Disability-adjusted life years (DALYs, in thousands): China**

Disease or injury (ICD 9 code)	Both sexes all ages	Males 0-4	Males 5-14	Males 15-44	Males 45-59	Males 60+	Males All ages	Females 0-4	Females 5-14	Females 15-44	Females 45-59	Females 60+	Females All ages
II. *Noncommunicable* (140-628,680-759) (minus 320-322,460-465,466,480-487, 614-616)	116,774	7,664	2,590	16,508	13,906	20,259	60,928	8,368	2,141	17,008	9,979	18,350	55,846
A. Malignant neoplasms (140-208)	18,605	205	481	3,322	3,831	3,511	11,350	286	262	2,209	2,268	2,230	7,255
A1. Mouth and oropharynx (140-149)	560	7	8	162	117	83	376	-	-	78	63	43	185
A2. Oesophagus (150)	1,702	6	-	167	452	543	1,168	-	-	40	187	307	535
A3. Stomach (151)	3,092	-	-	259	816	903	1,985	-	8	285	346	468	1,107
A4. Colorectal (152,153,154)	969	-	-	184	168	178	531	-	9	119	148	163	439
A5. Liver (155)	3,638	6	24	1,088	1,057	564	2,739	16	-	270	338	274	899
A6. Pancreas (157)	295	-	-	40	63	82	185	-	-	11	32	67	110
A7. Lung (162)	1,960	6	15	143	508	685	1,358	-	-	72	240	290	602
A8. Melanoma and other skin (172-173)	15	-	-	3	3	3	9	-	-	2	2	2	6
A9. Breast (174)	397	-	-	-	-	-	-	-	-	175	143	79	397
A10. Cervix (180)	313	-	-	-	-	-	-	-	-	83	127	94	313
A11. Corpus uteri (179,181-182)	91	-	-	-	-	-	-	-	-	20	52	19	91
A12. Ovary (183)	178	-	-	-	-	-	-	-	-	83	55	29	178
A13. Prostate (185)	35	-	-	-	8	27	35	-	-	-	-	-	-
A14. Bladder (188)	183	-	-	22	41	78	142	-	-	4	10	27	41
A15. Lymphoma (200-202)	374	-	32	111	61	53	258	-	-	42	48	25	116
A16. Leukemia (204-208)	1,525	90	192	406	88	38	814	96	101	390	82	43	711
B. Other neoplasm (210-239)	346	32	16	72	35	29	184	31	26	52	23	30	162
C. Diabetes mellitus (250)	766	6	-	111	127	111	355	8	9	97	137	160	411
D. Nutritional/endocrine (240-285, minus 250)	6,644	1,595	264	606	190	123	2,778	2,044	311	1,178	166	168	3,867
D1. Protein-energy malnutrition (260-263)	1,657	616	8	12	5	11	651	948	7	21	3	27	1,006
D2. Iodine deficiency (243)	984	393	28	62	9	5	497	390	26	58	8	4	487
D3. Vitamin A deficiency (264)	989	494	-	-	-	-	494	495	-	-	-	-	495
D4. Anaemias (280-285)	2,678	79	201	494	156	87	1,017	186	242	984	143	106	1,661
E. Neuro-psychiatric (290-359, minus 320-322)	16,008	259	564	4,822	1,234	1,273	8,151	200	426	4,976	935	1,322	7,857
E1. Major affective disorder	4,843	-	-	1,414	182	53	1,648	-	-	2,747	334	114	3,195
E2. Bipolar affective disorder (296)	321	-	-	144	15	4	164	-	-	138	15	5	158
E3. Psychoses (295, 291-294,297-299)	1,803	-	-	997	11	13	1,021	-	-	757	14	10	782
E4. Epilepsy (345)	1,703	133	371	434	55	24	1,017	91	240	291	42	21	685
E5. Alcohol dependence (303)	1,898	-	-	929	513	217	1,659	-	-	133	74	32	239
E6. Alzheimer & other dementias (330,331,333-336,290)	2,609	11	6	29	341	861	1,248	11	3	22	330	996	1,361
E7. Parkinson disease (332)	191	-	-	-	40	54	94	-	-	-	38	58	97
E8. Multiple sclerosis (340)	317	-	-	138	6	4	148	-	-	146	15	8	169
E9. Drug dependence (304)	296	-	-	195	26	4	225	-	-	62	6	1	72
E10. Post-traumatic stress disorder	1,138	12	8	316	-	5	443	-	-	498	37	8	695
F. Sense organ (360-389)	1,655	62	-	58	374	261	754	19	-	-	496	239	901
F1. Glaucoma-related blindness (365)	484	-	-	-	95	50	145	-	-	32	234	72	338
F2. Cataract-related blindness (366)	763	10	-	25	214	153	403	12	-	25	209	114	360
G. Cardiovascular diseases (390-459)	28,369	496	219	2,712	3,916	7,593	14,936	341	129	2,596	3,068	7,299	13,434
G1. Rheumatic heart disease (390-398)	2,126	-	42	499	184	182	907	24	42	587	296	270	1,219
G2. Ischaemic heart disease (*)	4,246	53	34	616	657	1,123	2,482	28	11	298	308	1,118	1,764
G3. Cerebrovascular disease (430-438)	12,653	84	82	901	1,904	3,869	6,840	66	32	691	1,450	3,575	5,813
G4. Inflammatory cardiac disease (+)	956	50	12	126	135	194	517	45	8	128	96	162	439
H. Chronic respiratory dis. (460-519, minus 460-466,480-487)	18,224	730	466	1,453	1,602	5,393	9,644	978	368	1,185	1,160	4,888	8,580
H1. Chronic obstructive lung dis. (490-492,495-496)	11,168	52	4	256	1,151	4,618	6,081	58	3	269	789	3,967	5,087
H2. Asthma (493)	3,532	112	432	928	223	130	1,824	102	347	828	234	197	1,708

Annex Table 7. **Disability-adjusted life years (DALYs, in thousands): China**

Disease or injury (ICD 9 code)	Both sexes all ages	Males 0-4	5-14	15-44	45-59	60+	All ages	Females 0-4	5-14	15-44	45-59	60+	All ages
I. Diseases of the digestive system (520-579)	8,870	993	236	1,618	1,174	1,013	5,034	1,152	225	921	712	827	3,836
I1. Peptic ulcer disease (531-533)	1,124	13	35	295	216	172	731	24	1	204	77	87	393
I2. Cirrhosis of the liver (571)	3,207	54	28	889	722	511	2,205	17	28	285	344	328	1,002
J. Genito-urinary (580-629)	3,452	71	104	850	737	411	2,172	77	69	629	225	281	1,280
J1. Nephritis/nephrosis (580-589)	2,591	52	104	814	241	269	1,479	77	69	582	174	210	1,111
J2. Benign prostatic hypertrophy (600)	540	-	-	8	453	73	540	-	-	-	-	-	-
K. Skin disease (680-709)	146	6	23	10	11	20	77	15	-	36	6	12	69
L. Musculo-skeletal system (710-739)	5,340	13	31	430	522	352	1,335	16	104	2,542	637	706	4,005
L1. Rheumatoid arthritis (714)	754	-	-	124	83	23	230	-	86	264	126	49	524
L2. Osteoarthritis (715)	3,962	-	-	251	407	190	848	-	-	2,112	456	546	3,114
M. Congenital abnormalities (740-759)	7,032	3,128	173	189	5	-	3,495	3,103	183	246	6	-	3,537
N. Oral health (520-529)	1,297	75	13	254	147	163	653	72	12	236	139	185	644
N1. Dental caries (521.0)	231	75	13	17	9	4	118	72	12	16	8	4	113
N2. Periodontal disease (523)	512	-	-	237	19	9	265	72	12	220	17	9	247
N3. Edentulism (520)	554	-	-	-	119	150	269	-	-	-	114	171	285
III. Injuries (E800-999)	33,624	3,934	2,146	11,047	1,554	1,085	19,766	4,153	1,486	6,069	1,000	1,150	13,858
A. Unintentional (E800-949)	23,321	3,528	1,960	7,495	1,078	779	14,841	3,399	1,288	2,378	552	862	8,480
A1. Road traffic accidents (E810-819, 826-829)	4,533	158	316	2,428	293	107	3,302	109	250	687	134	51	1,231
A2. Poisoning (E850-869)	1,459	177	66	380	130	46	799	55	93	439	35	37	660
A3. Falls (E880-888)	4,264	500	219	1,045	222	355	2,341	761	185	221	175	581	1,923
A4. Fires (E890-899)	1,371	282	80	337	42	66	807	198	118	132	43	73	564
A5. Drowning (E910)	4,417	1,020	835	802	64	38	2,758	865	415	311	32	35	1,659
A6. Occupational (#)	612	-	-	423	73	4	500	-	-	87	23	1	111
B. Intentional (E950-969,990-999)	10,303	406	186	3,552	477	306	4,926	754	197	3,691	448	288	5,378
B1. Self-inflicted (E950-959)	6,982	-	91	2,220	393	277	2,981	-	67	3,285	393	256	4,001
B2. Homicide and violence (E960-969)	3,321	406	95	1,332	84	29	1,945	754	130	406	55	32	1,377
B3. War (E990-999)	-	-	-	-	-	-	-	-	-	-	-	-	-
Population (in millions)	1,133.7	60.2	97.0	306.3	72.7	49.0	585.2	57.9	90.4	284.1	64.4	51.7	548.5

Notes

A dash (-) symbol indicates less than 1,000 DALYs.

* ICD 9 codes for ischaemic heart disease are as follows: 410-414, 440.9, plus: at ages 45-59: 50% of 427.1, 427.4, 427.5, and 33% of 428; at ages 60+: 80% of 427.1, 427.4, 427.5 and 50% of 428.

+ ICD 9 codes for inflammatory cardiac diseases are as follows: 420, 421, 422, 425 plus: at ages 0-44: 50% of 428; at ages 45-59: 25% of 428; at ages 60+: 20% of 428.

There are no established ICD 9 codes specific for occupational injuries.
 Estimates have been based on reported occupational injuries and deaths tabulated by the International Labour Organisation.

Annex Table 8. **Disability-adjusted life years (DALYs, in thousands): Other Asia and Islands**

Disease or injury (ICD 9 code)	Both sexes all ages	Males						Females					
		0-4	5-14	15-44	45-59	60+	All ages	0-4	5-14	15-44	45-59	60+	All ages
All Causes	176,423	36,589	14,957	24,519	9,929	8,963	94,958	30,211	11,646	22,666	7,882	9,060	81,465
I. Communicable, maternal & perinatal (001-139,320-322,460-465,466,480-487,614-616, 630-676,760-779)	85,654	27,467	8,114	5,395	1,631	1,090	43,697	22,274	7,083	10,579	1,032	989	41,957
A. Infectious & parasitic dis. (001-139,320-322,614-616)	48,594	12,064	6,984	4,685	1,461	543	25,737	10,075	6,002	5,616	817	347	22,857
A1. Tuberculosis (010-018,137)	8,935	207	768	2,572	1,170	449	5,165	180	749	2,149	503	189	3,771
A2. STDs excluding HIV (090-099,614-616)	1,328	2		58	2		63	2	4	1,251	8		1,265
a. Syphilis (090-097)	12	2		4			7	2		3			5
b. Chlamydia	276			43	1		45		3	219	7		231
c. Gonorrhoea (098)	29			11			12			16			17
d. Pelvic inflammatory disease (614-616)	1,012									1,012			1,012
A3. HIV infection	1,287	6	2	757	32	3	801	6		471	4		486
A4. Diarrhoeal diseases (001,002,004,006-009)	14,737	6,624	819	340	54	16	7,852	5,723	719	366	57	19	6,885
a. Acute watery	8,020	3,280	647	278	42	12	4,259	2,835	568	299	45	15	3,761
b. Persistent	4,416	2,337	32				2,369	2,019	28				2,047
c. Dysentery	2,301	1,006	140	63	12	4	1,224	869	124	67	12	4	1,077
A5. Childhood cluster (032-33,037,045,050,055-56,138)	7,989	3,533	773	17	7		4,334	2,986	636	21	7	5	3,655
a. Pertussis (133)	1,267	564	144				709	442	117				559
b. Poliomyelitis (045,138)	410	74	171				244	50	116				166
c. Diphtheria (032)	44	9	13				22	6	14	2			22
d. Measles (055)	4,161	1,871	360				2,230	1,616	315				1,931
e. Tetanus (037)	2,106	1,016	85	17	7	4	1,130	871	74	19	7	5	977
A6. Meningitis (036,320-322)	1,380	412	514	29	6	4	965	243	115	51	3	3	415
A7. Hepatitis (070)	282	31	72	24	8	3	138	27	63	41	9	5	144
A8. Malaria (084)	2,539	176	569	455	71	21	1,292	154	498	494	75	25	1,247
A9. Tropical cluster (085,086,120,125)	294	6	71	93	38	2	210	3	37	17	21	5	84
a. African trypanosomiasis (086.3,086.4,086.5)													
b. Chagas disease (086.0,086.1,086.2)													
c. Schistosomiasis (120)	105	4	52	13	1		71	2	25	7			35
d. Leishmaniasis (085)	78	2	19	32	8		54	1	11	10	3		24
e. Lymphatic filariasis (125.0, 125.1)	111			48	37	1	86				20	5	25
f. Onchocerciasis (125.3)													
A10. Leprosy (030)	161	8	61	11	1		81	8	59	12	1		80
A11. Trachoma (076)	931			177	37	21	235			523	98	74	695
A12. Intestinal helminths (126-129)	5,809		2,836	98	8		2,957	9	2,730	100	8	5	2,852
a. Ascaris (127.0)	3,207	10	1,621	3			1,634	9	1,560	3			1,573
b. Trichuris (127.3)	2,359	10	1,195	5			1,202	9	1,150	6			1,157
c. Hookworm (126)	243		20	90	6	4	121		20	91	7	5	122
B. Respiratory infections (381-382,460-466,480-487)	19,640	7,788	1,130	710	170	547	10,341	6,751	994	731	178	642	9,296
B1. Acute lower respiratory inf. (460-465)	18,471	7,409	1,070	570	150	537	9,737	6,401	939	605	159	630	8,734
B2. Acute upper respiratory inf. (466,480-487)	474	17	59	140	20	10	246	15	55	126	19	12	227
B3. Otitis media (381-382)	696	361					361	335					335
C. Maternal conditions (630-676)	4,357									4,233	37		4,357
C1. Haemorrhage (666,667)	749									717	6		749
C2. Sepsis (670)	1,581								18	1,549	14		1,581
C3. Eclampsia (642.4-642.6)	204									194	1		204
C4. Hypertension (642 minus 642.4-642.6)	254								11	241	2		254
C5. Obstructed labour (660)	1,017								9	999	9		1,017
C6. Abortion (630-639)	264								4	257	2		264
D. Perinatal causes (760-779)	13,062	7,615					7,615	5,447					5,447

Annex Table 8. Disability-adjusted life years (DALYs, in thousands): Other Asia and Islands

Disease or injury (ICD 9 code)	Both sexes all ages	Males						Females					
		0-4	5-14	15-44	45-59	60+	All ages	0-4	5-14	15-44	45-59	60+	All ages
II. Noncommunicable (140-628,680-759)	70,760	7,441	4,277	9,408	7,239	7,511	35,877	6,614	3,603	10,277	6,574	7,816	34,883
(minus 320-322,460-465,466,480-487, 614-616)													
A. Malignant neoplasms (140-208)	7,876	90	531	768	1,467	1,314	4,169	135	93	1,181	1,386	912	3,707
A1. Mouth and oropharynx (140-149)	629	2	12	75	90	197	376	3	2	76	54	118	254
A2. Oesophagus (150)	198	-	1	11	57	63	131	-	-	10	29	29	67
A3. Stomach (151)	540	-	1	51	144	138	334	1	-	48	79	79	207
A4. Colorectal (152,153,154)	380	-	4	40	42	101	188	-	-	50	50	90	192
A5. Liver (155)	659	3	15	100	230	134	481	3	2	40	70	64	178
A6. Pancreas (157)	83	-	-	8	19	24	50	-	-	4	13	16	33
A7. Lung (162)	744	-	5	50	227	265	547	1	-	28	76	91	197
A8. Melanoma and other skin (172-173)	24	-	-	3	4	3	10	-	-	4	5	5	15
A9. Breast (174)	396									154	171	70	396
A10. Cervix (180)	470									158	232	81	470
A11. Corpus uteri (179,181-182)	44									8	20	15	44
A12. Ovary (183)	157							4	3	83	45	23	157
A13. Prostate (185)	91			1	14	73	91						
A14. Bladder (188)	93			6	22	40	67			4	7	16	26
A15. Lymphoma (200-202)	289	9	54	47	27	44	182	6	4	39	20	38	107
A16. Leukemia (204-208)	430	25	147	58	14	24	268	34	24	66	16	22	162
B. Other neoplasm (210-239)	475	10	36	30	22	12	111	16	264	55	17	13	364
C. Diabetes mellitus (250)	1,147			106	187	166	460			122	276	289	687
D. Nutritional/endocrine (240-285, minus 250)	8,149	2,472	247	1,079	145	81	4,024	2,281	374	1,139	202	130	4,125
D1. Protein-energy malnutrition (260-263)	930	409	51	17	5	6	488	372	41	14	3	12	442
D2. Iodine deficiency (243)	1,284	577	34	29	6	3	648	568	29	29	6	3	636
D3. Vitamin A deficiency (264)	2,509	1,287					1,287	1,221					1,221
D4. Anaemias (280-285)	2,334	115	240	476	78	38	947	65	357	806	101	58	1,387
E. Neuro-psychiatric (290-359, minus 320-322)	12,475	440	1,605	3,073	876	714	6,707	357	1,061	3,092	578	681	5,768
E1. Major affective disorder	2,629			745	87	23	855			1,540	184	51	1,774
E2. Bipolar affective disorder (296)	174			76	8	2	86			77	8	2	88
E3. Psychoses (295, 291-294,297-299)	896			457	11	4	472		11	401	8	3	424
E4. Epilepsy (345)	1,689	129	539	250	55	19	992	90	347	214	32	14	697
E5. Alcohol dependence (303)	1,075			520	293	125	938			75	43	19	136
E6. Alzheimer & other dementias (330,331,333-336,290)	1,413	30	60	15	182	397	685	30	32	16	185	465	728
E7. Parkinson disease (332)	114				22	36	59				22	33	55
E8. Multiple sclerosis (340)	203		1	75	14	6	96			85	13	7	107
E9. Drug dependence (304)	915		36	548	77	19	682		10	192	27	5	234
E10. Post-traumatic stress disorder	697	8	73	166	12	2	262	14	118	280	20	3	436
F. Sense organ (360-389)	1,333	34	10	44	307	189	585	31	12	66	460	179	748
F1. Glaucoma-related blindness (365)	420			16	90	23	128			35	225	32	292
F2. Cataract-related blindness (366)	839	11		25	217	166	419	12		28	234	146	420
G. Cardiovascular diseases (390-459)	17,267	396	395	1,675	2,374	3,713	8,554	292	596	1,566	1,970	4,290	8,714
G1. Rheumatic heart disease (390-398)	592	4	50	83	32	30	200	5	59	132	102	94	392
G2. Ischaemic heart disease (*)	6,209	3	6	591	1,177	1,767	3,543	2	4	246	624	1,790	2,666
G3. Cerebrovascular disease (430-438)	3,789	37	58	207	421	891	1,614	21	96	330	541	1,188	2,175
G4. Inflammatory cardiac disease (+)	1,900	114	119	305	209	212	959	114	183	258	168	219	941
H. Chronic respiratory dis. (460-519, minus 460-466,480-487)	4,033	569	590	403	229	384	2,174	447	377	497	246	293	1,859
H1. Chronic obstructive lung dis. (490-492,495-496)	848	42	31	23	105	276	478	26	18	26	114	186	370
H2. Asthma (493)	1,447	67	346	261	54	21	749	56	262	289	65	26	698

Annex Table 8. **Disability-adjusted life years (DALYs, in thousands): Other Asia and Islands**

Disease or injury (ICD 9 code)	Both sexes all ages	Males 0-4	Males 5-14	Males 15-44	Males 45-59	Males 60+	Males All ages	Females 0-4	Females 5-14	Females 15-44	Females 45-59	Females 60+	Females All ages
I. Diseases of the digestive system (520-579)	5,572	728	284	884	731	441	3,068	705	339	697	440	323	2,504
I1. Peptic ulcer disease (531-533)	477	2	7	138	96	45	288	2	7	94	55	31	189
I2. Cirrhosis of the liver (571)	1,628	15	25	424	439	191	1,094	12	35	215	185	89	534
J. Genito-urinary (580-629)	2,393	90	361	170	388	229	1,238	38	264	331	265	257	1,155
J1. Nephritis/nephrosis (580-589)	1,419	30	325	130	120	124	728	14	241	193	117	124	691
J2. Benign prostatic hypertrophy (600)	265	-	-	-	226	39	265	-	-	-	-	-	-
K. Skin disease (680-709)	115	17	8	5	3	7	40	13	5	36	2	18	74
L. Musculo-skeletal system (710-739)	2,802	3	41	648	302	101	1,095	8	46	903	503	246	1,707
L1. Rheumatoid arthritis (714)	261	-	-	68	23	8	98	-	-	68	75	20	163
L2. Osteoarthritis (715)	2,172	-	-	561	265	59	886	-	-	721	394	171	1,286
M. Congenital abnormalities (740-759)	5,330	2,576	146	51	2	2	2,777	2,278	147	117	10	1	2,553
N. Oral health (520-529)	1,777	15	21	471	205	156	868	14	20	473	220	181	909
N1. Dental caries (521.0)	255	15	21	55	26	11	128	14	20	55	27	12	128
N2. Periodontal disease (523)	518	-	-	208	36	15	258	-	-	206	37	17	260
N3. Edentulism (520)	1,004	-	-	209	143	130	482	-	-	212	157	153	521
III. Injuries (E800-999)	20,009	1,682	2,566	9,715	1,059	362	15,384	1,323	960	1,810	276	255	4,625
A. Unintentional (E800-949)	14,401	1,521	2,298	6,058	756	291	10,924	1,155	833	1,077	192	220	3,477
A1. Road traffic accidents (E810-819, 826-829)	4,106	159	535	2,316	196	52	3,259	108	233	433	51	24	847
A2. Poisoning (E850-869)	521	53	38	242	49	10	392	33	25	57	10	5	129
A3. Falls (E850-869)	2,832	343	456	981	203	122	2,105	287	156	101	47	136	727
A4. Fires (E890-899)	800	204	113	157	24	11	509	141	83	51	8	8	291
A5. Drowning (E910)	1,351	183	405	426	31	9	1,054	117	110	57	8	4	297
A6. Occupational (#)	459	-	-	335	55	2	392	-	-	55	12	-	67
B. Intentional (E950-969,990-999)	5,608	161	268	3,658	303	71	4,460	168	127	733	84	35	1,148
B1. Self-inflicted (E950-959)	1,933	-	72	1,215	154	48	1,489	-	25	346	50	23	444
B2. Homicide and violence (E960-969)	3,285	128	173	2,245	140	22	2,709	135	87	314	29	11	576
B3. War (E990-999)	390	32	23	197	9	1	263	33	15	73	6	1	128
Population (in millions)	682.5	43.8	84.0	160.8	34.1	20.2	343.0	42.0	80.2	159.6	35.1	22.7	339.6

Notes

A dash (-) symbol indicates less than 1,000 DALYs.

* ICD 9 codes for ischaemic heart disease are as follows: 410-414, 440.9, plus: at ages 45-59: 50% of 427.1, 427.4, 427.5, and 33% of 428; at ages 60+: 80% of 427.1, 427.4, 427.5 and 50% of 428.

+ ICD 9 codes for inflammatory cardiac diseases are as follows: 420, 421, 422, 425 plus: at ages 0-44: 50% of 428; at ages 45-59: 25% of 428; at ages 60+: 20% of 428.

There are no established ICD 9 codes specific for occupational injuries.

‡ Estimates have been based on reported occupational injuries and deaths tabulated by the International Labour Organisation.

Annex Table 9. Disability-adjusted life years (DALYs, in thousands): Sub-Saharan Africa

Disease or injury (ICD 9 code)	Both sexes all ages	Males 0-4	5-14	15-44	45-59	60+	All ages	Females 0-4	5-14	15-44	45-59	60+	All ages
All Causes	292,632	83,665	19,717	36,499	7,763	5,204	152,848	73,167	17,466	35,897	6,977	6,277	139,784
I. Communicable, maternal & perinatal (001-139,320-322,460-465,466,480-487,614-616, 630-676,760-779)	208,744	70,741	13,063	17,689	2,155	1,133	104,781	61,714	12,515	27,155	1,565	1,015	103,964
A. Infectious & parasitic dis. (001-139,320-322,614-616)	148,231	45,183	11,645	16,951	2,016	672	76,467	40,555	10,890	18,553	1,337	427	71,764
A1. Tuberculosis (010-018,137)	13,673	442	1,154	4,039	1,327	503	7,464	405	1,321	3,582	674	227	6,209
A2. STDs excluding HIV (090-099,614-616)	7,465	1,172	20	1,622	68	6	2,888	1,055	24	3,426	67	6	4,578
a. Syphilis (090-097)	5,111	1,109	18	1,522	66	6	2,720	1,012	14	1,298	62	5	2,391
b. Chlamydia	183			28			29		2	147	5		154
c. Gonorrhoea (098)	299	63	1	73			138	43	7	110			161
d. Pelvic inflammatory disease (614-616)	1,872									1,872			1,872
A3. HIV infection	18,360	1,255	34	7,918	157	9	9,374	1,158	198	7,525	101	2	8,985
A4. Diarrhoeal diseases (001,002,004,006-009)	30,356	13,940	1,415	329	38	11	15,733	12,723	1,474	368	45	14	14,624
a. Acute watery	16,292	7,032	1,079	261	30	9	8,411	6,419	1,124	291	36	11	7,881
b. Persistent	9,341	4,819	60				4,880	4,398	63				4,461
c. Dysentery	4,723	2,088	275	68	8	3	2,442	1,906	287	76	9	3	2,281
A5. Childhood cluster (032-33,037,045,050,055-56,138)	28,093	12,345	2,417	35	9		14,811	10,915	2,307	42	12		13,282
a. Pertussis (133)	4,806	2,155	453				2,609	1,775	422				2,197
b. Poliomyelitis (045,138)	1,427	296	532				827	212	388				600
c. Diphtheria (032)	29	5	8				14	4	10				15
d. Measles (055)	16,051	7,037	1,268				8,305	6,422	1,323				7,746
e. Tetanus (037)	5,781	2,851	156	35	9	5	3,057	2,502	164	40	12	7	2,724
A6. Meningitis (036,320-322)	1,793	521	534	93	3	1	1,153	330	168	138	2	2	640
A7. Hepatitis (070)	235	31	53	19	5	1	109	29	55	33	6	3	126
A8. Malaria (084)	31,504	12,346	2,372	1,277	78	24	16,096	11,388	2,466	1,428	95	30	15,407
A9. Tropical cluster (085,086,120,125)	6,681	227	2,260	1,161	271	85	4,004	186	1,379	835	214	63	2,677
a. African trypanosomiasis (086.3,086.4,086.5)	1,782	51	395	362	82	9	899	94	356	371	57	5	883
b. Chagas disease (086.0,086.1,086.2)													
c. Schistosomiasis (120)	3,490	163	1,675	444	24	6	2,312	79	833	245	17	5	1,178
d. Leishmaniasis (085)	583	13	186	90	1		291	12	188	91	2		292
e. Lymphatic filariasis (125.0, 125.1)	184			90	40	3	132			45	7		51
f. Onchocerciasis (125.3)	641		4	176	124	66	370		3	128	94	47	272
A10. Leprosy (030)	227	9	93	9	2		116	9	86	10	3	4	111
A11. Trachoma (076)	901			168	29	14	210			558	79	53	690
A12. Intestinal helminths (126-129)	852	2	381	37			423	2	385	38	3		429
a. Ascaris (127.0)	440	2	217				219	2	219				221
b. Trichuris (127.3)	304		151				151		152				153
c. Hookworm (126)	108		13	36	2	1	53		14	37	3	2	55
B. Respiratory infections (381-382,460-466,480-487)	31,639	13,496	1,418	738	139	461	16,252	12,338	1,476	819	167	587	15,387
B1. Acute lower respiratory inf. (460-465)	30,560	13,096	1,356	670	130	455	15,707	11,952	1,415	749	157	580	14,853
B2. Acute upper respiratory inf. (466,480-487)	328	18	61	68	9	6	163	17	61	70	10	7	165
B3. Otitis media (381-382)	751	382					382	369					369
C. Maternal conditions (630-676)	7,992								148	7,783	60		7,992
C1. Haemorrhage (666,667)	1,430								44	1,377	9		1,430
C2. Sepsis (670)	2,753								30	2,700	24		2,753
C3. Eclampsia (642.4-642.6)	418								15	401	2		418
C4. Hypertension (642 minus 642.4-642.6)	204								7	195	1		204
C5. Obstructed labour (660)	1,897								15	1,865	17		1,897
C6. Abortion (630-639)	788								22	760	5		788
D. Perinatal causes (760-779)	20,882	12,062					12,062	8,821					8,821

Annex Table 9. **Disability-adjusted life years (DALYs, in thousands): Sub-Saharan Africa**

Disease or injury (ICD 9 code)	Both sexes all ages	Males						Females					
		0–4	5–14	15–44	45–59	60+	All ages	0–4	5–14	15–44	45–59	60+	All ages
II. Noncommunicable (140–628,680–759) (minus 320–322,460–465,466,480–487, 614–616)	56,554	9,624	3,767	6,594	4,777	3,931	28,694	8,348	3,283	6,121	5,093	5,014	27,860
A. Malignant neoplasms (140–208)	4,506	90	436	301	836	601	2,264	158	15	681	904	483	2,242
A1. Mouth and oropharynx (140–149)	215		4	19	33	61	118	5		28	22	42	98
A2. Oesophagus (150)	221			16	85	51	152			14	29	25	69
A3. Stomach (151)	323		2	18	81	61	162		2	36	81	44	161
A4. Colorectal (152,153,154)	141		2	12	19	33	65	3		22	19	35	76
A5. Liver (155)	591	2	12	111	184	77	386	3		79	76	47	206
A6. Pancreas (157)	70			4	18	11	33			10	18	9	36
A7. Lung (162)	179			11	65	49	126			10	27	17	54
A8. Melanoma and other skin (172–173)	83			3	16	11	30			8	23	22	52
A9. Breast (174)	249									85	110	53	249
A10. Cervix (180)	456									134	214	107	456
A11. Corpus uteri (179,181–182)	39									6	17	15	39
A12. Ovary (183)	109							4		40	44	21	109
A13. Prostate (185)	223			2	54	167	223						
A14. Bladder (188)	131			7	31	36	75			16	22	18	56
A15. Lymphoma (200–202)	452	39	187	31	30	35	321	38	5	45	22	22	131
A16. Leukemia (204–208)	131	7	33	10	6	12	68	16	2	22	13	10	63
B. Other neoplasm (210–239)	453	11	33	18	17	5	85	20	280	46	14	7	367
C. Diabetes mellitus (250)	324			23	51	43	117			27	87	93	208
D. Nutritional/endocrine (240–285, minus 250)	8,078	3,162	101	843	71	33	4,210	2,949	250	408	175	86	3,868
D1. Protein-energy malnutrition (260–263)	2,161	1,041	51	18	4	4	1,118	977	43	10	3	10	1,043
D2. Iodine deficiency (243)	1,670	748	42	27	5	2	823	767	40	31	6	2	846
D3. Vitamin A deficiency (264)	2,187	1,114					1,114	1,072					1,072
D4. Anaemias (280–285)	1,004	153	120	98	26	11	408	71	259	176	58	31	596
E. Neuro-psychiatric (290–359, minus 320–322)	9,763	531	1,458	2,361	800	465	5,615	426	989	1,991	382	360	4,148
E1. Major affective disorder	1,647			464	50	11	525			986	109	27	1,122
E2. Bipolar affective disorder (296)	109			47	4		53			50	5		56
E3. Psychoses (295, 291–294,297–299)	575		2	289	13	5	309		2	253	4	1	266
E4. Epilepsy (345)	1,348	129	456	170	34	8	797	94	302	129	19	7	551
E5. Alcohol dependence (303)	1,703			822	466	200	1,487			118	69	30	216
E6. Alzheimer & other dementias (330,331,333–336,290)	840	39	58	13	107	192	409	38	31	10	110	242	430
E7. Parkinson disease (332)	58				13	15	28				13	16	29
E8. Multiple sclerosis (340)	134		1	51	9	2	64		1	58	8	3	71
E9. Drug dependence (304)	375		17	225	30	8	280		5	77	10	2	94
E10. Post-traumatic stress disorder	505	9	61	107	7	1	186	16	103	186	13	2	319
F. Sense organ (360–389)	1,389	53	10	45	297	193	598	42	12	55	409	274	791
F1. Glaucoma-related blindness (365)	171				3		4				89	78	168
F2. Cataract-related blindness (366)	1,130	18		43	293	193	547	16		53	319	195	583
G. Cardiovascular diseases (390–459)	12,252	443	253	1,250	1,635	2,004	5,585	308	453	1,055	1,831	3,021	6,667
G1. Rheumatic heart disease (390–398)	852	8	31	83	65	50	238	9	46	141	226	192	614
G2. Ischaemic heart disease (*)	1,202			124	248	293	666			41	139	355	537
G3. Cerebrovascular disease (430–438)	4,272	45	38	236	532	890	1,742	22	73	291	725	1,420	2,530
G4. Inflammatory cardiac disease (+)	3,306	240	130	536	447	355	1,708	199	235	342	378	444	1,598
H. Chronic respiratory dis. (460–519, minus 460–466,480–487)	4,430	864	646	384	190	206	2,290	610	432	427	464	207	2,140
H1. Chronic obstructive lung dis. (490–492,495–496)	650	65	34	25	82	144	351	36	18	21	118	106	299
H2. Asthma (493)	1,781	84	384	243	53	15	780	74	318	278	277	55	1,001

Annex Table 9. Disability-adjusted life years (DALYs, in thousands): Sub-Saharan Africa

Disease or injury (ICD 9 code)	Both sexes all ages	Males 0-4	Males 5-14	Males 15-44	Males 45-59	Males 60+	Males All ages	Females 0-4	Females 5-14	Females 15-44	Females 45-59	Females 60+	Females All ages
I. Diseases of the digestive system (520-579)	5,508	1,088	260	882	482	209	2,920	1,009	334	643	412	190	2,588
I1. Peptic ulcer disease (531-533)	353	3	6	111	58	21	199	3	7	79	47	18	154
I2. Cirrhosis of the liver (571)	1,352	21	23	446	295	89	874	17	34	209	165	52	478
J. Genito-urinary (580-629)	2,120	128	367	148	335	117	1,094	49	274	221	287	195	1,026
J1. Nephritis/nephrosis (580-589)	1,179	41	332	106	89	55	622	15	252	122	99	69	557
J2. Benign prostatic hypertrophy (600)	233	-	-	-	210	22	233	-	-	-	-	-	-
K. Skin disease (680-709)	113	25	8	5	1	5	44	18	5	28	-	16	68
L. Musculo-skeletal system (710-739)	664	5	38	86	41	25	195	11	87	225	94	53	470
L1. Rheumatoid arthritis (714)	159	-	-	41	8	3	52	-	43	52	10	2	107
L2. Osteoarthritis (715)	223	-	-	30	22	5	57	-	-	99	54	12	166
M. Congenital abnormalities (740-759)	6,342	3,201	133	45	-	1	3,381	2,725	124	101	11	-	2,962
N. Oral health (520-529)	597	23	24	204	21	22	293	22	23	209	23	27	305
N1. Dental caries (521.0)	139	23	24	17	5	2	69	22	23	17	5	2	70
N2. Periodontal disease (523)	417	-	-	188	16	2	206	-	-	192	18	2	212
N3. Edentulism (520)	41	-	-	-	-	18	18	-	-	-	-	23	23
III. Injuries (E800-999)	27,333	3,299	2,887	12,216	831	141	19,373	3,105	1,668	2,621	319	247	7,960
A. Unintentional (E800-949)	15,067	2,360	2,160	5,699	490	89	10,799	2,119	1,181	635	143	190	4,267
A1. Road traffic accidents (E810-819, 826-829)	3,710	231	471	2,045	130	20	2,897	190	318	250	37	18	813
A2. Poisoning (E850-869)	535	84	36	236	32	4	391	61	35	36	8	4	144
A3. Falls (E850-869)	2,985	518	428	932	127	27	2,032	514	221	65	34	119	953
A4. Fires (E890-899)	1,006	313	107	150	15	3	588	255	119	30	6	7	417
A5. Drowning (E910)	1,554	292	392	425	20	3	1,133	219	160	32	6	4	421
A6. Occupational (#)	405	-	-	320	36	-	357	-	-	39	9	-	49
B. Intentional (E950-969,990-999)	12,266	939	726	6,516	341	52	8,574	987	487	1,986	176	57	3,692
B1. Self-inflicted (E950-959)	1,686	-	70	1,199	101	18	1,387	-	36	205	38	20	299
B2. Homicide and violence (E960-969)	2,598	158	131	1,756	73	7	2,124	196	99	154	17	8	474
B3. War (E990-999)	7,982	781	525	3,562	167	27	5,062	791	351	1,628	121	29	2,920
Population (in millions)	510.3	47.5	70.3	103.8	20.3	10.5	252.3	47.0	69.8	106.3	22.1	12.7	258.0

Notes

A dash (-) symbol indicates less than 1,000 DALYs.

* ICD 9 codes for ischaemic heart disease are as follows: 410-414, 440.9, plus: at ages 45-59: 50% of 427.1, 427.4, 427.5, and 33% of 428; at ages 60+: 80% of 427.1, 427.4, 427.5 and 50% of 428.

+ ICD 9 codes for inflammatory cardiac diseases are as follows: 420, 421, 422, 425 plus: at ages 0-44: 50% of 428; at ages 45-59: 25% of 428; at ages 60+: 20% of 428.

There are no established ICD 9 codes specific for occupational injuries.
Estimates have been based on reported occupational injuries and deaths tabulated by the International Labour Organisation.

Annex Table 10. Disability-adjusted life years (DALYs, in thousands): Latin America and the Caribbean

Disease or injury (ICD 9 code)	Both sexes all ages	Males						Females					
		0–4	5–14	15–44	45–59	60+	All ages	0–4	5–14	15–44	45–59	60+	All ages
All Causes	102,892	18,033	6,478	20,870	6,330	5,508	57,218	14,367	5,405	15,696	4,820	5,385	45,674
I. Communicable, maternal & perinatal (001-139,320-322,460-465,466,480-487,614-616,630-676,760-779)	43,415	12,627	3,289	5,686	702	344	22,649	9,713	2,954	7,282	516	301	20,766
A. Infectious & parasitic dis. (001-139,320-322,614-616)	25,851	4,784	2,867	5,317	601	215	13,783	3,925	2,583	4,996	396	167	12,067
A1. Tuberculosis (010-018,137)	2,569	59	132	904	314	100	1,508	56	141	685	137	41	1,061
A2. STDs excluding HIV (090-099,614-616)	2,403	53	1	181	8		244	50	3	2,094	10	1	2,159
a. Syphilis (090-097)	367	53		145	7		205	50		105	5		162
b. Chlamydia (098)	181			28			30		2	144	5		151
c. Gonorrhoea (098)	22			8			9			12			13
d. Pelvic inflammatory disease (614-616)	1,834									1,834			1,834
A3. HIV infection (090-099,614-616)	4,435	51	5	3,261	95	1	3,414	51	7	927	35	2	1,021
A4. Diarrhoeal diseases (001,002,004,006-009)	5,884	2,451	433	178	36	31	3,129	1,992	408	272	45	38	2,755
a. Acute watery	3,345	1,230	329	141	28	24	1,753	1,000	310	216	36	29	1,592
b. Persistent	1,574	852	15				867	692	14				706
c. Dysentery	965	369	88	37	7	7	509	300	83	56	9	8	457
A5. Childhood cluster (032-33,037,045,050,055-56,138)	1,605	601	242	10	2	1	857	526	190	28	4		748
a. Pertussis (133)	723	319	69				388	275	60				335
b. Poliomyelitis (045,138)	233	43	90				134	31	65	3			99
c. Diphtheria (032)	27	6	7				13	5	8	2			14
d. Measles (055)	384	144	47	3			194	130	48	11			190
e. Tetanus (037)	238	89	30	5	2		128	85	9	12			110
A6. Meningitis (036,320-322)	712	247	94	37	5	2	385	187	79	54	5	2	327
A7. Hepatitis (070)	160	18	30	16	3	2	69	15	22	47	5	2	91
A8. Malaria (084)	437	30	62	109	13	4	218	28	61	110	14	5	219
A9. Tropical cluster (085,086,120,125)	2,991	664	469	401	82	34	1,649	531	348	353	80	30	1,342
a. African trypanosomiasis (086.3,086.4,086.5)													
b. Chagas disease (086.0,086.1,086.2)	2,739	645	380	346	75	32	1,478	519	306	329	78	29	1,261
c. Schistosomiasis (120)	178	6	78	31	2		119	3	39	16	1		59
d. Leishmaniasis (085)	70	13	11	24	1		49	9	4	7			21
e. Lymphatic filariasis (125.0, 125.1)	3				3		3						
f. Onchocerciasis (125.3)	1			1			1						
A10. Leprosy (030)	66			28	5		33		3	27	2		33
A11. Trachoma (076)	110						38						72
A12. Intestinal helminths (126-129)	2,394	5	1,133	60	4	3	1,205	5	1,117	60	4	3	1,189
a. Ascaris (127.0)	1,347	5	671	2			678	5	662	2			669
b. Trichuris (127.3)	903		451	3			455		445	3			448
c. Hookworm (126)	144		10	55	4	3	72		10	55	4	3	72
B. Respiratory infections (381-382,460-466,480-487)	6,381	2,367	421	369	101	129	3,387	1,884	363	506	106	134	2,993
B1. Acute lower respiratory inf. (460-465)	5,662	2,111	390	300	91	123	3,015	1,655	333	437	95	128	2,647
B2. Acute upper respiratory inf. (466,480-487)	256	13	32	69	11	6	129	10	30	69	11	7	127
B3. Otitis media (381-382)	462	244					244	219					219
C. Maternal conditions (630-676)	1,800								6	1,779	14		1,800
C1. Haemorrhage (666,667)	250								1	247	2		250
C2. Sepsis (670)	406									402	4		406
C3. Eclampsia (642.4-642.6)	155								3	152			155
C4. Hypertension (642 minus 642.4-642.6)	71									70			71
C5. Obstructed labour (660)	571									565	5		571
C6. Abortion (630-639)	220									218	1		220
D. Perinatal causes (760-779)	9,383	5,476	1				5,478	3,905					3,905

Annex Table 10. **Disability-adjusted life years (DALYs, in thousands): Latin America and the Caribbean**

Disease or injury (ICD 9 code)	Both sexes all ages	Males						Females					
		0-4	5-14	15-44	45-59	60+	All ages	0-4	5-14	15-44	45-59	60+	All ages
II. Noncommunicable (140-628,680-759) (minus 320-322,460-465,466,480-487, 614-616)	44,030	4,551	1,768	6,803	4,860	4,865	22,847	4,003	1,689	6,550	4,059	4,882	21,183
A. Malignant neoplasms (140-208)	5,375	87	259	665	748	800	2,559	75	214	825	899	804	2,816
A1. Mouth and oropharynx (140-149)	167	-	1	30	59	36	126	-	1	9	14	15	40
A2. Oesophagus (150)	90	-	-	9	31	27	67	-	-	3	9	12	24
A3. Stomach (151)	375	-	-	41	89	105	236	-	-	27	47	65	139
A4. Colorectal (152,153,154)	258	-	-	29	42	53	125	-	-	25	47	60	133
A5. Liver (155)	51	-	2	6	10	10	28	-	-	4	8	10	23
A6. Pancreas (157)	58	-	-	5	12	16	33	-	-	3	9	14	25
A7. Lung (162)	288	-	-	32	90	95	218	-	-	12	27	30	69
A8. Melanoma and other skin (172-173)	49	-	-	10	8	5	23	-	-	10	8	6	26
A9. Breast (174)	469	-	-	-	-	-	-	-	-	181	195	93	469
A10. Cervix (180)	427	-	-	-	-	-	-	-	-	203	161	63	427
A11. Corpus uteri (179,181-182)	76	-	-	-	-	-	-	-	-	14	39	22	76
A12. Ovary (183)	81	-	-	-	-	-	-	1	4	34	28	14	81
A13. Prostate (185)	163	-	-	-	25	135	163	-	-	-	-	-	-
A14. Bladder (188)	93	-	-	2	23	40	71	-	-	3	7	12	22
A15. Lymphoma (200-202)	278	12	37	63	30	24	165	7	20	38	24	23	113
A16. Leukemia (204-208)	253	21	64	42	10	10	147	16	45	27	9	9	106
B. Other neoplasm (210-239)	160	9	19	25	12	11	77	8	17	29	17	13	83
C. Diabetes mellitus (250)	1,011	3	4	122	161	139	429	2	8	123	219	230	582
D. Nutritional/endocrine (240-285, minus 250)	4,710	1,619	226	285	84	93	2,307	1,492	213	477	101	120	2,403
D1. Protein-energy malnutrition (260-263)	985	440	25	25	12	22	523	380	26	21	10	25	461
D2. Iodine deficiency (243)	520	237	9	13	2	1	262	233	8	12	2	1	257
D3. Vitamin A deficiency (264)	1,414	721	-	-	-	-	721	693	-	-	-	-	693
D4. Anaemias (280-285)	978	58	137	136	35	25	391	46	131	338	40	31	586
E. Neuro-psychiatric (290-359, minus 320-322)	8,274	247	461	2,616	803	566	4,692	200	376	2,089	437	480	3,582
E1. Major affective disorder	1,749	-	-	490	60	17	567	-	-	1,016	127	39	1,182
E2. Bipolar affective disorder (296)	115	-	-	50	5	1	57	-	-	51	6	2	58
E3. Psychoses (295, 291-294,297-299)	584	-	-	299	9	6	315	-	-	259	5	5	269
E4. Epilepsy (345)	824	-	215	155	23	8	471	50	154	124	18	7	353
E5. Alcohol dependence (303)	1,607	70	-	786	436	184	1,405	-	-	112	62	27	201
E6. Alzheimer & other dementias (330,331,333-336,290)	864	-	-	8	114	275	397	-	-	4	123	340	467
E7. Parkinson disease (332)	123	-	-	-	27	32	59	-	-	-	29	34	64
E8. Multiple sclerosis (340)	89	-	-	41	1	-	43	-	-	43	2	-	46
E9. Drug dependence (304)	845	-	31	512	73	18	634	-	8	174	25	5	211
E10. Post-traumatic stress disorder	450	6	45	108	8	1	168	9	75	182	13	3	282
F. Sense organ (360-389)	637	28	4	29	151	98	309	22	5	29	176	96	328
F1. Glaucoma-related blindness (365)	60	-	-	-	11	10	21	-	-	-	25	14	39
F2. Cataract-related blindness (366)	511	2	-	23	139	88	252	2	-	25	151	81	259
G. Cardiovascular diseases (390-459)	9,538	168	144	1,168	1,400	2,036	4,916	106	133	1,130	1,132	2,121	4,622
G1. Rheumatic heart disease (390-398)	319	2	46	77	10	5	140	2	49	96	23	10	180
G2. Ischaemic heart disease (*)	2,733	4	7	331	534	726	1,602	2	4	169	297	659	1,132
G3. Cerebrovascular disease (430-438)	2,725	14	28	335	399	546	1,322	9	25	374	389	605	1,402
G4. Inflammatory cardiac disease (+)	1,581	84	58	321	196	207	866	91	50	235	143	197	715
H. Chronic respiratory dis. (460-519, minus 460-466,480-487)	3,268	559	227	410	207	344	1,747	478	216	401	170	255	1,520
H1. Chronic obstructive lung dis. (490-492,495-496)	699	43	6	25	93	246	412	29	6	19	71	162	286
H2. Asthma (493)	1,103	48	181	239	52	21	542	43	177	255	59	27	561

Annex Table 10. **Disability-adjusted life years (DALYs, in thousands): Latin America and the Caribbean**

Disease or injury (ICD 9 code)	Both sexes all ages	Males						Females					
		0-4	5-14	15-44	45-59	60+	All ages	0-4	5-14	15-44	45-59	60+	All ages
I. Diseases of the digestive system (520-579)	3,380	199	106	847	566	361	2,080	143	85	465	305	303	1,301
I1. Peptic ulcer disease (531-533)	196	1	3	60	34	24	123	1	2	32	20	18	73
I2. Cirrhosis of the liver (571)	1,166	5	8	404	314	137	868	4	7	112	107	67	298
J. Genito-urinary (580-629)	1,439	74	56	173	297	173	773	56	57	282	120	151	667
J1. Nephritis/nephrosis (580-589)	873	39	44	144	80	114	420	30	47	178	87	111	453
J2. Benign prostatic hypertrophy (600)	216	-	-	-	197	19	216	-	-	-	-	-	-
K. Skin disease (680-709)	63	7	4	6	4	4	25	7	3	16	5	7	38
L. Musculo-skeletal system (710-739)	2,191	5	93	281	343	161	883	4	204	509	385	205	1,308
L1. Rheumatoid arthritis (714)	710	-	-	76	137	39	253	-	107	238	87	25	458
L2. Osteoarthritis (715)	1,214	-	80	179	194	104	557	-	80	167	265	144	657
M. Congenital abnormalities (740-759)	3,107	1,527	51	38	3	2	1,621	1,392	47	39	5	2	1,486
N. Oral health (520-529)	870	18	114	137	82	76	426	17	111	137	87	92	444
N1. Dental caries (521.0)	436	18	114	84	3	2	220	17	111	83	4	2	216
N2. Periodontal disease (523)	285	-	-	54	59	26	139	-	-	54	62	31	146
N3. Edentulism (520)	149	-	-	-	20	48	68	-	-	-	22	59	81
III. Injuries (E800-999)	15,447	855	1,420	8,381	768	298	11,722	651	763	1,864	245	202	3,725
A. Unintentional (E800-949)	11,060	767	1,275	5,138	519	247	7,946	572	698	1,454	202	188	3,115
A1. Road traffic accidents (E810-819, 826-829)	5,910	182	644	2,999	230	66	4,122	128	457	1,053	124	28	1,789
A2. Poisoning (E850-869)	83	15	7	24	3	1	51	13	5	11	2	1	32
A3. Falls (E850-869)	990	78	131	360	67	82	719	55	53	42	14	107	271
A4. Fires (E890-899)	455	100	45	99	16	9	269	93	34	44	8	7	186
A5. Drowning (E910)	586	66	114	276	19	5	480	40	32	30	8	7	106
A6. Occupational (#)	334	-	-	242	41	2	284	-	-	40	3	1	50
B. Intentional (E950-969,990-999)	4,387	88	145	3,243	249	51	3,777	79	64	410	43	14	610
B1. Self-inflicted (E950-959)	383	-	8	229	34	15	286	-	5	75	12	5	97
B2. Homicide and violence (E960-969)	3,406	38	103	2,706	200	35	3,082	28	36	230	22	7	324
B3. War (E990-999)	598	51	34	309	14	2	409	51	23	104	8	2	188
Population (in millions)	444.3	28.7	52.1	104.3	22.2	14.2	221.6	27.7	50.7	104.1	23.4	16.8	222.7

Notes

A dash (-) symbol indicates less than 1,000 DALYs.

* ICD 9 codes for ischaemic heart disease are as follows: 410-414, 440.9, plus: at ages 45-59: 50% of 427.1, 427.4, 427.5, and 33% of 428; at ages 60+: 80% of 427.1, 427.4, 427.5 and 50% of 428.

+ ICD 9 codes for inflammatory cardiac diseases are as follows: 420, 421, 422, 425 plus: at ages 0-44: 50% of 428; at ages 45-59: 25% of 428; at ages 60+: 20% of 428.

There are no established ICD 9 codes specific for occupational injuries.
Estimates have been based on reported occupational injuries and deaths tabulated by the International Labour Organisation.

Annex Table 11. Disability-adjusted life years (DALYs, in thousands): Middle Eastern Crescent

Disease or injury (ICD 9 code)	Both sexes all ages	Males						Females					
		0-4	5-14	15-44	45-59	60+	All ages	0-4	5-14	15-44	45-59	60+	All ages
All Causes	144,246	38,002	9,284	14,611	6,232	5,863	73,992	36,180	8,158	15,536	4,594	5,787	70,255
I. Communicable, maternal & perinatal (001-139,320-322,460-465,466,480-487,614-616, 630-676,760-779)	73,614	27,997	3,379	2,129	729	550	34,785	27,156	3,675	6,993	486	519	38,829
A. Infectious & parasitic dis. (001-139,320-322,614-616)	37,088	12,650	2,725	1,807	648	249	18,080	13,077	2,874	2,513	366	179	19,009
A1. Tuberculosis (010-018,137)	4,045	139	340	987	500	198	2,165	144	427	1,020	207	82	1,880
A2. STDs excluding HIV (090-099,614-616)	663			30			32		1	628	2		632
a. Syphilis (090-097)	2						1						1
b. Chlamydia	85			25			26			55			58
c. Gonorrhoea (098)	10			4			4			6			6
d. Pelvic inflammatory disease (614-616)	566									566			566
A3. HIV infection	319	3		233	19		256	3		57	2		63
A4. Diarrhoeal diseases (001,002,004,006-009)	15,402	6,669	569	224	37	12	7,512	6,913	647	278	38	13	7,890
a. Acute watery	8,119	3,317	418	175	29	9	3,949	3,438	475	217	30	10	4,170
b. Persistent	4,822	2,338	27				2,366	2,424	32				2,456
c. Dysentery	2,461	1,013	124	49	8	3	1,197	1,050	141	62	8	3	1,264
A5. Childhood cluster (032-33,037,045,050,055-56,138)	8,593	3,538	699	10	4		4,255	3,608	708	15	5		4,339
a. Pertussis (133)	1,546	625	129				754	646	145				791
b. Poliomyelitis (045,138)	672	136	251				387	99	186				285
c. Diphtheria (032)	14	3	4				6	2	5				8
d. Measles (055)	3,872	1,627	256	10	4		1,883	1,687	303	15	5		1,990
e. Tetanus (037)	2,490	1,148	59	14			1,224	1,174	69	39			1,266
A6. Meningitis (036,320-322)	1,272	454	268	10	3	3	741	374	115	39	8	3	531
A7. Hepatitis (070)	173	24	39	10	3		77	24	45	20	3		96
A8. Malaria (084)	282	22	54	46	7	3	132	23	61	62	3		150
A9. Tropical cluster (085,086,120,125)	351	36	114	42	12	1	205	25	77	27	12	6	146
a. African trypanosomiasis (086.3,086.4,086.5)													
b. Chagas disease (086.0,086.1,086.2)													
c. Schistosomiasis (120)	75	3	36	10	4		50		17				25
d. Leishmaniasis (085)	253	33	78	32	3		146	23	59	22	1		107
e. Lymphatic filariasis (125.0, 125.1)	24						9			5			15
f. Onchocerciasis (125.3)													
A10. Leprosy (030)	38		14				19		13				19
A11. Trachoma (076)	576			161	39	18	218			235	69	54	358
A12. Intestinal helminths (126-129)	544	2	261	18	1		283	2	241	17	1		262
a. Ascaris (127.0)	497	2	256				259	2	236				238
b. Trichuris (127.3)	48		5	17									
c. Hookworm (126)													
B. Respiratory infections (381-382,460-466,480-487)	16,570	6,724	654	323	81	301	8,083	6,954	744	366	83	341	8,487
B1. Acute lower respiratory inf. (460-465)	15,780	6,366	640	303	79	298	7,686	6,600	731	347	80	337	8,094
B2. Acute upper respiratory inf. (466,480-487)	91	6	14	20	3	3	46	6	13	19	3	4	45
B3. Otitis media (381-382)	699	351					351	348					348
C. Maternal conditions (630-676)	4,208								58	4,114	37		4,208
C1. Haemorrhage (666,667)	471								14	453	3		471
C2. Sepsis (670)	1,749								12	1,721	16		1,749
C3. Eclampsia (642.4-642.6)	129								6	123			129
C4. Hypertension (642 minus 642.4-642.6)	181								9	171	1		181
C5. Obstructed labour (660)	1,332								6	1,314	13		1,332
C6. Abortion (630-639)	198								6	190	1		198
D. Perinatal causes (760-779)	15,748	8,623					8,623	7,125					7,125

Annex Table 11. Disability-adjusted life years (DALYs, in thousands): Middle Eastern Crescent

Disease or injury (ICD 9 code)	Both sexes all ages	Males						Females					
		0-4	5-14	15-44	45-59	60+	All ages	0-4	5-14	15-44	45-59	60+	All ages
II. Noncommunicable (140-628,680-759) (minus 320-322,460-465,466,480-487, 614-616)	51,842	7,869	3,189	5,446	4,825	5,076	26,406	7,201	2,912	6,352	3,875	5,095	25,436
A. Malignant neoplasms (140-208)	4,927	108	367	477	924	801	2,676	158	70	660	781	581	2,250
A1. Mouth and oropharynx (140-149)	302	2	5	42	50	91	190	2	1	35	29	44	112
A2. Oesophagus (150)	168	–	–	12	42	41	96	–	–	15	30	26	72
A3. Stomach (151)	358	–	2	32	88	87	210	–	–	33	52	62	148
A4. Colorectal (152,153,154)	227	–	2	25	27	58	112	–	–	29	26	58	115
A5. Liver (155)	146	1	4	13	36	34	89	–	–	12	22	21	57
A6. Pancreas (157)	77	–	–	7	20	19	45	–	–	5	13	14	32
A7. Lung (162)	504	2	6	41	183	170	402	–	–	18	39	42	102
A8. Melanoma and other skin (172-173)	24	–	–	3	6	3	13	–	–	5	3	2	11
A9. Breast (174)	313	–	–	–	–	–	–	–	–	124	127	61	313
A10. Cervix (180)	188	–	–	–	–	–	–	–	–	63	85	39	188
A11. Corpus uteri (179,181-182)	41	–	–	–	–	–	–	–	–	7	18	16	41
A12. Ovary (183)	91	–	–	–	–	–	–	–	–	42	30	15	91
A13. Prostate (185)	69	–	–	2	13	53	69	–	–	–	–	–	–
A14. Bladder (188)	171	–	–	18	48	66	135	–	–	7	14	14	36
A15. Lymphoma (200-202)	229	14	49	42	21	29	156	11	6	29	11	16	73
A16. Leukemia (204-208)	318	26	88	38	14	24	189	37	17	43	12	21	129
B. Other neoplasm (210-239)	329	11	24	17	12	9	74	18	189	30	–	8	255
C. Diabetes mellitus (250)	1,111	–	–	121	197	160	480	–	–	124	255	252	632
D. Nutritional/endocrine (240-285, minus 250)	5,152	1,672	252	476	82	46	2,529	1,536	332	597	97	61	2,624
D1. Protein-energy malnutrition (260-263)	1,033	476	31	7	2	3	519	472	28	7	1	5	514
D2. Iodine deficiency (243)	1,358	630	26	22	4	2	685	619	25	22	4	2	672
D3. Vitamin A deficiency (264)	549	288	–	–	–	–	288	261	–	–	–	–	261
D4. Anaemias (280-285)	1,518	129	237	202	39	20	628	80	320	415	48	27	890
E. Neuro-psychiatric (290-359, minus 320-322)	8,101	473	1,086	1,785	445	407	4,196	405	776	1,966	340	418	3,905
E1. Major affective disorder	1,791	–	15	530	58	16	603	–	8	1,036	117	34	1,188
E2. Bipolar affective disorder (296)	119	–	–	54	5	1	60	–	–	52	5	2	59
E3. Psychoses (295, 291,294,297-299)	608	–	–	319	5	2	327	–	–	267	3	2	281
E4. Epilepsy (345)	1,236	124	57	161	31	11	727	89	263	132	19	8	510
E5. Alcohol dependence (303)	429	–	–	207	117	50	375	–	–	30	17	7	54
E6. Alzheimer & other dementias (330,331,333-336,290)	947	34	–	8	116	260	456	36	–	116	116	306	490
E7. Parkinson disease (332)	67	–	–	–	14	20	34	–	–	9	14	19	33
E8. Multiple sclerosis (340)	126	–	–	50	7	8	61	–	5	55	7	3	66
E9. Drug dependence (304)	366	–	6	218	30	1	271	–	23	78	10	2	95
E10. Post-traumatic stress disorder	499	8	–	117	8	–	192	13	91	188	13	–	308
F. Sense organ (360-389)	699	31	–	29	194	126	386	28	8	21	165	90	313
F1. Glaucoma-related blindness (365)	38	–	–	–	20	5	25	–	–	–	10	2	13
F2. Cataract-related blindness (366)	597	7	–	27	173	121	329	–	–	19	154	88	268
G. Cardiovascular diseases (390-459)	12,782	707	345	1,011	1,741	2,651	6,454	562	500	1,044	1,298	2,925	6,329
G1. Rheumatic heart disease (390-398)	468	7	38	58	31	28	162	9	45	91	80	80	305
G2. Ischaemic heart disease (*)	2,607	3	2	206	551	786	1,549	2	2	85	233	736	1,058
G3. Cerebrovascular disease (430-438)	3,393	66	52	155	419	855	1,547	40	82	242	429	1,053	1,846
G4. Inflammatory cardiac disease (+)	1,836	205	107	227	208	202	949	221	156	188	132	190	887
H. Chronic respiratory dis. (460-519, minus 460-466,480-487)	3,838	844	478	304	198	314	2,138	726	272	310	165	227	1,700
H1. Chronic obstructive lung dis. (490-492,495-496)	715	64	23	15	93	225	419	44	14	16	76	145	296
H2. Asthma (493)	1,143	83	301	212	43	17	656	55	183	184	44	21	487

Annex Table 11. **Disability-adjusted life years (DALYs, in thousands): Middle Eastern Crescent**

Disease or injury (ICD 9 code)	Both sexes all ages	Males						Females					
		0-4	5-14	15-44	45-59	60 +	All ages	0-4	5-14	15-44	45-59	60 +	All ages
I. Diseases of the digestive system (520-579)	4,574	1,003	204	437	427	269	2,340	1,102	255	404	268	205	2,233
I1. Peptic ulcer disease (531-533)	281	3	5	77	54	27	165	3	5	56	32	19	116
I2. Cirrhosis of the liver (571)	726	16	17	159	179	83	454	14	25	110	83	40	272
J. Genito-urinary (580-629)	1,879	114	240	150	366	176	1,047	60	197	235	176	164	832
J1. Nephritis/nephrosis (580-589)	915	37	205	73	72	78	465	21	172	116	67	74	450
J2. Benign prostatic hypertrophy (600)	228	-	-	-	205	23	228	-	-	-	-	-	-
K. Skin disease (680-709)	81	18	5	3	2	5	33	15	4	20	1	8	48
L. Musculo-skeletal system (710-739)	920	4	29	92	40	32	197	11	153	386	111	61	723
L1. Rheumatoid arthritis (714)	412	-	-	43	5	2	50	-	118	209	27	8	362
L2. Osteoarthritis (715)	256	-	-	37	26	7	70	-	-	108	61	16	186
M. Congenital abnormalities (740-759)	5,684	2,841	102	27	2	1	2,974	2,536	106	62	5	1	2,709
N. Oral health (520-529)	1,755	42	49	517	193	78	880	41	47	494	202	92	875
N1. Dental caries (521.0)	335	42	49	52	17	10	170	41	47	49	17	11	165
N2. Periodontal disease (523)	303	-	-	147	6	3	155	-	-	138	6	3	147
N3. Edentulism (520)	1,117	-	-	318	170	66	554	-	-	306	179	78	563
III. Injuries (E800-999)	18,790	2,136	2,715	7,035	678	236	12,800	1,824	1,570	2,191	233	172	5,990
A. Unintentional (E800-949)	11,336	1,569	2,235	3,224	419	181	7,629	1,238	1,292	922	119	135	3,708
A1. Road traffic accidents (E810-819, 826-829)	4,760	267	1,019	1,657	137	43	3,122	175	851	557	38	17	1,638
A2. Poisoning (E850-869)	330	55	29	112	27	6	230	37	20	34	6	3	101
A3. Falls (E850-869)	1,427	250	240	327	84	68	970	224	88	44	22	80	458
A4. Fires (E890-899)	650	211	84	72	13	7	387	156	66	30	5	5	263
A5. Drowning (E910)	961	189	302	189	17	5	703	129	88	33	5	3	258
A6. Occupational (#)	227	-	-	155	31	1	186	-	-	33	7	-	41
B. Intentional (E950-969,990-999)	7,454	567	480	3,811	259	55	5,172	586	278	1,269	114	37	2,283
B1. Self-inflicted (E950-959)	987	-	54	548	85	29	716	-	20	204	31	15	270
B2. Homicide and violence (E960-969)	1,508	111	108	852	66	11	1,147	124	57	157	15	6	361
B3. War (E990-999)	4,960	457	318	2,411	107	15	3,308	461	201	907	67	16	1,652
Population (in millions)	503.1	41.2	65.3	113.9	22.3	13.7	256.4	39.7	62.0	107.2	22.3	15.5	246.7

Notes

A dash (-) symbol indicates less than 1,000 DALYs.

* ICD 9 codes for ischaemic heart disease are as follows: 410-414, 440.9, plus: at ages 45-59: 50% of 427.1, 427.4, 427.5, and 33% of 428; at ages 60+: 80% of 427.1, 427.4, 427.5 and 50% of 428.

+ ICD 9 codes for inflammatory cardiac diseases are as follows: 420, 421, 422, 425 plus: at ages 0-44: 50% of 428; at ages 45-59: 25% of 428; at ages 60+: 20% of 428.

\# There are no established ICD 9 codes specific for occupational injuries.

Estimates have been based on reported occupational injuries and deaths tabulated by the International Labour Organisation.

Annex Table 12. **Disability-adjusted life years (DALYs, in thousands): World**

Disease or injury (ICD 9 code)	Both sexes all ages	Males						Females					
		0-4	5-14	15-44	45-59	60 +	All ages	0-4	5-14	15-44	45-59	60 +	All ages
All Causes	1,361,803	273,211	77,474	186,774	84,165	91,782	713,406	254,791	68,262	174,650	60,359	90,335	648,397
I. Communicable, maternal & perinatal (001-139,320-322,460-465,466,480-487,614-616, 630-676,760-779)	624,700	202,693	39,448	46,910	10,312	6,767	306,130	185,584	38,458	81,879	6,820	5,828	318,570
A. Infectious & parasitic dis. (001-139,320-322,614-616)	372,539	99,802	34,186	42,525	9,066	3,661	189,241	94,328	32,627	48,529	5,354	2,461	183,299
A1. Tuberculosis (010-018,137)	46,450	1,227	3,099	13,362	6,156	2,623	26,468	1,330	3,796	10,906	2,786	1,164	19,982
A2. STDs excluding HIV (090-099,614-616)	21,081	1,349	27	2,371	108	10	3,864	1,229	41	15,799	132	15	17,217
a. Syphilis (090-097)	6,318	1,285	22	2,000	97	9	3,412	1,186	17	1,609	86	7	2,905
b. Chlamydia	1,549	–	3	255	9	1	269	–	14	1,215	45	7	1,280
c. Gonorrhoea (098)	414	63	2	116	2	–	183	44	10	176	–	–	231
d. Pelvic inflammatory disease (614-616)	12,800									12,799		1	12,800
A3. HIV infection	30,207	1,358	54	15,973	522	23	17,930	1,262	230	10,609	171	6	12,277
A4. Diarrhoeal diseases (001,002,004,006-009)	99,111	42,145	4,592	2,759	434	245	50,174	40,706	4,760	2,769	447	255	48,937
a. Acute watery	54,378	21,254	3,505	2,193	339	188	27,479	20,534	3,626	2,198	348	192	26,899
b. Persistent	29,076	14,585	188	4	1	–	14,780	14,084	199	7	2	4	14,296
c. Dysentery	15,658	6,305	898	561	94	56	7,915	6,088	935	564	97	58	7,743
A5. Childhood cluster (032-33,037,045,050,055-56,138)	67,611	28,479	6,117	155	59	26	34,836	26,738	5,762	181	65	28	32,775
a. Pertussis (133)	11,957	5,104	1,120	–	–	–	6,223	4,635	1,099	–	–	–	5,733
b. Poliomyelitis (045,138)	4,807	959	1,853	1	3	–	2,816	677	1,309	3	–	–	1,991
c. Diphtheria (032)	234	46	62	1	–	–	109	36	78	11	–	–	125
d. Measles (055)	34,118	14,689	2,571	4	–	–	17,263	14,089	2,754	12	–	–	16,855
e. Tetanus (037)	16,495	7,683	511	149	56	25	8,424	7,302	522	155	64	28	8,071
A6. Meningitis (036,320-322)	8,089	2,558	1,864	435	85	38	4,980	1,869	682	482	45	32	3,109
A7. Hepatitis (070)	1,928	212	266	345	164	58	1,044	191	280	275	69	70	884
A8. Malaria (084)	35,728	12,633	3,209	2,116	209	61	18,227	11,655	3,262	2,277	235	72	17,501
A9. Tropical cluster (085,086,120,125)	13,350	1,054	3,563	2,510	621	160	7,907	831	2,316	1,563	590	143	5,443
a. African trypanosomiasis (086.3,086.4,086.5)	1,783	51	395	362	82	9	900	94	356	371	57	5	883
b. Chagas disease (086.0,086.1,086.2)	2,739	645	380	346	75	32	1,478	519	306	329	78	29	1,261
c. Schistosomiasis (120)	4,529	193	2,019	722	40	18	2,992	96	1,019	312	103	6	1,536
d. Leishmaniasis (085)	2,813	165	766	648	23	6	1,608	122	633	422	24	4	1,205
e. Lymphatic filariasis (125.0, 125.1)	845	–	255	255	276	28	560	–	–	–	233	52	285
f. Onchocerciasis (125.3)	642	–	4	176	124	66	370	–	3	128	94	47	272
A10. Leprosy (030)	1,018	52	403	35	13	6	510	50	402	36	13	7	507
A11. Trachoma (076)	3,298	–	4	621	180	127	928	–	3	1,567	422	381	2,370
A12. Intestinal helminths (126-129)	17,968	40	8,593	483	40	25	9,180	39	8,222	460	40	26	8,788
a. Ascaris (127.0)	10,519	40	5,321	18	2	–	5,382	39	5,079	17	2	–	5,138
b. Trichuris (127.3)	6,305	–	3,186	26	3	–	3,216	–	3,059	25	3	1	3,089
c. Hookworm (126)	1,144	–	87	439	34	23	583	–	84	418	35	24	561
B. Respiratory infections (381-382,460-466,480-487)	122,790	47,711	5,259	4,384	1,246	3,106	61,706	46,783	5,374	4,370	1,189	3,368	61,084
B1. Acute lower respiratory inf. (460-465)	114,745	45,011	4,935	3,577	1,100	3,012	57,636	44,145	5,067	3,596	1,050	3,252	57,109
B2. Acute upper respiratory inf. (466,480-487)	2,925	109	324	807	146	93	1,480	109	307	775	139	116	1,445
B3. Otitis media (381-382)	5,120	2,590					2,590	2,529					2,529
C. Maternal conditions (630-676)	29,713												29,713
C1. Haemorrhage (666,667)	5,044												5,044
C2. Sepsis (670)	10,225												10,225
C3. Eclampsia (642.4-642.6)	1,380												1,380
C4. Hypertension (642 minus 642.4-642.6)	936												936
C5. Obstructed labour (660)	7,976												7,976
C6. Abortion (630-639)	2,565												2,565
D. Perinatal causes (760-779)	99,658	55,180	2				55,183	44,472	1				44,474

Annex Table 12. **Disability-adjusted life years (DALYs, in thousands): World**

Disease or injury (ICD 9 code)	Both sexes all ages	Males 0-4	5-14	15-44	45-59	60+	All ages	Females 0-4	5-14	15-44	45-59	60+	All ages
II. *Noncommunicable* (140-628,680-759) (minus 320-322,460-465,466,480-487, 614-616)	574,442	55,187	21,576	74,141	65,750	81,362	298,016	54,533	19,692	70,988	50,252	80,962	276,426
A. Malignant neoplasms (140-208)	80,015	843	2,774	9,130	15,777	16,178	44,701	1,385	895	9,119	12,148	11,767	35,314
A1. Mouth and oropharynx (140-149)	4,449	15	41	643	1,008	1,296	3,003	24	9	380	431	602	1,446
A2. Oesophagus (150)	3,746	7	1	306	1,077	1,138	2,529	-	-	147	467	602	1,217
A3. Stomach (151)	7,556	2	14	652	1,952	2,115	4,735	-	8	609	953	1,250	2,821
A4. Colorectal (152,153,154)	5,079	2	10	500	820	1,306	2,638	5	11	415	721	1,288	2,440
A5. Liver (155)	5,702	16	62	1,367	1,713	1,007	4,166	29	5	429	569	504	1,536
A6. Pancreas (157)	1,398	-	-	116	305	395	815	2	3	60	185	334	582
A7. Lung (162)	8,847	10	29	608	2,764	3,279	6,690	5	3	251	806	1,092	2,157
A8. Melanoma and other skin (172-173)	576	1	3	97	106	86	294	2	1	95	94	91	282
A9. Breast (174)	4,514	-	-	-	-	-	-	3	1	1,414	1,876	1,219	4,514
A10. Cervix (180)	3,248	-	-	-	-	-	-	9	-	1,093	1,447	698	3,248
A11. Corpus uteri (179,181-182)	621	-	-	-	-	-	-	1	-	92	271	256	621
A12. Ovary (183)	1,376	-	-	-	-	-	-	22	15	466	487	385	1,376
A13. Prostate (185)	1,555	-	-	-	255	1,277	1,555	-	-	-	-	-	-
A14. Bladder (188)	1,454	4	6	99	350	626	1,085	5	2	46	107	208	369
A15. Lymphoma (200-202)	3,165	105	459	600	394	468	2,026	92	51	347	267	382	1,139
A16. Leukemia (204-208)	4,128	235	723	824	258	291	2,332	340	251	728	229	248	1,796
B. Other neoplasm (210-239)	2,950	105	181	293	199	155	933	161	1,200	345	153	157	2,017
C. Diabetes mellitus (250)	7,968	11	7	891	1,319	1,243	3,473	12	22	841	1,656	1,964	4,495
D. Nutritional/endocrine (240-285, minus 250)	53,183	16,484	1,820	5,880	1,069	762	26,017	16,412	2,329	5,986	1,345	1,094	27,167
D1. Protein-energy malnutrition (260-263)	12,680	5,685	198	126	39	63	6,111	6,117	208	104	25	115	6,569
D2. Iodine deficiency (243)	7,214	3,226	164	188	35	16	3,629	3,191	161	187	30	16	3,585
D3. Vitamin A deficiency (264)	11,757	5,990	-	-	-	-	5,990	5,767	-	-	-	-	5,767
D4. Anaemias (280-285)	13,896	800	1,553	2,409	617	339	5,717	673	2,129	4,197	709	471	8,179
E. Neuro-psychiatric (290-359, minus 320-322)	92,768	2,969	7,355	24,842	7,915	7,056	50,137	2,826	5,434	22,189	4,857	7,326	42,632
E1. Major affective disorder	18,996	-	-	5,366	717	216	6,299	-	-	10,720	1,460	517	12,697
E2. Bipolar affective disorder (296)	1,230	-	-	536	60	17	613	-	-	526	64	27	617
E3. Psychoses (295, 291-294,297-299)	7,481	2	5	3,738	100	70	3,915	3	24	3,418	50	70	3,566
E4. Epilepsy (345)	10,157	842	2,831	1,817	355	130	5,975	615	1,892	1,355	215	104	4,182
E5. Alcohol dependence (303)	13,313	-	-	6,426	3,639	1,550	11,616	-	140	925	539	234	1,698
E6. Alzheimer & other dementias (330,331,333-336,290)	13,995	194	235	131	1,609	4,190	6,360	241	-	104	1,645	5,504	7,635
E7. Parkinson disease (332)	1,189	-	1	3	218	348	571	-	-	3	225	389	618
E8. Multiple sclerosis (340)	1,454	-	6	577	80	34	696	-	6	619	88	44	758
E9. Drug dependence (304)	5,258	-	195	3,199	430	108	3,933	-	54	1,092	151	28	1,325
E10. Post-traumatic stress disorder	5,162	62	478	1,289	112	22	1,964	102	776	2,101	179	40	3,198
F. Sense organ (360-389)	8,240	276	40	327	1,963	1,316	3,923	253	74	374	2,311	1,305	4,318
F1. Glaucoma-related blindness (365)	1,639	-	-	35	395	143	573	-	-	67	727	272	1,066
F2. Cataract-related blindness (366)	5,708	60	-	234	1,500	1,113	2,906	58	-	238	1,527	978	2,802
G. Cardiovascular diseases (390-459)	147,920	3,008	1,748	13,332	21,403	36,893	76,384	2,584	2,569	10,431	15,022	40,930	71,536
G1. Rheumatic heart disease (390-398)	6,711	35	295	1,068	557	501	2,456	73	354	1,387	1,234	1,207	4,255
G2. Ischaemic heart disease (*)	42,460	69	53	3,624	8,085	13,132	24,963	38	24	1,194	3,207	13,034	17,498
G3. Cerebrovascular disease (430-438)	42,982	319	318	2,686	5,445	11,544	20,311	238	410	2,691	5,083	14,251	22,672
G4. Inflammatory cardiac disease (+)	17,388	1,081	575	2,695	2,394	2,515	9,261	1,247	998	1,831	1,643	2,409	8,127
H. Chronic respiratory dis. (460-519, minus 460-466,480-487)	47,406	5,014	3,218	4,255	3,637	9,207	25,331	5,115	2,267	4,114	3,078	7,501	22,075
H1. Chronic obstructive lung dis. (490-492,495-496)	18,325	378	139	430	2,100	7,338	10,384	311	94	415	1,546	5,575	7,941
H2. Asthma (493)	12,402	496	2,141	2,601	662	334	6,234	431	1,684	2,594	952	507	6,167

Annex Table 12. **Disability-adjusted life years (DALYs, in thousands): World**

Disease or injury (ICD 9 code)	Both sexes all ages	Males 0-4	Males 5-14	Males 15-44	Males 45-59	Males 60 +	Males All ages	Females 0-4	Females 5-14	Females 15-44	Females 45-59	Females 60 +	Females All ages
I. Diseases of the digestive system (520-579)	45,332	5,739	1,399	7,417	6,046	4,286	24,887	7,006	1,756	4,697	3,505	3,481	20,445
I1. Peptic ulcer disease (531-533)	4,134	27	71	1,200	817	481	2,596	40	36	744	413	307	1,539
I2. Cirrhosis of the liver (571)	12,926	146	126	3,420	3,366	1,791	8,849	115	181	1,392	1,419	970	4,076
J. Genito-urinary (580-629)	17,610	694	1,515	2,032	3,141	2,210	9,592	434	1,265	2,437	1,761	2,122	8,018
J1. Nephritis/nephrosis (580-589)	10,390	274	1,354	1,662	975	1,181	5,446	211	1,151	1,604	833	1,146	4,944
J2. Benign prostatic hypertrophy (600)	2,239	6	-	9	1,776	448	2,239						-
K. Skin disease (680-709)	842	-	58	54	30	69	330	121	26	218	23	124	512
L. Musculo-skeletal system (710-739)	18,490	119	355	2,389	1,968	1,099	5,839	81	736	6,763	2,979	2,092	12,651
L1. Rheumatoid arthritis (714)	4,456	28	-	575	452	159	1,186	-	384	1,952	658	275	3,270
L2. Osteoarthritis (715)	11,218	-	156	1,600	1,379	598	3,733	-	117	4,007	2,026	1,336	7,486
M. Congenital abnormalities (740-759)	40,859	19,689	822	601	32	19	21,164	17,941	823	843	72	17	19,695
N. Oral health (520-529)	10,733	205	281	2,691	1,240	841	5,257	197	276	2,620	1,336	1,046	5,476
N1. Dental caries (521.0)	1,940	205	281	336	99	56	977	197	276	325	100	65	963
N2. Periodontal disease (523)	3,228	-	-	1,338	215	89	1,642	-	-	1,274	216	97	1,587
N3. Edentulism (520)	5,564	-	-	1,017	926	695	2,639	-	-	1,021	1,021	884	2,926
III. Injuries (E800-999)	162,662	15,331	16,450	65,723	8,103	3,654	109,261	14,674	10,112	21,783	3,287	3,545	53,401
A. Unintentional (E800-949)	112,562	13,034	14,377	39,326	5,629	2,856	75,222	12,020	8,752	11,521	2,099	2,949	37,340
A1. Road traffic accidents (E810-819, 826-829)	31,739	1,286	3,630	16,120	1,587	506	23,129	969	2,610	4,189	583	259	8,610
A2. Poisoning (E850-869)	4,337	468	230	1,670	468	110	2,948	250	224	719	120	76	1,389
A3. Falls (E850-869)	19,874	2,652	2,369	5,014	1,175	1,204	12,413	3,022	1,316	737	457	1,929	7,461
A4. Fires (E890-899)	6,730	1,721	616	1,150	213	155	3,855	1,216	833	561	109	156	2,875
A5. Drowning (E910)	11,438	1,998	2,553	2,829	253	93	7,727	1,620	1,146	780	97	68	3,711
A6. Occupational (#)	3,444	-	-	2,226	425	19	2,670	-	-	643	125	7	774
B. Intentional (E950-969,990-999)	50,100	2,297	2,072	26,397	2,474	798	34,039	2,655	1,360	10,263	1,188	596	16,061
B1. Self-inflicted (E950-959)	17,530	-	444	8,210	1,345	598	10,596	-	305	5,463	733	432	6,934
B2. Homicide and violence (E960-969)	18,340	950	713	11,554	824	154	14,195	1,293	453	2,036	249	114	4,145
B3. War (E990-999)	14,230	1,347	916	6,633	305	46	9,247	1,362	601	2,765	206	50	4,983
Population (in millions)	5,267.4	321.3	551.2	1,249.9	312.4	218.9	2,653.7	309.3	525.5	1,198.6	311.1	269.2	2,613.7

Notes

A dash (-) symbol indicates less than 1,000 DALYs.

* ICD 9 codes for ischaemic heart disease are as follows: 410-414, 440.9, plus: at ages 45-59: 50% of 427.1, 427.4, 427.5, and 33% of 428; at ages 60 +: 80% of 427.1, 427.4, 427.5 and 50% of 428.

+ ICD 9 codes for inflammatory cardiac diseases are as follows: 420, 421, 422, 425 plus: at ages 0-44: 50% of 428; at ages 45-59: 25% of 428; at ages 60+: 20% of 428.

There are no established ICD 9 codes specific for occupational injuries.
Estimates have been based on reported occupational injuries and deaths tabulated by the International Labour Organisation.

Health expenditures and intervention packages: a global overview

Dépenses de santé et modules d'intervention: analyse mondiale

Comparative assessments of financial resources available to the health sector and the range of intervention options that can be purchased with these resources should be an integral part of health policy debate. The preparation of the World development report 1993: investing in health *(WDR) by the World Bank stimulated the development of the first comparative assessments of national health expenditures and external assistance to the health sector. Four papers are presented here: the first reports in detail on the methods, materials and new results for assessing national health expenditures in all countries, while the second provides a detailed analysis of external assistance to the health sector over the last two decades. With the development of the Global Burden of Disease study and the expanding database on the cost-effectiveness of health interventions, information is now available to directly analyse the content of the health sector's activities. The third paper describes the basis for the packages of essential clinical and public health care proposed in the WDR. An alternative method of using information on burden and cost-effectiveness to identify packages of cost-effective health care, which also includes investments in improving the health system, is provided in the fourth paper.*

* * *

Il est souhaitable que la comparaison des ressources financières disponibles pour le secteur de santé et des diverses possibilités d'intervention susceptibles d'être achetées avec ces ressources fasse partie intégrante du débat sur les politiques de santé. La rédaction du Rapport sur le développement dans le monde 1993: investir dans la santé *par la Banque mondiale a stimulé le développement des premières évaluations comparées des dépenses nationales de santé et de l'aide extérieure au secteur de santé. Quatre articles sont présentés ici; le premier rend compte en détail des matériels, des méthodes et des résultats nouveaux utilisés pour évaluer les dépenses nationales de santé dans tous les pays, tandis que le deuxième contient une analyse détaillée de l'aide extérieure au secteur de santé pendant les vingt dernières années. L'étude du poids de la morbidité dans le monde et l'extension des bases de données sur le rapport coût-efficacité des interventions sanitaires ont apporté des informations qui permettent d'analyser directement le contenu des activités du secteur de santé. Dans le troisième article sont indiqués les principes de base des modules de soins cliniques et de santé publique essentiels proposés dans le* Rapport. *Une autre méthode d'utilisation des données sur le poids de la morbidité et le rapport coût-efficacité pour identifier les modules de soins de santé à bon rapport coût-efficacité, qui tient compte également des fonds investis dans l'amélioration du système de santé, est indiquée dans le quatrième article.*

National health expenditures: a global analysis

C.J.L. Murray,[1] R. Govindaraj,[2] & P. Musgrove[3]

As part of the background research to the World development report 1993: investing in health, *an effort was made to estimate public, private and total expenditures on health for all countries of the world. Estimates could be found for public spending for most countries, but for private expenditure in many fewer countries. Regressions were used to predict the missing values of regional and global estimates. These econometric exercises were also used to relate expenditure to measures of health status. In 1990 the world spent an estimated US$ 1.7 trillion (1.7×10^{12}) on health, or $ 1.9 trillion (1.9×10^{12}) in dollars adjusted for higher purchasing power in poorer countries. This amount was about 60% public and 40% private in origin. However, as incomes rise, public health expenditure tends to displace private spending and to account for the increasing share of incomes devoted to health.*

Interest in health expenditures is rising, both in poor countries facing the challenge of maintaining health services during global recession and structural adjustment, and in the richer countries trying to limit health expenditures that are growing faster than the GDP. Due to the lack of standardized estimates of national health expenditure with which to make meaningful international comparisons, the present study on national health expenditures was commissioned as a key preparatory step for the *World development report 1993: investing in health (1)*.

Past studies

Extensive reviews of both descriptive and analytical studies on national health expenditures in developing and industrialized countries have been prepared periodically (*2–4*). Four themes from past studies are important to put this work in context. First, information on health expenditure has evolved considerably in the past three decades in the industrialized countries but not in the developing countries. The earliest comprehensive international study, published by the International Labour Organisation (ILO) in 1959, compared medical payments under social insurance programmes with payments provided under voluntary insurance in the USA (*5*). Abel-Smith (*6, 7*) was the first to try to standardize cross-national data by defining the constituent components of health ser-

vices, listing the main sources of finance, and laying down a standard classification of expenditures which he applied to several industrialized countries. His efforts were followed by a series of comparative studies that led to the development of an annual database on OECD (Organisation for Economic Co-operation and Development) health expenditures, prepared using standard definitions and approaches (*8–10*).[a]

The development of health expenditure data for the developing countries has been less successful. WHO, PAHO, USAID and the Sandoz Institute for Health and Socioeconomic Studies have attempted to improve information by promoting household surveys and publishing manuals for estimating national health expenditures (*3, 11–13*).[b] Despite these efforts, most estimates of national health expenditure have come from *ad hoc* studies or development agency missions to countries, often conducted over a short period of time. Consequently, the unpublished literature from agencies such as the World Bank remains an important but difficult to obtain source of expenditure estimates for the developing countries. Regional reviews drawing largely on these sources have been prepared for Asia (*14*), Africa (*15*), and Latin America (*16*).

Second, many cross-sectional studies have explored the determinants of national health expenditure, particularly in OECD countries (e.g. *17–31*). Taken together, these studies show that income per capita explains most of the variance in health expenditure per capita; Newhouse (*21*), for example, found that 90% of the variance in OECD health expendi-

[1] Associate Professor of International Health Economics, Harvard Center for Population and Development Studies, 9 Bow Street, Cambridge, MA 02138, USA. Requests for reprints should be sent to this author.

[2] Research Associate, Harvard Center for Population and Development Studies, Cambridge, MA, USA.

[3] Senior Economist, Population, Health and Nutrition Department, The World Bank, Washington, DC, USA.

[a] **Poullier J-P, Sandier S.** *Cost containment in OECD countries.* Paper presented at the European Health Policy Forum, Paris, 25–26 February 1988.

[b] **Rice D.** *Financing health services: a manual for developing countries.* Unpublished WHO document No. SHS/SPM/80.3, 1980.

Reprinted from *Bulletin of the World Health Organization*, 1994, 72 (4): 623–637.

141

ture was explained by GDP per capita. Some studies report that other variables such as reimbursement methods, institutional variables, and the inpatient/outpatient mix can explain some of the variance in health expenditure (23, 29, 32–35). Nevertheless, the strongest factor in nearly all studies, including those few which examined the developing countries (33, 36, 37), has been income per capita.

Most studies have also found that health expenditure has an income elasticity greater than one: for a 10 percent increase in income per capita, the health expenditure per capita increases more than 10 percent. Goods or services with an income elasticity greater than one are defined in economics to be a luxury. On this basis, Newhouse concluded that health expenditure in OECD countries must be purchasing *caring* (which is more of a luxury) than *curing* (which seems to be more of a necessity). However, others have taken issue with the empirical observation that health expenditure has an income elasticity greater than one and challenge the interpretation of health care as a luxury item (38).

Third, most studies at the household level in developed countries do not show a greater-than-one elasticity for health expenditure with respect to income. The discrepancy between the relations at the national level and at the household level has been attributed in Canada to non-price rationing, so that consumers buy less health care than they want and can afford (39). However, this would imply that high-income consumers are more rationed than those with lower incomes. A more plausible explanation is that large health care expenditures are financed primarily by insurance rather than by individuals, and insurance spending rises less rapidly with income.

Finally, few studies in either the OECD countries or the developing countries have examined public health expenditures and private health expenditures and their determinants separately. Musgrove's study (40), using household survey data from six Latin American countries, is a noteworthy exception. In these countries, private care had a higher income elasticity than public sector health expenditures, suggesting that private care is a luxury relative to public care and that consumption shifts from public to private, other things being equal, as household incomes rise. This may partly be attributed to differences in real or perceived quality which make private and public health care only imperfect substitutes. The finding that a higher income shifts expenditure to the private sector is not generally observed at the aggregate level, when countries outside Latin America are also studied.

The objectives of the present study are fourfold: (*a*) to assess existing information on national health expenditures and identify gaps in it; (*b*) to explore the relation between national health expenditures and important social, economic and demographic variables using econometric analysis; (*c*) to estimate, using equations from (*b*), the level of national health expenditures in every country of the world for 1990; and (*d*) to analyse patterns of expenditure disaggregated by activity, type, and source of finance. The last objective is treated elsewhere (4); the other three are discussed here.

Definitions, methods and materials

The first objective, that of assessing what is known about health spending, required a consistent definition of expenditure and agreement on how to group spending by different agents and express its value in internationally comparable terms.

Defining and valuing health expenditure

To define health expenditure requires defining *health*, the set of health-promoting *activities*, and the subset of such activities to be included in the health *sector*. Many definitions of health have been proposed. WHO's Constitution defines health as a state of complete physical, mental, and social well-being and not merely the absence of disease or infirmity (41). Such a broad definition may be conceptually appealing, but it makes health almost equivalent to a utility or welfare and poses many practical measurement problems (42). A negative definition, such as the absence of dysfunction or death, is more practical and closer to what is involved in health *care*.

This raises the question of which expenditures on the various health-improving activities should be included as health sector expenditures. Programmes such as primary school education often contribute significantly to health, but these interventions also have objectives other than health status improvement. One could rank activities by the proportion of their intended outcome in terms of health improvement; for example, 100% of measles immunization benefits are expected to improve health, while perhaps only 20% of the benefits of indoor piped water supply contribute to health improvement. Where do we draw the line defining health expenditure?

For this study, the operational definition includes all expenditures incurred by the preventive and curative health services for individuals, and on population-based public health programmes, as well as some programmes with a direct impact on health status (e.g., family planning programmes, nutrition programmes, and health education but not other kinds of education). Programmes that only indirectly affect health, such as relief and food programmes, and environmental programmes related to water and sanitation, were excluded.

We hoped to estimate health expenditure according to who pays for it and also who provides it. Categorizing health expenditure according to both financing and provision of services by the government, parastatal agencies (i.e., social security and social insurance programmes of the government), and the private sector defines a 3×3 matrix (Table 1). Typically, data were available for the total financing provided by each of the three subsectors. The breakdown of government financing for services provided by the government itself, by parastatal agencies and by the private sector was also often available. However, data were rarely found for the other cells in the matrix. The study was therefore restricted to the *financing* of health services by the various sectors. This focus is consistent with the approach of the U.S. Health Care Financing Administration (HCFA) (29), and facilitates comparisons of health expenditures in the OECD countries.

While estimates for individual countries are the main objective of the study, for some purposes countries have been grouped, as in the *World development report 1993*, into eight regions: Established Market Economies (EME), Formerly Socialist Economies of Europe (FSE), Middle Eastern Crescent (MEC), India (IND), China (CHN), Other Asia and Islands (OAI), Latin America and the Caribbean (LAC), and Sub-Saharan Africa (SSA). The first two groups together are referred to as "demographically developed" since they have largely completed the transition to low fertility and mortality levels.

The base year for the study is 1990. For countries with estimates prior to 1990 but not for 1990, we assumed that spending on health as a share of GDP was the same in 1990 as in the year of the most recent estimate. Estimates of the 1990 expenditure in local currency have been converted into US dollars (US$) using the 1990 official exchange rates. The results were also calculated in "International dollars" (I$) using purchasing-power parity (PPP) ratios from the World Bank's modification of the United Nations international comparisons project (43). Purchasing-power parity ratios calculated specifically for the

health sector would be preferable to those based on total GDP, but as these are available for so few countries (4) the GDP PPPs were used for all countries. In the calculation of expenditures in international dollars, external assistance (primarily paid in US dollars or other hard currency) was assumed to fund only tradable goods, so it was not corrected for purchasing-power parity.

Domestic expenditures for each country are classified as government, parastatal, or private sector spending. Total health expenditure comprises these expenditures and external assistance. Government health expenditure is what has been spent on health by the government at various administrative levels or by institutions wholly controlled by the government. Parastatal expenditures consist of the health components of social security and social insurance programmes, and the expenditures on health of other parastatal agencies. Public expenditures are defined as the sum of government and parastatal expenditures, to permit comparisons with the OECD countries where expenditures on health-related social insurance and social security programmes are not distinguished from government expenditure. Private sector health expenditure refers to spending by all nongovernmental entities, including individuals, households, private corporations and non-profit organizations. Private expenditures are the sum of private institutional and individual expenditures (including both direct or incidental costs and purchase of insurance by institutions and individuals or households).

Data sources, coverage and limitations

Substantial effort was invested in obtaining data on government, parastatal and private health expenditure directly from governments, supplemented with reports and data from WHO, the World Bank, the International Labour Organisation, regional development banks, and the United Nations Statistics Division as well as the published literature. The collection includes material from nearly 1000 different reports, articles and budgets, much of which is not published.

Information on government health expenditures was available for 138 countries. These expenditures were for the years from 1977 to 1990, with the majority (119 countries) having data for the period 1986–90. Information for the 24 OECD countries for 1990 was obtained from the HCFA national health accounts. Data on government health expenditures from 43 other countries came from national budgets. Information for another 45 countries was taken from an IMF yearbook (44). Data for 21 countries not covered by these sources were obtained through the World Bank health and public sector studies. Finally, data for five countries came from *ad hoc* studies.

Table 1: **Availability of health data, financing vs. provision**

	Financing			Total health
	Government	Parastatal	Private	
Provision				
Government	X			
Parastatal				
Private	X			
Total health	X	X	X	X

Information on parastatal spending was available from 111 countries for the period from 1983 to 1990; 1988 was the latest year for which there was comprehensive information for most countries. Data on social security in 100 countries were obtained from ILO studies, and for eleven countries from the World Bank and *ad hoc* studies.

Even using multiple sources, reasonable data on private sector spending were available for only 73 countries for the period 1974 to 1990. Information came from household surveys (some conducted by the ILO), national accounts, as well as World Bank, HCFA and *ad hoc* studies. Unfortunately, even when these assessments were based on surveys—either institutional or at the household level—many estimates were suspect. Household surveys, although widely acknowledged to provide the most reliable assessment of private spending on health, often exhibited systematic sampling and non-sampling bias. For some household consumption surveys, total household expenditure, expanded to all households in the country, exceeded estimated private consumption in the national accounts data for the same year, which made the estimated private household expenditure on health for the country unrealistically high. For example, in a household survey in the Republic of Korea in 1990, calculated private health spending was 11–12% of GDP. Even more strikingly, a survey in Fiji in 1977 gives a figure for private health spending that exceeds GDP.

For several reasons, including non-representative sampling, many household surveys in developing countries may overestimate per capita private consumption. However, private health expenditures as a *share* of total private expenditure may not be biased if the income elasticity across households is close to one (and any bias in the data is independent of income). To estimate private sector financing, the household survey results were therefore adjusted by applying the percentage of household spending on health from these surveys to the total private consumption numbers from the national accounts. This adjustment yielded far more believable estimates of private health spending; in the above examples, the figure for the Republic of Korea was adjusted down to 2.9% of GDP and the corresponding figure for Fiji was 1.4%.

Comparability across data sources was a major issue for all three subsectors. For several countries there is a wide divergence in the quoted expenditure figures for the same year across data sources, and over fairly short periods of time (which may be explained by radical changes in the levels of spending from one year to the next for some countries, but seems very unlikely for others). Discussions with the country officers at the World Bank or with people familiar with those countries led to a choice of which estimate was most plausible.

Estimating out-of-sample

One of the objectives of this study is to estimate total health expenditures for *every* country in 1990. Estimates of public sector expenditures for 12 countries and of private sector expenditures in a further 118 countries were not available. This section therefore develops predictive equations to estimate these expenditures for these 130 countries. We have assumed that public sector expenditure is not a function of private sector health expenditure, while the latter could be a function of the former. This hypothesis is grounded in the belief that most governments are largely unaware of the magnitude of the private health sector, or at least do not take it into account in determining their health budgets. The health services that people are willing to buy for themselves, in contrast, may depend on what the public sector is already financing.

Estimating public sector expenditure. We examined the relation between public sector expenditure and GDP per capita, government consumption as percent GDP, private consumption as percent GDP, life expectancy at birth, infant mortality rate, percent urban population, average years of schooling completed, and regional dummy variables.[c] Regressions were estimated in both US dollars and International dollars; in each case the dependent variable, public sector health spending, was measured both per capita and as a percent of GDP. The independent variables were derived primarily from sources at the World Bank, with some augmentation from the OECD, the IMF (government and international financial statistics) and United Nations agencies.

For the per-capita specification, univariate tests with the different independent variables showed closer association with the logarithm of expenditure than with the expenditure itself. Strong univariate relations were observed, among others, for public sector expenditures per capita as a function of GDP per capita in US and International dollar terms (R^2 of 0.91 and 0.85, respectively), and of health status indicators such as infant mortality rate and life expectancy at birth. However, close relations between public sector expenditure denominated in per capita terms and income per capita are not so impressive as one might assume, as the following experiment demonstrates.

---

[c] Each region is represented as a binary (dummy) variable. If a country is a member of a particular regional group, its value for that regional variable is 1. If it is not a member, that value is zero.

Take a set of countries with a range of income per capita equal to that in the dataset (US$ 44 to 34 135; I$ 402 to 21 701) and randomly assign each country a share of GDP spent on health between 1% and 8%, the range of shares of GDP found in the dataset. Estimated public health expenditure per capita is then calculated as the share of GDP times income per capita. Regressing this *randomly generated* estimate against income per capita (in a linear model) yields a surprisingly high R^2. This Monte Carlo simulation has been repeated 8000 times. The expectation of the distribution of R^2 is 0.55 (max=0.79; min=0.24) for the US$ simulation and 0.54 (max=0.76; min=0.3) for the I$ simulation. The corresponding expectations for the regression using the logarithms of per capita expenditures and income are 0.76 (max=0.91; min=0.41) for the US$ simulation and 0.70 (max=0.85; min=0.42) for the I$ simulation. These results confirm that even randomly generated expenditure shares can suggest a close fit between per capita expenditure and per capita income. A more exacting test of the relation between public health expenditure and income as well as other independent variables that are highly collinear with income is to examine public health expenditure as a share of GDP, which is the specification used in the regressions.

We tested the most general model first, using all the independent variables. Non-significant independent variables were dropped until the most parsimonious form was generated. Groups of independent variables were F-tested, and retained if the F-test was significant. Four parsimonious regressions were estimated for the share of GDP: linear forms with independent variables in US$ and in I$, and double-log forms with independent variables in US$ and in I$.

For prediction, we chose the form with the highest adjusted R^2. This equation:

Public health expenditure as % GDP = 0.02 + 1.10E-6 GDP per capita + 0.09 government consumption as % GDP – 0.03 dummy for MEC – 0.03 dummy for OAI – 0.02 dummy for LAC – 0.03 dummy for SSA

shows public expenditure on health as a share of GDP to be a linear function of GDP per capita in I$, government consumption as a percent of GDP, and dummy variables for MEC, OAI and SSA (which are indistinguishable from one another) and LAC. (All coefficients are non-zero with P values less than 0.01). The adjusted R^2 was 0.79. Higher income was associated with a higher share of income spent on health—the elasticity from the double-log form was 1.43 (1.34 in US$). Governments that consumed a larger share of GDP in total also had a higher

expenditure on health. The significant dummy variables indicate greater regional differences in share of GDP spent on health than can be explained by income per capita alone. However, the infant mortality rate and life expectancy at birth were not related to public sector health expenditure. Thus the equation says nothing about causal relations between expenditure and health status. (We will return to this question in the final section).

Estimating private health expenditure. We hypothesized that while the public sector is relatively insensitive to private sector spending in health, the private sector is sensitive to the size of government financing of health services. We therefore used public sector expenditures as an independent variable in the private sector equation. There are, however, two reasons why observed private spending cannot simply be regressed on observed public expenditure. First, the private sector estimates span 16 years from 1974 to 1990. Estimates of public sector expenditures are not always available for the same years. Second, if private sector expenditure is a function of GDP per capita, other socioeconomic variables, and public sector health expenditure—while public health expenditure is also a function of GDP per capita, the parameter estimates from OLS regression will be biased. To deal with both problems, we used the public sector regression developed above to *predict* public sector expenditure in the same year as the private sector expenditure estimate, effectively creating an instrumental variable for public sector health expenditure. Of course, the independent variables, GDP per capita, and government consumption as a share of GDP were also taken from the same year as the private sector estimate in generating the instrumental variable. We have assumed, in effect, that the functional relationship between the share of GDP spent by the public sector on health and GDP per capita and government consumption has not changed over the last 16 years.

Private sector health expenditures per capita and private expenditures as a percent of GDP were analysed as dependent variables. As before, regressions were run using US dollar and PPP-adjusted incomes. All independent variables were from the same year as the private expenditure estimate, for each country. In addition to those variables included in the public sector regressions, we added a dummy variable for former British colonies which gained independence after the Second World War and another for former French colonies, on the assumption that colonial history might play a significant role in explaining the variance in private health expenditures.

Parsimonious forms were estimated for eight different models, using three binary choices: per capita expenditure versus share of GDP, US$ versus I$, and linear versus double-log functional forms. The highest adjusted R^2 (0.86) was for private sector expenditure per capita in the double-log form using US$ for the independent variables, so this equation was used for prediction:

Natural log of private health spending per capita = – 4.34 + 1.03 natural log GDP per capita

The only significant (P <0.01) variable in any specification was GDP per capita. The elasticity is 1.03 or indistinguishable from unity. In other words, the share of GDP privately spent on health is nearly constant over the range of GDP per capita. Notably, public sector expenditure was not significant in any of these regressions. Nor were there any significant regional dummy variables. The dummy variables for colonial history, meant to capture potential institutional effects, were also not significant. Separate regressions were undertaken for private sector estimates from each source (OECD, national accounts, household surveys, etc.) but the relations did not change. The lack of relation between private sector expenditure as a share of GDP, and GDP per capita (or any of the other independent variables) is confirmed in the regressions using share of GDP as the dependent variable. The adjusted R^2 for the linear form was less than 0.08 in both US$ and I$ forms.

Results

Global and regional spending on health care in 1990 was estimated by combining the observed values with those predicted by the regressions for the public and private subsectors. These regression estimates were used for 12 and 87 countries, respectively, but they account for only 0.03% and 2.0% of the estimated total expenditure in the two subsectors, because the great bulk of spending occurs in countries for which data were available and it was not necessary to predict values from the equations. There were 153 such countries for public spending and 78 for private spending.[d] Expenditure estimated from the regressions is of course a larger share of the estimated total spending in the poorer regions. Only in Sub-Saharan Africa was more than 1% of the estimated regional public spending derived from the regressions, but the shares for private expenditure are 31% in Africa, 39% in the Middle Eastern Crescent, 15% in Latin America and the Caribbean, 6.2% in the Formerly Socialist Economies, and 3.6% in Asia.

---

[d] A total of 138 and 73 countries were used for the public and private sector regressions, respectively. Data for additional countries were obtained after completion of the regression analyses.

Estimates of public, private and total health expenditures are provided in the Annex for every country: estimates derived from the regression analysis are in bold-face italics. For a few countries there was no information even on public spending, so the total health expenditure was estimated by using the same share of GDP, or the same level per capita, as in the other countries of the same region. Public and private shares can then be estimated by the same ratio as in the rest of the region. These estimates are used only to complete the regional and global totals and are not reported in the Annex. Estimates of public expenditure only, disaggregated by function and activity, are presented in Murray et al. (4).

The world as a whole is estimated to have spent US$ 1.7 trillion (1.7×10^{12}) on health in 1990 (Table 2), which constituted 8% of the global GDP. The Established Market Economies accounted for over 87% of the total; inclusion of the Formerly Socialist Economies of Europe, which are also demographically developed, raises the share to 90% or US$ 1532 billion (1532×10^9). It is even more striking that spending on health in the US alone is 41% of global health expenditures. In contrast, spending in developing regions was only 10% or US$ 167 billion (167×10^9), even counting external assistance.

When expenditures are corrected for purchasing power parity, global spending amounted to a little under I$ 1.9 trillion (1.9×10^{12}) (Table 3). This makes developing country expenditure much larger (380 versus 167 billion dollars), but there is little change in estimated spending by the EME and FSE countries. They appear to spend 80% of the total while the USA still spends 37%. External assistance to the health sector is only 0.7% of the total health expenditure in developing countries measured in International dollars, as opposed to 1.7% in US$.

Approximately 60% of global health spending is from the public sector (inclusive of external assistance), while private sector financing constitutes the other 40%. The picture is very similar in the PPP-adjusted calculations. Because the EME countries dominate world health expenditure, the global public share is close to what it is in those countries (61%: it is higher if the USA is left out). Public expenditure is relatively more important in the FSE countries (71%), and much less important in the developing regions. This is particularly clear if expenditure is examined exclusive of external assistance: the public share is only 38% in OAI, 44% in SSA and 20% in India. With much variation among countries, the trend is for the public share of health financing to rise with income, reflecting high levels of spending on social insurance and public health programmes by governments in richer countries and much reliance on out-of-pocket purchases in poor countries.

Table 2: **Regional total health expenditures in 1990 United States dollars**

Region	1990 GDP (1990 US$ × 10⁶)	1990 Public health expenditures (1990 US$ × 10⁶)	1990 Private health expenditures (1990 US$ × 10⁶)	1990 Aid flows for health (1990 US$ × 10⁶)	Total health expenditures (1990 US$ × 10⁶)	Total health expenditures	
						As % GDP	Per capita (1990 US$)
Established Market Economies	15 974 547	905 998	577 287	0	1 483 285	9.29	1 869
Middle Eastern Crescent	1 248 990	25 414	18 887	330	44 631	3.57	88
Formerly Socialist Economies of Europe	1 380 409	34 864	14 250	0	49 114	3.56	142
India	291 561	3 499	13 703	286	17 488	6.00	20
China	365 557	7 494	5 248	77	12 819	3.51	11
Other Asia and Islands	817 304	13 972	22 303	542	36 817	4.50	53
Latin America and the Caribbean	1 106 035	26 218	17 065	542	43 825	3.96	98
Sub-Saharan Africa	275 580	5 102	5 432	1 072	11 607	4.21	22
All regions	21 459 983	1 022 561	674 175	2 848	1 699 585	7.92	320

Total health expenditures as a share of GDP reach a high of more than 9% in the EME region. Including external assistance to the health sector, the share of GDP spent on health is remarkably similar in most other regions, ranging from 3.5% to 4.5% in US dollars and 3.5% to 3.9% in PPP terms. The exception is India, which spends 6% (Fig. 1). If external assistance is subtracted from the total, the shares are more varied and more correlated with income: poorer countries spend a smaller share of GDP out of their own resources. Sub-Saharan Africa spends the lowest share of GDP on health, and for many African countries such as Burkina Faso, Guinea-Bissau, Liberia and Mozambique, aid exceeds half of the total health expenditures.

Since EME has the highest incomes and a relatively large share of GDP devoted to health, there is a great dichotomy between per capita health spending in this region and the rest of the world. In EME, on average, US$ 1859 per capita is spent on health. In FSE, which has the second highest level of health expenditures per capita, spending is only US$ 144. Spending in the other regions is $103 in Latin America, $97 in the Middle Eastern Crescent, $61 in Asia, $23 in Sub-Saharan Africa, $21 in China, and only $11 in India. Using purchasing-power parity ratios to compare expenditures narrows the gap between the North and South. While the EME region spends about I$ 1793 per capita, the FSE region, which still has the second highest level, spends about I$ 241 per capita. Latin America spends I$ 181 per capita, the Middle Eastern Crescent about I$ 167, Other Asia and Islands about I$ 111, and Sub-Saharan Africa approximately I$ 50.

Table 3: **Regional total health expenditures in 1990 International dollars**

Region	1990 GDP (1990 I$ × 10⁶)	1990 Public health expenditures (1990 I$ × 10⁶)	1990 Private health expenditures (1990 I$ × 10⁶)	1990 Aid flows for health (1990 I$ × 10⁶)	Total health expenditures (1990 I$ × 10⁶)	Total health expenditures	
						As % GDP	Per capita (1990 I$)
Established Market Economies	15 202 504	864 110	565 850	0	1 429 961	9.41	1 802
Middle Eastern Crescent	1 514 707	33 401	27 668	1 097	62 166	4.10	122
Formerly Socialist Economies of Europe	2 208 580	58 643	22 911	0	81 554	3.69	235
India	878 687	10 544	41 298	861	52 703	6.00	62
China	2 346 464	48 103	33 685	494	82 281	3.51	72
Other Asia and Islands	1 752 350	23 630	42 678	2 161	68 469	3.91	98
Latin America and the Caribbean	1 987 172	45 075	31 589	1 344	78 009	3.93	174
Sub-Saharan Africa	649 021	10 783	12 164	3 441	26 388	4.07	50
All regions	26 539 483	1 094 289	777 843	9 398	1 881 530	7.09	354

Fig. 1. **Sectoral composition of estimated regional health expenditures in 1990, as percentage of regional GDP.**

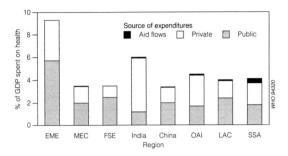

Discussion

This study has demonstrated large gaps in our knowledge of health expenditures. Neither the World Health Organization nor the World Bank has devoted resources to maintaining a database on national health expenditures. Costly *ad hoc* studies could be avoided in the future, if data collection were more systematized.

Government health expenditures are not difficult to obtain once the most appropriate source of data in each country has been identified. The International Monetary Fund already maintains a database of government expenditure. With some extra investment of resources, WHO or the World Bank could supplement this routinely collected information and generate more complete information on national health expenditures. For relatively little cost, government expenditures could be monitored annually.

Despite attempts by the ILO to collect information on a regular basis for parastatal expenditures on health (chiefly through social security systems), the figures suffer many critical problems, including that of double counting. Reporting should be coordinated with a system such as the one just discussed for the collection of government expenditures. Parastatal expenditure data, divorced from an analysis of government action and expenditure in the health sector, are at best incomplete and at worst misleading.

Measurement of private sector expenditures is clearly inadequate in the developing world. Even for those countries with detailed *ad hoc* studies, the data are subject to doubt. For example, the high level of private expenditures estimated for India, which is at odds with the pattern in the rest of the developing world, may be real or may be a measurement artifact. One way forward would be the development of national health accounting akin to the OECD health expenditure database. However, the majority of developing countries probably cannot institute such information systems in the near future. Rapid assessment

techniques therefore need to be developed and implemented, in conjunction with an international database on government expenditures, to fill the information gap in the short term.

Income and health status as determinants of health expenditure. The data reviewed in this study suggest that private sector expenditure on health depends on nothing but income, and moreover that the share of GDP is constant across countries. Private health spending relative to GDP is unrelated to income, mortality, the size of government, geographical region, education or public health expenditure. It is particularly surprising to find no association with education or with public expenditure, since the former was expected *a priori* to influence people's understanding of their health needs and their demand for health care, while the latter should provide an alternative to private expenditures. Apparently public and private spending are not simply substitutes, because they finance services that differ in kind, or quality, or in utilization by different population groups. And education may have effects on health status and even on the use of health care which do not show up in aggregate private spending. Of course, private health expenditure may be determined partly by historical, cultural and institutional factors not captured in this analysis; and errors or mis-specifications in the data may reduce the statistical significance of the variables tested.

In contrast to private spending, public health expenditure has an elasticity substantially greater than one. Total health expenditure, however, also includes external assistance that flows primarily to low-income countries (45). Is total health expenditure a luxury item? For all developing countries with observed data (not derived from our estimating equations), a double-log regression of total health expenditure per capita against income per capita gives an elasticity of 1.003, which is indistinguishable from unity. In other words, the *share* of GDP spent on health does not increase with income. As noted above, however, average total health expenditure in EME is substantially higher than in all other regions, so a regression including these countries shows health care to be a luxury item. Compared with the pattern in poorer countries, high health expenditure in EME is not accounted for simply by higher average income.

How do we expect health expenditures to change with income per capita? More income means more resources with which to deal with health problems. We suspect, however, that there are two separate factors involved in the "health problems" which generate demand for health care: *observed or objective* health status and *perceived or subjective* health status. Murray & Chen (46) draw a fundamental distinction between health status as observed by a medical professional and that perceived by the individual. Numerous interview surveys in poor developing countries have recorded higher rates of self-reported morbidity and disability in rich than in poor households (47). Such counter-intuitive patterns of reported morbidity may be at least partly explained by changing expectations of health status. If expectations of good health increase faster than the actual health status—because people have more access to health care, or because more education makes them understand more about health—then the perception of ill health may increase with income. The result will be increasing expenditure which is only loosely related to objective health problems.

The importance of perceived health status may help explain why health expenditure is so much higher in the EME countries and why it continues to rise as a share of income. In poor countries, it may also explain why the rich treat health care as a luxury. However, it is private health spending that seems most likely to respond to this perceived need, whereas government health expenditure might be expected to derive more from observed need as measured by mortality and disability. This would be the case particularly for public health measures that do not respond to subjective demand. This explanation would predict a higher elasticity for private than for public expenditure on health, just the reverse of what we observe.

The relation between total health expenditure and income per capita will be some combination of the effects of both kinds of health status, among other things. If perceived health status is more of a luxury whereas treatment for observed health problems is more of a necessity, then the elasticity of the combined tendencies to spend might increase with the income per capita as "health status" comes to be more a matter of subjective perception. However, as a population ages and develops chronic health problems which are costly to treat, even objective health status may generate pressure to spend an increasing share of the income on health care. And because objective health problems can be life-threatening, people may reasonably be willing to spend increasing shares of their income on health care as they become richer, even with no changes in the underlying demographic or epidemiological situation or in their subjective perceptions.

The relation between income and expenditure on health cannot be understood without taking account of the expanding role for the public sector in financing health care, as observed in nearly all OECD countries and a number of middle-income countries as well. This makes public spending respond to per-

ceived health status and the demand for health services from the population and not only to objective needs. But because that leads to rapidly increasing total expenditure, greater public involvement in financing care also tends to stimulate greater public control of spending, at least to keep the share of GDP from continuing to grow. Any understanding of what accounts for health expenditure and how it is related to health status that goes beyond the superficial will have to disentangle these effects.

What does health expenditure buy? The relations studied here raise the perennial question about what health expenditures actually purchase, in particular whether they buy improved objective health ("curing") or something more subjective ("caring"), or whether they are largely wasted through inefficiency in the production of services and the choice of which services to provide. Using the improved estimates of national health expenditures including external assistance provided in this study, we can examine some relations between health expenditures and measures of health status.

One such analysis is shown in Fig. 2. GDP per capita and a human capital variable summarizing schooling levels were used to predict for 58 countries both the observed total national health expenditure (as a share of GDP) and the life expectancy at birth:

> Total health expenditure as % GDP = −0.0485 + 0.0119 natural log GDP per capita − 0.0055 natural log human capital

and

> Life expectancy at birth (years) = 41.98 + 3.120 natural log GDP per capita + 5.316 natural log human capital

Estimates of expenditures derived from the regressions reported earlier were not used in this exercise, which was limited chiefly by the availability of estimates for private health spending and the human capital variable. (Human capital was just significant at the 0.05 confidence level in explaining health expenditure; otherwise all variables were significant at the 0.01 level. In a similar analysis for 73 countries (1), human capital did not contribute significantly to explaining health spending.) The values of expenditure and life expectancy predicted from these equations were then compared with the observed values, and the differences or *residuals* plotted (Fig. 2).

The result shows for each country whether it spends more or less than might be expected, given its income and education level, and whether its population lives longer or less than might be anticipated. Although income, education and health expenditure are not the only factors influencing life expectancy,

Fig. 2. **Life expectancies and health expenditures in developing countries: deviations from estimates based on GDP and schooling.**

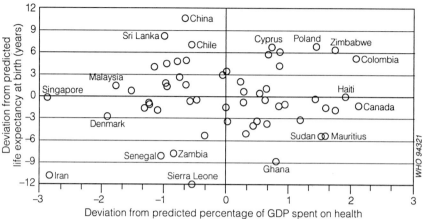

this comparison indicates, roughly, whether health expenditure in a given country is buying increased life to the same degree as in other countries with similar resources and human capital. Points in the upper right and lower left quadrants in Fig. 2 correspond to countries showing a systematic relation between more health expenditure and longer life: that is, spending on health appears to be buying more years of life. Countries in the upper left quadrant achieve gains in life expectancy without spending so much—their health expenditure appears to translate more effectively into improved health status. The data do not indicate, of course, whether this occurs for reasons directly related to how resources are spent in health care, or because the population takes better care of its health through diet and other habits and therefore needs less medical care to achieve the same result. Countries shown in the lower right quadrant are in the opposite situation, with a shorter-than-expected life despite spending more on health care than would be expected on the basis of income and schooling.

Similar relations could be explored using other indicators of health status such as child mortality. The most interesting comparison would relate health expenditure to the total burden of disease in a country, including the effects of disability as well as premature mortality, as described elsewhere (*48*). We cannot provide a parallel analysis to that given in Fig. 2, however, for two reasons. One is that the disease burden has so far been estimated only for the eight regions of the world and for a few individual countries. The other is that even the regional estimates now available describe only the burden of disease *remaining* as a result of everything that has been done, including the expenditure on health care,

to improve health. Comparison should really be made with the *reduction* in disease burden that can be attributed to health spending, which implies a comparison with the situation that would exist in the absence of that expenditure.

Since no such estimates exist, we can only compare the current estimated health spending with the current disease burden: if the expenditure is effective in reducing the burden, the relation should be inverse. Table 4 shows regional disease burdens, in millions of disability-adjusted life years (DALYs), and total health expenditure in International dollars. Across all eight regions, more health spending is clearly associated with better health. However, this relation depends very much on regions with an extremely high disease burden (India and Sub-Saharan Africa) or high expenditure (EME); no inverse relation is apparent among the intermediate regions.

Table 4: **DALY loss and public health expenditures in 1990, by region**

Region	DALY loss (millions)	1990 Public health expenditure (1990 I$ × 10⁶)
Established Market Economies	94	1 429 961
Middle Eastern Crescent	144	62 166
Formerly Socialist Economies of Europe	58	81 554
India	292	52 703
China	201	82 281
Other Asia and Islands	177	68 469
Latin America and the Caribbean	103	78 009
Sub-Saharan Africa	293	26 388
All regions	1 362	1 881 530

As shown in Fig. 2, there is some unknown mixture of varying effectiveness in health care spending, and differences in health status due to other factors such as income, education, and historical and cultural influences. When the burden of disease is estimated for more countries, it should be possible to separate these effects and begin to assess the overall contribution of health care expenditure to improved health.

Acknowledgements

Research assistance for this paper was provided by Robert V. Ashley and William Whang. The authors are grateful to Dr G. Chellaraj of the World Bank for his contribution to the *World development report 1993* background study on global health expenditures, on which this paper is based. The authors also gratefully acknowledge the contribution of colleagues at Harvard University, The World Bank (particularly Ms Karima Saleh, Dr Abdo Yazbeck and Ms Anna Maripuu), U.N. agencies, and various Ministries of Health, whose input and assistance made this study possible.

Résumé

Dépenses nationales de santé: analyse mondiale

Plus de 1000 sources de données, publiées et non publiées, ont été examinées concernant les dépenses publiques, parapubliques (sécurité sociale et programmes publics d'assurance sociale) et privées en soins de santé. Les estimations des dépenses publiques (publiques et parapubliques) ont été obtenues pour 153 pays et les dépenses privées pour 78 pays; un ajustement de ces estimations est souvent nécessaire pour pouvoir prédire les dépenses en 1990 à partir des dépenses des années précédentes. Ces valeurs ont ensuite été soumises à l'analyse économétrique et rapportées aux pays (revenu par habitant, degré de scolarisation, consommation publique totale) et aux régions. Plusieurs modèles ont été testés, les dépenses et les revenus étant évalués en dollars au taux de change et en dollars internationaux ajustés sur le pouvoir d'achat. Les dépenses publiques dans 12 pays et les dépenses privées dans 87 pays ont été évaluées par régression. Les valeurs observées et les valeurs attendues ont ensuite été additionnées pour estimer les dépenses de santé totales dans le monde. L'estimation ainsi obtenue montre qu'en 1990 US$ $1,7 \times 10^{12}$ ont été consacrés dans le monde à la santé, dont 60% par financement public et 40% par financement privé. Quatre-vingt sept pour cent de l'ensemble de ces dépenses ont eu lieu dans les pays les plus riches; les Etats-Unis d'Amérique comptent à eux seuls pour 41%. Les pays en développement ne représentent que US$ 167 milliards, soit 380 milliards de dollars ajustés sur le pouvoir d'achat, aide extérieure comprise.

Pour l'ensemble de la planète, les dépenses de santé sont manifestement un luxe, vu la part importante du revenu consacrée à la santé dans les pays les plus riches. Dans le monde en développement, la part du revenu total prélevée pour la santé est cependant presque constante. Ce résultat concorde avec l'observation que les dépenses publiques, lesquelles sont plus importantes dans les pays riches que dans les pays pauvres, tendent à augmenter plus que les dépenses privées à la suite de l'augmentation du revenu. Les dépenses privées semblent ne dépendre que du niveau de revenu et, en particulier, être indépendantes du niveau des dépenses pour la santé du secteur public. Il apparaît ainsi que ces deux catégories de dépenses ne peuvent pas exactement se substituer l'une à l'autre, en partie probablement parce qu'elles répondent de manière différente aux besoins objectifs de santé et à la perception qu'ont les personnes de leur état de santé.

Ces estimations des dépenses nationales peuvent servir à analyser les achats réels des pays avec les ressources consacrées à la santé et, en particulier, à rechercher si les dépenses sont étroitement associées aux indicateurs que sont l'espérance de vie et le poids de la morbidité dans le pays. L'énorme disparité entre les pays et les régions concernant cette relation, même en tenant compte du revenu et du degré de scolarisation, montre que l'«efficacité» des dépenses à générer une amélioration de l'état de santé est extrêmement variable.

References

1. **World Bank.** *World development report 1993: investing in health.* New York, Oxford University Press, 1993.
2. **Maxwell RJ.** *Health and wealth: an international study of health care spending.* Lexington, Lexington Books, 1981.
3. **Griffiths A, Mills M.** *Money for health: a manual for surveys in developing countries.* Geneva, Sandoz Institute for Health and Socio-economic Studies and the Ministry of Health of the Republic of Botswana, 1982.
4. **Murray CJL et al.** *Global domestic expenditures on health.* Washington, World Bank, 1994.
5. **International Labour Organisation.** *The cost of medical care.* Geneva, 1959.
6. **Abel-Smith B.** *Paying for health services.* Geneva, World Health Organization, 1963 (Public Health Papers, No. 17).

7. **Abel-Smith B.** *An international study of health expenditure.* Geneva, World Health Organization, 1967 (Public Health Papers, No. 32).

8. **Simanis JG.** National expenditures on social security and health in selected countries. *Social security bulletin,* 1990, **53**: 12–16.

9. **Simanis JG.** Medical care expenditures in seven countries. *Social security bulletin,* 1973, **36**: 112–116.

10. **OECD.** Health care expenditure and other data: an international compendium from the OECD. *Health care financing review, 1989 annual supplement,* 1989: 111–194.

11. **Zschock D et al.** *How to study health sector financing in developing countries.* Washington, U.S. Department of Health, Education and Welfare, 1977.

12. **Mach EP, Abel-Smith B.** *Planning the finances of the health sector—a manual for developing countries.* Geneva, World Health Organization, 1983.

13. **Robertson RL et al.** *Guidelines for analysis of health sector financing in developing countries.* Bethesda, U.S. Department of Health, Education, and Welfare, 1979.

14. **Griffin CC.** *Health care in Asia: comparative study of cost and financing.* Washington, World Bank, 1992.

15. **Vogel RJ.** *Trends in health expenditures and revenue sources in sub-Saharan Africa.* Washington, World Bank, 1989.

16. **McGreevy P.** *Social security in Latin America: issues and options for the World Bank.* Washington, World Bank, 1992 (World Bank discussion paper 110).

17. **Fraser RD.** An international study of health and general systems of financing health care. *International journal of health services,* 1973, **3**: 369–397.

18. **Kleiman E.** The determinants of national outlay on health. In: Perlman M, ed. *The economics of health and medical care.* London, Macmillan, 1974.

19. **Newhouse JP.** Medical care expenditure: a cross-national survey, *Journal of human resources,* 1977, **12**: 115–125.

20. **Newhouse JP.** Cross-national differences in health spending—what do they mean? *Journal of health economics,* 1987, **6**: 159–162.

21. **Leu RE.** The public-private mix and international health care costs. In: Culyer A, Jonsson B, eds. *Public and private health services.* Oxford, Blackwell, 1986.

22. **OECD.** *Measuring health care 1960–1983: expenditure, costs, performance.* Paris, 1985 (OECD social policy studies, No. 2).

23. **Gerdtham U-G et al.** *Econometric analysis of health care expenditures: a cross-section study of the OECD countries.* Linkoping, Center for Medical Technology, University of Linkoping, 1988.

24. **Jonsson B.** What can Americans learn from Europeans? *Health care financing review, 1989 annual supplement,* 1989: 79–110.

25. **Gerdtham U-G, Jonsson B.** Conversion factor instability in international comparisons of health care expenditures. *Journal of health economics,* 1991, **10**: 227–234.

26. **Gerdtham U-G, Jonsson B.** Price and quantity in international comparisons of health care expenditure. *Applied economics,* 1991, **23**: 1519–1528.

27. **Pfaff M.** Differences in health care spending across

countries: statistical evidence. *Journal of health politics, policy and law,* 1990, **15**: 1–65.

28. **Getzen TE.** Macro forecasting of national health expenditure. *Advances in health economics and health services research,* 1990, **11**: 1127–1148.

29. **Poullier JP.** Health data file: overview and methodology. *Health care financing review, 1989 annual supplement,* 1989: 111–118.

30. **Gerdtham U-G et al.** An economic analysis of health care expenditure: a cross-section study of the OECD countries. *Journal of health economics,* 1992, **11**: 1163–1184.

31. **Vogel RJ.** *Trends in health expenditures and revenue sources in sub-Saharan Africa.* Washington, World Bank, 1989.

32. **Anderson O.** *Health care: can there be equity? The United States, Sweden, and England.* New York, John Wiley, 1972.

33. **White KL.** International comparisons of medical care. *Scientific American,* 1975, **233**(8): 17–25.

34. **Glaser WA.** *Paying the hospital.* San Francisco, Jossey-Bass Publishers, 1987.

35. **Culyer A.** Cost supplement in Europe. *Health care financing review, 1989 annual supplement.* 1989: 21–32.

36. **Vogel RJ.** *Financing health care in sub-Saharan Africa: a policy study.* Phoenix, University of Arizona, 1992.

37. **Gertler P, van der Gaag J.** *The willingness to pay for medical care: evidence from two developing countries.* Baltimore, World Bank, 1990.

38. **Parkin D et al.** Aggregate health care expenditures and national income, *Journal of health economics,* 1987, **6**: 109–127.

39. **Culyer A.** *Health expenditures in Canada, myth and reality; past and future.* Toronto, Canadian Tax Foundation, 1988. (Canadian Tax Paper No. 82).

40. **Musgrove P.** Family health spending in Latin America. *Journal of health economics,* 1983, **2**: 2245–2257.

41. **World Health Organization.** *Basic documents.* Geneva, 1984.

42. **Breslow L.** A quantitative approach to the World Health Organization definition of health: physical, mental, and social well-being. *International journal of epidemiology,* 1972, **4**: 347–355.

43. **International comparison project.** *World comparisons of purchasing power and real product for 1980 (ICP phase iv).* New York, United Nations, 1986.

44. **International Monetary Fund.** *Government financial statistics yearbook.* Washington, IMF, 1991.

45. **Michaud C, Murray CJL.** External assistance to the health sector in developing countries: a detailed analysis, 1972–90. *Bulletin of the World Health Organization,* 1994, **72**(4): 639–651.

46. **Murray CJL, Chen LC.** Understanding morbidity change. *Population and development review,* 1992, **18**: 481–503.

47. **Murray CJL et al.** Adult mortality: levels, patterns, and trends. In: Feachem R et al. eds. *Adult health in the developing world,* Washington, World Bank, 1993.

48. **Murray CJL.** Quantifying the burden of disease: the technical basis for disability-adjusted life years. *Bulletin of the World Health Organization,* 1994, **72**(3): 429–445.

Annex

1990 Total health expenditures: public, private, and aid flows (1990 US$)

Regions and countries	Public health expenditures: As % GDP[a]	Private health expenditures: As % GDP[a]	Aid flows for health: As % GDP[b]	Total health expenditures As % GDP	Total health expenditures 1990 US$ (x10^6)	Total health expenditures 1990 US$ per capita	Public: As % total	Private: As % total	Aid flows: As % total[b]
Established Market Economies:	5.67	3.61		9.29	1 483 285	1 958	61.1	38.9	
Australia	5.34	2.33		7.67	22 736	1 294	69.6	30.4	
Austria	5.57	2.82		8.38	13 193	1 711	66.4	33.6	
Belgium	6.19	1.31		7.50	14 428	1 449	82.5	17.5	
Canada	6.70	2.34		9.05	51 594	1 945	74.1	25.9	
Denmark	5.30	1.00		6.30	8 160	1 588	84.2	15.8	
Finland	6.52	1.30		7.82	10 200	2 046	83.3	16.7	
France	6.97	2.43		9.40	105 467	1 869	74.2	25.8	
Germany	6.34	2.38		8.73	120 072	1 511	72.7	27.3	
Greece	4.10	1.29		5.39	3 609	359	76.0	24.0	
Iceland	7.29	1.04		8.34	480	1 884	87.5	12.5	
Ireland	5.85	1.37		7.22	3 068	876	81.1	18.9	
Italy	5.85	1.68		7.54	82 214	4 655	77.7	22.3	
Japan	4.81	1.64		6.45	189 930	1 538	74.5	25.5	
Luxembourg	6.00	0.56		6.56	628	1 662	91.4	8.6	
Netherlands	5.83	2.20		8.03	22 423	1 501	72.6	27.4	
New Zealand	6.02	1.35		7.37	3 150	925	81.7	18.3	
Norway	7.04	0.32		7.35	7 782	1 835	95.7	4.3	
Portugal	4.31	2.68		6.99	3 970	383	61.7	38.3	
Spain	5.17	1.42		6.59	32 375	831	78.4	21.6	
Sweden	7.85	0.94		8.79	20 055	2 343	89.3	10.7	
Switzerland	5.15	2.37		7.52	16 916	2 520	68.5	31.5	
United Kingdom	5.19	0.92		6.11	59 623	1 039	84.9	15.1	
United States	5.60	7.11		12.71	691 211	2 765	44.1	55.9	
Middle Eastern Crescent:	2.03	1.51	0.02	3.53	44 131	97	57.6	42.8	0.7
Algeria	5.34	1.60	0.00	6.95	3 738	149	76.9	23.0	0.1
Armenia	2.50	*1.68*		4.17	505	152	59.8	40.2	
Azerbaijan	2.62	*1.66*		4.27	785	99	61.2	38.8	
Bahrain	2.91	*1.71*	0.00	4.62	163	324	63.0	36.9	0.1
Cyprus	2.49	1.06	0.41	3.96	45	64	62.9	26.8	10.3
Egypt	0.79	*1.61*	0.20	2.61	1 443	28	30.3	62.0	7.7
Georgia	2.78	*1.67*		4.45	830	152	62.5	37.5	
Islamic Rep. of Iran	1.45	1.10	0.00	2.54	13 618	244	56.9	43.1	0.0
Israel	2.07	2.13	0.01	4.20	2 236	480	49.3	50.6	0.1
Jordan (East Bank)	1.39	1.97	0.41	3.77	170	55	36.9	52.3	10.8
Kazakhstan	2.77	*1.67*		4.44	2 573	154	62.3	37.7	
Kirghizstan	3.32	*1.65*		4.97	517	118	66.7	33.3	
Kuwait	3.12	*1.73*	0.01	4.86	1 160	541	64.2	35.6	0.1
Malta	3.68	*1.70*	0.00	5.38	123	349	68.3	31.7	0.0
Morocco	0.86	*1.61*	0.08	2.55	642	26	33.6	63.3	3.1
Oman	2.51	*1.69*	0.02	4.22	325	209	59.5	40.1	0.5
Pakistan	1.65	1.64	0.19	3.48	1 382	12	47.4	47.1	5.5
Qatar	2.98	*1.75*	0.00	4.73	276	630	63.0	36.9	0.0
Saudi Arabia	3.06	*1.70*	0.00	4.76	3 846	260	64.3	35.7	0.0
Syrian Arab Republic	0.34	*1.64*	0.08	2.07	506	41	16.6	79.4	4.0
Tadzhikistan	4.35	*1.64*		5.98	532	100	72.6	27.4	
Tunisia	3.13	*1.63*	0.15	4.91	614	76	63.8	33.3	3.0
Turkey	1.43	2.50	0.02	3.94	4 276	76	36.2	63.3	0.5
Turkmenistan	3.31	*1.66*	0.02	4.99	458	125	66.4	33.2	0.4
United Arab Emirates	0.90	*1.75*	0.00	2.66	752	472	34.0	66.0	0.1
Uzbekistan	4.25	*1.64*		5.90	2 391	116	72.1	27.9	
Yemen	1.11	1.72	0.36	3.19	223	20	34.7	54.1	11.3

Annex Table: continued

Formerly Socialist Economies of Europe:	2.53	1.03		3.55	48 942	144	71.2	29.1
Albania	*3.36*	0.64		4.00	94	26	84.0	16.0
Belarus	2.19	*1.00*		3.19	1 613	157	68.7	31.3
Bulgaria	4.36	*1.00*		5.36	1 068	121	81.4	18.6
Czechoslovakia	5.04	0.90		5.94	2 642	169	84.9	15.1
Estonia	1.92	*1.70*		3.62	361	228	53.0	47.0
Hungary	5.02	0.93		5.95	1 957	185	84.4	15.6
Latvia	2.17	*1.70*		3.87	590	220	56.1	43.9
Lithuania	2.58	*1.00*		3.58	594	159	72.0	28.0
Moldova	2.91	*1.00*		3.91	623	143	74.4	25.6
Poland	4.07	*1.00*		5.07	3 206	84	80.3	19.7
Romania	2.38	1.49		3.87	1 355	58	61.4	38.6
Russian Federation	2.02	*1.00*		3.02	23 527	159	66.8	33.2
Ukraine	2.30	*1.00*		3.30	6 804	131	69.7	30.3
Yugoslavia	4.11	*1.00*		5.11	4 518	264	80.4	19.6
India	1.20	4.70	0.10	6.00	17 488	21	20.0	78.4	1.6
China	2.05	1.44	0.02	3.51	12 819	11	58.5	40.9	0.6
Other Asia and Islands:	1.71	2.73	0.07	4.50	36 817	61	38.0	60.6	1.5
Bangladesh	0.79	1.81	0.59	3.19	693	6	24.8	56.7	18.5
Bhutan	2.08	*1.54*	1.44	5.05	15	10	41.1	30.4	28.5
Fiji	2.06	1.44	0.26	3.76	52	70	54.9	38.3	6.9
Hong Kong	1.11	4.58	0.00	5.69	3 988	687	19.5	80.5	0.0
Indonesia	0.52	1.34	0.15	2.01	2 073	12	25.6	66.7	7.7
Lao People's Dem. Rep.	0.44	*1.54*	0.56	2.53	22	5	17.4	60.7	21.9
Malaysia	1.30	*1.65*	0.01	2.96	1 259	71	44.0	55.8	0.2
Mongolia	5.51	*1.00*	0.13	6.63	124	58	83.0	15.1	1.9
Nepal	1.04	2.34	1.15	4.54	131	7	23.0	51.7	25.4
Papua New Guinea	2.63	*1.60*	0.21	4.44	145	37	59.1	36.1	4.8
Philippines	1.00	1.00	0.15	2.15	1 001	16	46.7	46.4	6.9
Republic of Korea	2.71	3.89	0.01	6.61	15 634	365	40.9	58.9	0.2
Samoa	*0.18*	*1.59*	1.17	2.94	3	20	6.1	54.2	39.7
Singapore	1.09	0.78	0.00	1.87	647	215	58.3	41.6	0.1
Solomon Islands	0.94	*1.10*	0.14	2.18	37	117	43.2	50.5	6.3
Sri Lanka	1.51	1.91	0.32	3.74	305	18	40.4	51.1	8.6
Taiwan, China	2.28	2.02	0.00	4.30	6 559	323	53.0	47.0	0.0
Thailand	1.01	3.92	0.05	4.98	3 994	72	20.4	78.7	0.9
Tonga	3.90	*1.61*	0.95	6.46	6	63	60.3	25.0	14.8
Vanuatu	2.93	1.46	1.29	5.68	10	67	51.5	25.7	22.8
Viet Nam	0.83	1.00	0.28	2.11	191	3	39.3	47.4	13.3
Latin America & Caribbean:	2.37	1.54	0.05	3.96	43 825	103	59.8	38.9	1.2
Antigua and Barbuda	2.69	*1.70*	0.16	4.55	19	241	59.1	37.3	3.6
Argentina	2.53	*1.67*	0.01	4.21	4 437	137	60.1	39.7	0.2
Barbados	3.24	*1.70*	0.10	5.04	83	323	64.3	33.8	1.9
Belize	2.85	2.41	0.63	5.88	23	120	48.4	41.0	10.7
Bolivia	1.60	*1.59*	0.82	4.01	180	25	39.9	39.6	20.5
Brazil	2.76	1.42	0.02	4.20	21 887	146	65.7	33.9	0.4
British Virgin Islands	1.54	*1.73*		3.27	5	375	47.1	52.9	
Cayman Islands	2.03	*1.75*		3.78	14	657	53.8	46.2	
Chile	3.32	1.38	0.03	4.73	1 315	100	70.1	29.1	0.7
Colombia	1.75	2.17	0.06	3.98	1 636	51	44.0	54.4	1.6
Costa Rica	4.79	*1.64*	0.08	6.51	371	132	73.6	25.2	1.2
Dominica	5.25	*1.65*	1.17	8.06	14	192	65.1	20.4	14.5
Dominican Republic	1.96	*1.61*	0.15	3.72	272	38	52.7	43.3	4.0
Ecuador	2.31	1.55	0.28	4.14	450	44	55.9	37.3	6.8
El Salvador	1.74	3.26	0.86	5.86	300	58	29.7	55.6	14.7
Grenada	4.10	*1.65*	0.21	5.96	12	133	68.8	27.8	3.5
Guatemala	1.63	*1.60*	0.46	3.70	251	27	44.2	43.2	12.6
Guyana	4.22	*1.57*	4.58	10.37	33	42	40.7	15.1	44.2

Annex Table: continued

Haiti	1.84	3.83	1.33	6.99	173	27	26.3	54.8	19.0
Honduras	2.57	*1.62*	0.35	4.54	264	52	56.7	35.7	7.7
Jamaica	2.89	1.67	0.48	5.04	200	83	57.4	33.2	9.5
Mexico	1.56	1.58	0.03	3.17	7 525	89	49.3	49.8	0.9
Nicaragua	4.90	*1.93*	1.77	8.61	129	34	56.9	22.5	20.6
Panama	5.18	*1.65*	0.31	7.13	343	142	72.6	23.1	4.3
Paraguay	0.98	*1.62*	0.19	2.79	153	35	35.1	58.2	6.7
Peru	1.80	1.34	0.07	3.21	1 312	61	56.1	41.7	2.2
St Kitts and Nevis	3.48	*1.67*	0.85	5.99	8	212	58.1	27.8	14.1
St Lucia	5.43	*1.65*	0.10	7.18	25	169	75.6	23.0	1.4
St Vincent	3.90	*1.64*	0.15	5.69	11	102	68.5	28.8	2.7
Suriname	0.09	*1.67*	0.12	2.88	41	93	37.9	58.0	4.1
Trindad and Tobago	2.83	*1.68*	0.03	4.54	222	180	62.4	36.9	0.6
Uruguay	2.49	2.07	0.06	4.62	380	123	53.8	44.8	1.4
Venezuela	1.95	1.64	0.01	3.60	1 735	88	54.2	45.6	0.1
Sub-Saharan Africa:	1.85	1.97	0.39	4.23	11 648	22	43.8	46.6	9.2
Benin	1.14	*1.57*	1.61	4.32	88	19	26.3	36.4	37.3
Botswana	3.83	1.34	1.02	6.19	174	139	61.8	21.6	16.5
Burkina Faso	0.83	*1.52*	6.12	8.46	59	7	9.8	17.9	72.3
Burundi	1.39	*1.59*	0.30	3.28	165	30	42.4	48.3	9.3
Cameroon	0.69	*1.61*	0.31	2.62	321	27	26.4	61.7	11.9
Cape Verde	1.31	*1.61*	3.40	6.32	24	64	20.7	25.5	53.7
Central African Republic	*1.11*	*1.57*	1.51	4.19	55	18	26.5	37.5	36.0
Chad	*1.72*	*1.54*	2.97	6.22	69	12	27.6	24.7	47.7
Comoros	*2.50*	*1.57*	1.32	5.40	13	28	46.3	29.2	24.5
Congo	*1.88*	*1.62*	0.48	3.99	114	50	47.1	40.7	12.1
Côte d'Ivoire	1.63	*1.60*	0.11	3.35	332	28	48.7	47.9	3.4
Equatorial Guinea	*2.78*	*1.57*	3.25	7.60	11	28	36.6	20.7	42.7
Ethiopia	1.57	*1.52*	0.71	3.80	229	4	41.3	39.9	18.8
Gabon	*2.16*	*1.68*	0.26	4.10	186	164	52.7	40.9	6.4
Gambia	2.13	*1.56*	3.84	7.53	19	22	28.3	20.7	51.0
Ghana	1.23	1.81	0.46	3.50	219	15	35.0	51.8	13.2
Guinea	*1.55*	*1.57*	0.78	3.90	99	17	39.7	40.3	20.0
Guinea-Bissau	*2.55*	*1.54*	4.06	8.15	16	16	31.3	18.9	49.8
Kenya	1.73	1.64	0.96	4.33	379	16	40.0	37.9	22.1
Lesotho	3.19	2.20	2.93	8.32	45	26	38.3	26.5	35.2
Liberia	1.64	*0.97*	5.63	8.24	9	4	19.9	11.8	68.3
Madagascar	0.74	1.27	0.55	2.56	79	7	29.0	49.6	21.4
Malawi	1.74	2.08	1.16	4.98	93	11	35.0	41.7	23.3
Mali	1.30	2.42	1.47	5.19	127	15	24.9	46.7	28.4
Mauritania	1.08	*1.58*	1.14	3.80	36	18	28.5	41.5	30.0
Mauritius	2.10	1.72	0.58	4.40	108	100	47.8	39.0	13.3
Mozambique	1.23	*1.50*	3.12	5.86	84	5	21.0	25.7	53.3
Namibia	1.88	*1.62*	0.43	3.92	80	45	47.8	41.3	10.9
Niger	1.72	*1.56*	1.70	4.98	126	16	24.5	31.3	34.1
Nigeria	0.99	*1.56*	0.17	2.72	944	10	36.5	57.4	6.1
Rwanda	0.52	*1.56*	1.37	3.44	73	10	15.0	45.2	39.8
São Tome and Principe	2.66	*1.57*	4.99	9.22	4	38	28.8	17.0	54.2
Senegal	1.65	1.39	0.62	3.66	214	29	45.1	38.0	16.9
Seychelles	3.03	*1.69*	1.32	6.03	20	289	50.2	28.0	21.9
Sierra Leone	0.48	0.75	1.20	2.43	15	4	19.6	30.9	49.5
Somalia	*0.11*	0.62	0.78	1.51	60	8	7.3	41.1	51.6
South Africa	3.20	2.36	0.00	5.56	5 048	77	57.5	42.5	0.0
Sudan	0.37	2.81	0.15	3.33	860	34	11.0	84.5	4.5
Swaziland	3.15	*1.61*	2.47	7.22	51	64	43.6	22.2	34.2
Tanzania (United Rep. of)	*0.68*	*1.49*	2.55	4.73	97	4	14.4	31.6	54.0
Togo	1.65	*1.58*	0.87	4.10	66	18	40.4	38.5	21.2
Uganda	0.45	1.80	1.15	3.40	136	8	13.3	53.0	33.7
Zaire	0.20	*1.54*	0.63	2.38	179	5	8.5	64.8	26.7
Zambia	2.07	0.97	0.13	3.16	139	17	65.4	30.6	4.1
Zimbabwe	2.51	3.03	0.69	6.23	379	39	40.3	48.7	11.0

[a] Figures in bold-face italics indicate that the value was predicted using the regression equation.
[b] Blank space indicates that the country receives no foreign aid for health.

External assistance to the health sector in developing countries: a detailed analysis, 1972–90

C. Michaud[1] & C.J.L. Murray[2]

This study, which was conducted for the World Bank's World development report 1993: investing in health, *provides an objective analysis of the external assistance to the health sector by quantifying in detail the sources and recipients of such assistance in 1990, by analysing time trends for external assistance to the health sector over the last two decades, and, to the extent possible, by describing the allocation of resources to specific activities in the health sector. The main findings of the study are that total external assistance to the health sector in 1990 was US$ 4800 million, or only 2.9% of total health expenditures in developing countries. After stagnation in real terms during the first half of the 1980s, health sector assistance has been increasing since 1986. Despite their small volume, external assistance at the margins may play a critical role in capital investment, research and strategic planning. The study confirms prior findings that health status variables* per se *are not related to the amount of aid received. Comparing investments to the burden of disease shows tremendous differences in the funding for different health problems. A number of conditions are comparatively under-financed, particularly noncommunicable diseases and injuries.*

Introduction

Discussions of international health priorities and responses often focus on external assistance to the health sector. Although such assistance accounts for only a small share (less than 3%) of health sector expenditures in developing countries (1), its impact could be critical in the areas of capital investment, research and strategic planning in these countries. Donor agencies, using minimal resources, have sometimes influenced government health sector policies by drawing attention to special problems or interventions. The success of UNICEF, WHO, and several bilateral donor agencies on the Expanded Programme of Immunization due to their influence on the developing countries' health agendas. Considering its potential importance in determining policy, external assistance to the health sector has been poorly quantified.

The objectives of the present study were specifically to: (1) quantify in detail the sources and recipients of external assistance to the health sector in 1990; (2) analyse time trends for external assistance to the health sector over the last two decades in as much detail as possible; and, (3) to the extent possible, describe the allocation of resources to specific activities in the health sector.

This study is not the first attempt to measure external assistance to the health sector. Two general databases on development assistance are maintained by the OECD (Organization for Economic Cooperation and Development) and are described more fully below. A number of *ad hoc* studies have used these databases, supplemented with other sources, to examine external assistance to the health sector or a component of the health sector (2–9).[a, b] Taken together, these studies have defined the rough order of magnitude of such external assistance but the likely government sources, the channels, recipients and activities funded remain poorly delineated.

Definitions, materials and methods

There are no clear boundaries defining the components that should be included in estimates of external assistance to the health sector. In previous studies,

[1] Research Associate, Center for Population and Development Studies, Cambridge, MA, USA.

[2] Associate Professor of International Health Economics, Centre for Population and Development Studies, Harvard University, 9 Bow Street, Cambridge MA 02138, USA. Requests for reprints should be sent to this author.

[a] **Howard L.** *A new look at development cooperation for health: a study of official donor policies, programmes and perspectives in support of Health for All by the Year 2000.* Unpublished WHO document No. COR/HRG/INF.1, 1981.

[b] **Orivel F et al.** *L'aide extérieure publique à la santé en Afrique sub-Saharienne.* Paper presented at Journées d'Economie Sociale, Caen, 28–29 September 1989 (in French).

Reprinted from *Bulletin of the World Health Organization*, 1994, **72** (4): 639–651.

157

Howard included all water and sanitation investments while the OECD did not (3).[a] In the present analysis, the health sector was narrowly defined and included two major components — health and population. *Health* activities include promotive, preventive, curative and rehabilitative interventions to improve the health status of individuals and population groups; programme food aid; vector control, training of health manpower and health research. *Population* activities pertain to family planning programmes, and the collection and analysis of demographic survey data. Water and sanitation, emergency food aid, and general education activities were excluded. We believe it is useful to analyse expenditures whose primary purpose is health improvement as distinct from all expenditures that contribute to health. Our definition is also consistent with the components included in the parallel study on national health expenditures (1) and facilitates comparison of the two results.

Total external assistance to the health sector has three main parts: official development assistance (ODA), multilateral loans, and nongovernmental flows. ODA is defined as those resources provided to developing countries and multilateral institutions by official agencies. Such resources must be administered with promotion of economic development as their main objective, and must be concessional in character, containing a grant element of at least 25%. Official contribution to private voluntary organizations are recorded as ODA, but private contributions are not. ODA excludes any kind of military assistance.

Governments and private households from the established market economies and some oil-exporting countries are the ultimate sources of external assistance for health. This assistance is then channelled to the developing countries through three main types of institutions — bilateral and multilateral agencies and nongovernmental organizations. For the purpose of this paper, bilateral agencies are the aid arms of OECD governments, often attached to the ministry of foreign affairs. Multilateral agencies include members of the United Nations system, the major development banks (MDBs), the European Community, and the Organization of Petroleum-Exporting Countries (OPEC). International, national and local nongovernmental organizations (NGOs) utilize a combination of publicly-provided funds and privately-contributed resources for health.

External assistance can be measured in terms of commitments or disbursements. Commitments show the intention of the donor agency at the time of agreement. They are a useful indicator of future disbursements and funding trends. Disbursements capture the amount of funds actually expended in any given year and provide the best information to assess time trends and to make comparisons. The estimates reported in our study are for disbursements exclusively.

Data sources and quality

Unfortunately no single database yet exists that provides a comprehensive view of health sector external assistance. The primary means of data collection was through a questionnaire and follow-up visits or telephone contacts to all major bilaterals, multilaterals and large nongovernmental agencies. For reasons of space, the citations for the extremely extensive set of annual reports and other budgetary documents are not provided but can be obtained on request. Where direct responses were not received or were insufficient, we resorted to using the three major databases on development assistance: the OECD Development Assistance Committee (DAC) annual tables, the Creditor Reporting System (CRS) from OECD, and the Register of Development Activities of the United Nations system compiled by the Advisory Committee for the Co-ordination of Information Systems (ACCIS) (10–13).

The two OECD databases — DAC and the CRS — are extensively used and form the basis for most sectoral studies. DAC is based on annual reports sent by each OECD government. CRS is based on project-specific reports forwarded to the OECD. Because information is collected on each project by donor, recipient and content, the CRS has greater potential in analysing health sector external assistance in detail.

Unfortunately, careful comparison of DAC and CRS commitment data reveal major discrepancies. In aggregate for all OECD countries, commitments recorded over the last decade in the CRS cover only 38% to 61% of those recorded by DAC. The variation in CRS coverage compared to DAC is from 0% to over 200% if individual donor reports for specific years are examined. Reporting in the CRS was even worse for population activities (39% on average) than for the health sector (47% on average). While the extent of discrepancies between CRS and DAC remain difficult to understand, it is clear that without major adjustments the CRS data are unreliable for estimating the level of health sector external assistance and, given the variation in coverage from one year to another, even more unreliable for assessing time trends.

Based on the comparison of DAC and CRS, it appears that DAC has better coverage. Since the DAC information is the basis on which donor's performances are assessed by the OECD, it is important to validate the DAC figures with commitments reported directly through bilateral accounts. Three countries (USA, Japan and Netherlands) provided direct information on commitments in addition to disbursement data that could be compared to DAC commitments. With the exception of the Netherlands in 1989, the concordance for each country ranged from 93% to 99% in 1990, indicating a much better fit between data reported to DAC and national consolidated accounts than those we observed between CRS and DAC. As mentioned, however, DAC does not provide more than a sector total for bilateral ODA.

Commitments and disbursements differ by the time at which they occur. In addition, the total amounts for a given project may differ because funds which were initially committed may be cancelled, reduced or increased during the project's lifetime. Based on detailed project reports, the budget execution was 82% for the World Bank IDA (International Development Association) health sector loans for 1975–90 and 72% for IBRD (International Bank for Reconstruction and Development) health sector loans for the same period. Both the Asian and Inter-American Development Banks disbursed 82% of commitments in closed loans. Budget execution data for the only bilateral, the Canadian International Development Agency (CIDA), that could provide such detailed information was 93% for the period 1975–90. When disbursement data were not directly available, disbursements were estimated using these observed budget execution rates. The formula for estimating disbursements from commitments also incorporated phased implementation of most projects during their life-cycle and the average duration of projects for different types of institutions.

All estimated commitments and disbursements for the health sector have been converted into 1990 US dollars. For time trends we have used a two-stage procedure. First we have converted commitments or disbursements reported in local currency to current US dollars, using official exchange rates. Second, total amounts disbursed from all sources combined, expressed in current dollars, were converted into 1990 US dollars using the United States GDP deflator (14).

Direct information provided by NGOs, as well as information from bilaterals have been used to estimate the total disbursements of NGOs to the health sector. Not all NGO disbursements are new funds; bilateral agencies channel funds through NGOs. Where information on NGO income was not available, direct information provided by donor countries on the amount of bilateral assistance to the health sector channelled through NGOs in 1990 was used.

Some bilaterals and multilaterals provided detailed information on recipient countries and/or specific health sector activities. For those agencies not providing detail, we have developed a method to estimate the allocation by recipient or health sector activity. Although the CRS has low overall coverage

of external assistance, we have assumed that the recipient and activity allocations for those funds included in the CRS are representative of all assistance for a specific donor. Thus, distributions of external assistance by topical area have been applied to corrected total external assistance by donor.

Results

External assistance to the health sector, 1990

A cross-sectional picture of external assistance to the health sector in developing countries is summarized in Fig. 1. Health external assistance totalled $4800 million, 82% of which originated from public coffers in developed countries and 18% from private households. The middle row in the figure indicates the institutional mechanism through which resources flow to the health sectors of developing countries: 40% is through bilateral development agencies, 33% through United Nations agencies (most notably WHO, UNICEF and the United Nations Population Fund (UNFPA)), and 8% through the World Bank and the regional development banks such as the Asian Development Bank. NGOs account for 17% and a small share (1.5%) flows through foundations.

The overall share of external assistance going to the health sector was 8.8% in 1990. This amount ($4800 million), however, represented only 2.8% of total health expenditures in the developing world ($170 000 million).

The allocation of aid for health, by recipient region (Table 1), shows that Africa receives the largest share of donor support (38.5%) and has the highest per capita allocation ($2.45 per person), while China receives the least (6% and $0.07, respectively). The importance of aid flows for health in Africa is particularly striking: $1200 million, or 10% of all health expenditures in Africa, comes from external sources. In Sub-Saharan Africa excluding South Africa, 20% of health expenditure is from external assistance. While Latin America and Other Asian countries also receive substantial external assistance for health, these funds account for less than 2% of health expenditure.

Total external assistance for population was $936 million in 1990, almost 20% of the total health sector external assistance. All bilaterals combined contributed 60%, United Nations agencies (mostly UNFPA) 22%, the development banks 13%, and private sources 5%. The amount allocated from private sources is probably an underestimate, but sufficient information was not available to allocate total NGO health sector expenditure between health and population.

Fig. 1. **External assistance to the health sector, 1990 (in millions of $).**

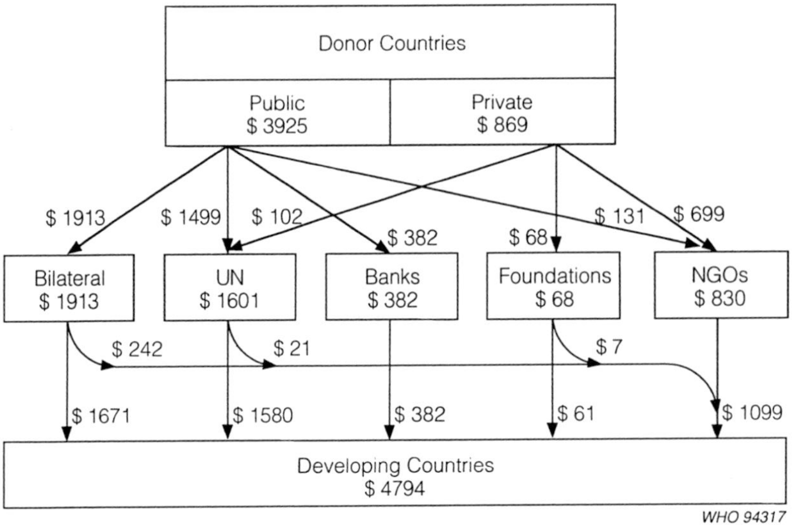

WHO 94317

External assistance to the health sector, 1972–90

Time trends in total health sector external assistance are difficult to assess because of the lack of documentation of time trends in private flows through nongovernmental organizations over the last two decades. Data on bilateral and multilateral disbursements, however, were successfully obtained for the period 1972–90. The following discussion of time trends is, therefore, restricted to external assistance from public sources. Fig. 2 and Table 2 summarize the aggregate trends for nearly two decades in 1990 US dollars.

Three periods of external assistance can be identified. From 1972 to 1980, there was a sustained increase in external assistance to the health sector, increasing over 305% or 14% per year. With the

onset of the global recession, external assistance remained constant in real terms from 1980 to 1985. Beginning in 1986, we have again entered a period of sustained growth in real terms to the health sector. The pace of increase is lower than in the 1970s but has averaged 7% per year. The increase is present in both bilateral and multilateral agencies.

The share of the total official development assistance (ODA) going to the health sector was 8% for the period of 1981–85, and decreased to 6.5% on average for the period 1986–90. The share of bilateral ODA going to the health sector has declined the most, from an average of 7% during 1980–85 to 5% in 1986–90, while the share of multilateral ODA going to the health sector increased from 10% to 12% on average during the same period. In other words, much of the increase in real assistance to the health sector beginning in 1986 has been due not to a

Table 1: **Official development assistance to the health sector by region, 1990**

Region	Total (millions of $)	Health aid Per capita ($)	As % of health expenditures
Sub-Saharan Africa (SSA)	1251	2.45	10.4
SSA excluding South Africa	1251	2.66	19.5
Other Asia and islands (OAI)	594	0.87	1.4
Latin America and the Caribbean (LAC)	591	1.33	1.3
Middle Eastern Crescent (MEC)	453	1.31	1.3
India	286	0.34	1.6
China	77	0.07	0.6
Total	3252	0.81	1.9

Fig. 2. **Disbursements by bilateral and multilateral agencies to the health sector, 1972–1990.**

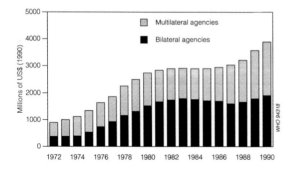

re-allocation of aid to health from other sectors, but instead to an increase in total ODA accompanied by a decrease in the relative share claimed by the health sector.

External assistance should also be assessed in comparison with the number of recipients. Health sector external assistance per person in the developing world indicates that external assistance has barely kept pace with population growth during most of the 1980s. Per capita health sector assistance was $0.84 in 1981 and $0.82 in 1988. In 1989 and 1990 the per capita health sector assistance outpaced population growth, reaching $0.95 in 1990.

Time trends for bilateral and multilateral agencies differ substantially. Bilateral health ODA fluctuated from year to year during the 1980s, but increased very little in real terms, growing from $1800 million in 1983 to $1900 million in 1990 (Fig. 2). A large part of the year-to-year fluctuations can be attributed to changes in the real exchange rates for the US dollar. Multilateral health ODA remained stationary during the early 1980s, but grew in the second part of the decade to $2000 million in 1990 (Fig. 2). As a result, the multilateral share of total health ODA grew from about 44% at the beginning of the 1980s to around 51% in 1990.

External assistance for population activities increased only slowly during the 1970s from $400 million in 1972 to $540 million in 1980, stagnated at $550 million on average until 1987, and then increased to $860 million in 1990, despite the withdrawal of the United States from UNFPA.

Examination of the time trends for each agency shows three patterns. (1) Australia, Austria, Belgium, Canada, Finland, Italy, Japan, Norway, Switzerland, and the United Kingdom increased their assistance through bilateral channels to the health sector in real terms. (2) Denmark, France, Netherlands, and New Zealand recorded major declines in their bilateral health sector external assistance. (3) The remainder,

Germany, Sweden and the United States showed no clear trend in bilateral disbursements.

Of the multilateral agencies for which data were available, all have demonstrated growth. UNICEF's health expenditure increased 120% over the period 1981–83 to 1988–90 and WHO's by 36% over the same period. UNDP increased but its total health sector budget is extremely small, totalling only $14 million in 1990 or 0.2% of total health sector external assistance. United Nations agencies have increased their contributions from $1100 million in 1980 to $1500 million in 1990. Their total share of health sector official development assistance remained constant at around 40% during that period.

Disbursements from the multilateral development banks grew rapidly, from $79 million in 1981 to nearly $400 million in 1990. Most of the increase came from the World Bank, whose disbursements for health rose from about $33 million to $263 million during the same period. In this case, disbursements do not tell the whole story. New commitments by the World Bank for health and population amounted to $933 million in 1990 and $1500 million in 1991, implying that by the mid-1990s, Bank disbursements for health are likely to be four or five times the $263 million spent in 1990. A trend towards an expanded role for the multilateral agencies in external assistance for health thus appears to be emerging.

Table 2: **Disbursements by bilateral and multilateral agencies to the health sector, 1972–1990**

| Year | Disbursements (in million of 1990 $) | | |
	Bilaterals	Multilaterals	Total
1972	372	527	899
1973	378	623	1 001
1974	389	732	1 122
1975	540	801	1 341
1976	736	899	1 635
1977	936	924	1 860
1978	1 167	1 088	2 255
1979	1 315	1 182	2 496
1980	1 525	1 214	2 739
1981	1 669	1 167	2 837
1982	1 735	1 159	2 893
1983	1 790	1 120	2 909
1984	1 760	1 132	2 892
1985	1 710	1 187	2 897
1986	1 690	1 259	2 949
1987	1 599	1 437	3 036
1988	1 662	1 551	3 213
1989	1 786	1 790	3 577
1990	1 907	1 983	3 890

Expanded external assistance can be expected from a number of United Nations agencies. And the momentum of fresh lending for health from the development banks will lead to larger disbursements in the coming years.

In absolute terms, the USA was and still remains the single largest bilateral donor to population activities. USAID disbursed $350 million, on average, each year from 1972 to 1986. These contributions decreased by 30% to $270 million, on average, for the period 1987–90. With increasing direct contributions from other bilateral agencies during the 1980s, the share of total population assistance provided by USAID decreased from 88% in 1972 to 55% in 1980, and was only 32% in 1990.

Sources and recipients of health sector external assistance, 1990

Developed country governments are able to channel external assistance to the health sector through bilateral and multilateral channels. In terms of total contributions, three donors account for more than half of all assistance: the USA (27.5%), France (12.9%), and Japan (11.5%) (Fig. 3). The figures for France include assistance given to French territories overseas, so they are not comparable with the contributions of other countries. One quarter of all health

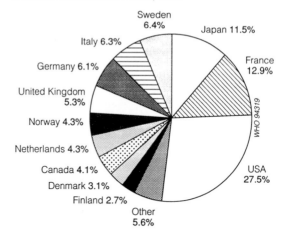

Fig. 3. **Official development assistance from OECD countries to the health sector, 1990.**

sector assistance is paid for by Sweden, Italy, Germany and the United Kingdom.

Contributions to health sector external assistance by developed country governments should be assessed relative to the size of each country's economy. Table 3 provides estimates of the share of GDP devoted to health sector assistance. Norway, Swe-

Table 3: **OECD countries' disbursements to the health sector channelled through multilaterals and bilaterals, 1990**

	Disbursements to multilaterals (in millions of $)		Disbursements to bilaterals (in millions of $)	Total (in millions of $)	Total (as % GDP)
Norway	103	(61)[a]	66	169	0.159
Sweden	174	(70)	75	249	0.109
Denmark	79	(65)	42	121	0.093
Finland	70	(68)	33	103	0.075
Netherlands	110	(66)	56	166	0.059
France	152	(30)	350	502	0.042
Belgium	31	(40)	47	78	0.041
Canada	102	(64)	57	159	0.028
Switzerland	42	(69)	18	60	0.027
Ireland	8	(77)	2	10	0.023
Italy	114	(47)	129	243	0.022
United Kingdom	124	(60)	82	206	0.021
USA	445	(41)	629	1074	0.020
Australia	29	(54)	25	54	0.018
Germany	145	(61)	91	237	0.016
Japan	248	(55)	202	450	0.015
Austria	8	(65)	4	13	0.008
New Zealand	2	(69)	1	3	0.006

[a] Figures in parentheses are percentages of total.

den, Denmark, Finland and the Netherlands (in that order) provide the largest shares of GDP to health sector assistance. New Zealand, Austria, Japan and Germany provide the least. Norway contributes over 25 times more, in terms of the share of GDP, than New Zealand. Italy, the United Kingdom and the USA all contribute similar shares (0.02% of GDP).

As mentioned, the proportions of external assistance for health channelled through bilateral and multilateral agencies vary enormously among the OECD countries. The USA, Italy, France and Belgium disburse the majority of funds primarily through direct bilateral channels. Most other countries contribute about two-thirds through multilateral agencies and one-third through direct bilateral projects.

Country-specific estimates of external assistance in total dollars, dollars per capita, and in terms of percent GDP and percent health expenditure are provided in the Annex. Per capita assistance in 1990 ranges from $0.10 in Algeria, Malaysia, Qatar, Saudi Arabia and Venezuela to $63 in Seychelles. The impact of external assistance can also be assessed in terms of the share it represents of the total health sector expenditure. Estimates have been developed of total health sector expenditure for nearly every country in 1990 (1). In 23 sub-Saharan African countries, Guyana, Bhutan and Nepal, health assistance represents greater than 25% of the health sector expenditure. Donor agencies in eight countries — Burkina-Faso, Cape Verde, Gambia, Liberia, Mozambique, São Tome & Principe, Somalia and United Republic of Tanzania — are more important funders of the health sector than all domestic sources, both public and private.

Health sector external assistance directed to specific activities

Although more tentative than other results in this study, we present the known allocation of health sector external assistance by health sector activity in Table 4. These are minimum estimates, as there is always the potential for omission in the analysis of detailed budgets. Disbursements can be classified into general programmes or infrastructure and activities targeted to specific health problems. The health problems have been classified into three groups along the lines of the Global Burden of Disease system: communicable, maternal and perinatal; noncommunicable; and injuries (15). According to our data, almost half (44.5%) of all external assistance is spent on hospitals and health services; of the other half, 18.8% is allocated to specific health problems, 9.4% to nutrition programmes, 7.6% to maternal and child health programmes, and 19.6% to popula-

tion activities. The allocation, however, is not proportionate to the burden of each of these conditions.

Some health problems get a disproportionate share of external assistance compared to their contribution to the burden of disease (Table 4). With the results of the Global Burden of Disease study (16), we can compare health sector external assistance for particular problems per disability-adjusted life year (DALY) caused by that problem. Leprosy receives $75 per DALY, followed by onchocerciasis ($55), blinding conditions ($6.90), and sexually transmitted diseases and HIV combined ($4). A glaring imbalance is the paltry $0.15 per DALY spent on acute respiratory infections. Perhaps reflecting an outdated view about the epidemiological profile of developing countries, virtually all noncommunicable diseases and injuries receive less than $0.05 per DALY. As noncommunicable diseases and injuries now account for 49.6% of the burden of disease in developing countries, this is a startling distribution of resources. Further evidence of the neglect of noncommunicable disease and injuries in developing countries is the relative importance given by WHO, where no programme is specifically devoted to chronic respiratory, digestive or genitourinary diseases.

Discussion

In aggregate, external assistance forms only 2.8% of the total health sector expenditure in developing countries. Given its small size, what is the appropriate role for external assistance? In some regions, its share of total health expenditure is higher, but only in a few countries does external assistance play a major financing role. If resource transfers or general financing of health services is not the primary role of external assistance, where can such aid have the biggest impact? At the very least, external assistance is likely to have a bigger role in altering the priorities or policies of institutions in developing countries rather than paying for programmes in their entirety. A marginal view of the role of external assistance would probably put more of a premium on research, operational research, capacity building and policy analysis. In addition, there probably is a role for external assistance to finance capital investments. Unfortunately, the degree of detail for both national health expenditures and external assistance was not sufficient to allow for a direct analysis of the proportion of capital investments financed in each country by external assistance.

Considering all donors together, what factors determine the allocation of external assistance to the health sector? Is external assistance donor- or need-driven? Drager has argued that health assistance is

Table 4: **Disbursements from all sources by groups and components, and their relationship to DALYs**

	Sources of funds (in $ x 1000):				Total funding	Share of external funding (%)	DALYs (hundreds of thousands lost)	$ / DALY
	Bilaterals	Multilaterals	NGOs	Foundations				
Communicable diseases (Gr. I)								
Tuberculosis	11 694	4 165			15 859	0.3	459.4	0.35
STD and HIV infection	64 043	120 006	622	90	184 761	3.9	474.7	3.89
Diarrhoea	31 604	23 402			55 006	1.2	986.6	0.56
Vaccine-preventable childhood infection	39 654	160 109			199 763	4.2	674.8	2.96
Malaria	36 745	10 087			46 832	1.0	357.3	1.31
Worm infection							179.7	
Respiratory infection	7 986	4 525			12 511	0.3	1 188.8	0.11
Other:	69 530	31 970			101 500	2.1		
Hepatitis	990				990	0.0	18.2	0.54
Tropical cluster:	4 831	58 848		10 815	74 494	1.6	127.1	5.86
Trypanosomiasis	471				471	0.0	17.8	0.26
Chagas disease							27.4	
Schistosomiasis	4 360			199	4 559	0.1	45.3	1.01
Leishmaniasis							28.1	
Lymphatic filariasis							8.4	
Onchocerciasis	4 835	22 720	4 518	3 041	35 114	0.7	6.4	54.67
Leprosy	2 770	3 108	71 000		76 878	1.6	10.2	75.56
Trachoma	453			3 150	3 603	0.1	33.0	1.09
Subtotal	275 135	438 939	76 140	17 096	807 310	17.0	6 105.7	1.32
Noncommunicable diseases (Gr. II)								
Malignant neoplasms	1 737		725		2 462	0.1	533.3	0.05
Blindness	2 080	22 720	30 661		55 461	1.2	81.0	6.85
Neuropsychiatric diseases	2 838	2 838			5 676	0.1	604.0	0.09
Cerebrovascular diseases							330.8	
Cardiovascular disease	961				961	0.0	757.2	0.01
Pulmonary obstruction							157.8	
Drug/alcohol dependence	6 950	2 785	7		9 742	0.2	120.6	0.81
Other	391							
Subtotal	14 957	28 343	31 393		74 693	1.6	4 576.0	0.16
Injuries (Gr. III)								
Unintentional		984			984	0.0	983.2	0.01
Intentional	8 024	546			8 570	0.2	436.2	0.20
Subtotal	8 024	546			8 570	0.2	1 419.3	0.06
Other								
Nutrition	39 910	406 533			446 443	9,4		
Maternal and child health	199 863	159 606	4 149	5 800	369 418	7.8		
Population activities	558 000	332 000	22 000	24 000	936 000	19.7		
Hospitals	178 905	44 546			223 451	4.7		
Health services	396 034	547 904	938 378	13 959	1 896 275	39.8		
Subtotal	1 372 712	1 490 589	964 527	43 759	3 871 587			
Total	1 670 828	1 958 417	1 072 060	60 855	4 762 160			

essentially unrelated to need and thus entirely political (2). In an ideal world, one might hope that health
assistance is targeted to poor countries and those
with the worst health problems. Using our more
refined dataset on bilateral and multilateral assistance to the health sector by recipient country, we
have examined the relationship between health sector
assistance and various socioeconomic determinants
in the recipient country using regression analysis.
The following variables were included in the analysis: population, GDP per capita in US dollars and
International dollars, domestic health expenditures
per capita and in percentage GDP terms, under-five
(0–4 years) mortality, and adult (15–59 years) mortality by sex.

There is no clear relationship between external
assistance per capita and GDP per capita or measures
of health status including child and adult mortality
levels. There is a relationship with population size
where the elasticity is close to −0.5 (depending on
precise functional form). In other words, smaller
countries get more aid, with a 10% increase in population aid per capita decreases 5%.

Various models relating external assistance per
capita and socioeconomic variables were tested. The
best fit multivariate equation (log-log) has an adjusted R^2 of 0.48, and coefficients of −0.49 for the natural log of population and −0.75 for the natural log of
GDP per capita. Both coefficients are significant at
the $P=0.0005$ level. Dummy variables were also
included for all regions; only two (Middle Eastern
Crescent and Other Asia and Islands) were negative
and significant.

External assistance measured as a share of GDP
was examined in relation to various socioeconomic
variables. The proportion of variance explained in
the regression models for external assistance as a
share of GDP was much higher than for external
assistance per capita. The best fit equation gave an
adjusted R^2 of 0.76. The above equation indicates
that with a 10% increase in population, external
assistance as a share of GDP decreases 5.2%; likewise, a 10% increase in GDP per capita leads to a
14.5% decline in external assistance as a share of
GDP per capita. No health status variables were statistically related to external assistance per capita. In
other words, donors appear to give more assistance
to poor small countries but simultaneously take into
account the relative cost of operating in each country.

The regression equations identified here are at
odds with previous analyses of the determinants of
health aid allocation by country (2).[c] Three-quarters

of variation in the allocation of external assistance
by country can be explained by population size and
income per capita. We confirm earlier findings that
health status variables *per se* are not related to the
amount of aid received. When population size and
income per capita are taken into account, patterns of
external assistance do not differ very significantly
among different regions. The data show more aid to
sub-Saharan Africa than to any other region, whether
expressed in absolute amounts, or per capita, or as a
percentage of total disbursements to the health
sector, but this appears to be fully explained by the
tendency of donors to allocate assistance preferen-
tially to smaller, poorer countries.

Conclusions

The main findings of this study can be summarized
in the following points.

(1) Studies on health sector external assistance, disaggregated by recipient or activity, have to date
depended on the creditor reporting system (CRS).
This system is only 63% complete for health and less
than 50% for the health sector (i.e., combination of
health and population). CRS coverage is variable
across donors and years. Further improvements in
the information system monitoring external assistance to the health sector will have to address the
poor coverage of the CRS. Despite its current limitations, CRS is probably the best hope for a better
system because of the detail that can be gained in
such a project-based information system.

(2) Total external assistance to the health sector was
$4800 million in 1990. This is only 2.9% of the total
health expenditure in developing countries. The role
of external assistance must be viewed at the margin,
in terms of its impact on capital formation and policy
formulation.

(3) Health sector assistance, after stagnating in real
terms during the first half of the 1980s, has been
increasing since 1986 through both bilateral and
multilateral channels. The increase from 1986 to
1990 only offset the population growth until 1988; in
1989–90, external assistance slightly outpaced population growth. Future directions will depend on the
balance of increasing multilateral expenditure and
potentially declining bilateral flows, given the recent
political developments in the USA and Scandinavia.

(4) During the 1980s multilateral institutions, particularly UNICEF and the World Bank, played a
larger role in financing health sector assistance than
previously. This pattern of growth is expected to
accelerate in the 1990s as the World Bank emerges

---

[c] See footnote *b* on page 157.

as the single largest donor agency in the health sector, probably outstripping USAID in bilateral assistance in the near future.

(5) While in absolute terms, the USA, France and Japan are the largest donor countries, the Nordic countries and the Netherlands give the largest share of GDP to health sector external assistance.

(6) Almost half of health assistance is spent on development of infrastructure through grants for health services and hospitals. The other half is allocated to specific health programmes. Comparing investments to the burden of disease, there are striking differences in the funding for different health problems. The best funded health problems are leprosy, onchocerciasis, other tropical diseases, STDs and HIV infection, and blinding conditions; all these receive more than $4 per DALY. EPI, malaria and trachoma receive more than $1 per DALY. A number of important conditions are comparatively underfinanced: acute respiratory infections, nearly all noncommunicable diseases, and all injuries receive less than $0.10 per DALY.

(7) Smaller and poorer countries receive more health sector assistance than larger and richer countries measured in terms of per capita or the share of GDP. Despite widespread perception to the contrary, sub-Saharan Africa does not receive more aid than other regions, after taking into consideration income and population size.

Résumé

Aide extérieure au secteur de santé dans les pays en développement: analyse détaillée, 1972–1990

Cette étude a pour but d'examiner quantitativement en détail les sources et les bénéficiaires de l'aide extérieure apportée au secteur de santé en 1990, d'analyser dans le temps l'évolution de cette aide à ce secteur sur les vingt dernières années de façon aussi détaillée que possible, et, dans la mesure du possible, de décrire l'allocation de ressources à des activités spécifiques du secteur de santé.

Les principaux résultats sont les suivants:

1) Les études sur l'aide extérieure au secteur de santé, ventilée par bénéficiaire ou par activité, sont jusqu'à présent dépendantes du *creditor reporting system* (CRS). Ce système couvre la santé qu'à 63% seulement et le secteur de santé (c'est-à-dire une association entre santé et population) à moins de 50%. La couverture du CRS varie avec le donateur et l'année. Le système d'information utilisé pour contrôler l'aide extérieure apportée au système de santé aura besoin d'être amélioré pour remédier à la faiblesse de la couverture par le CRS. Malgré ses limites actuelles, et grâce aux données détaillées que permet d'obtenir un système d'information basé sur un projet tel que le CRS, ce système est probablement celui qui offre le maximum de possibilités d'amélioration.

2) L'aide extérieure totale au secteur de santé s'est élevée à US$4,8 milliards en 1990. Cette somme ne représente que 2,9% du total des dépenses de santé dans les pays en développement. Le rôle de l'aide extérieure doit être considéré marginalement, en fonction de son impact sur la formation de capital et la formulation de politiques.

3) Après avoir stagné en valeur réelle pendant la première moitié des années 1980, l'aide au secteur de santé augmente depuis 1986, à la fois bilatéralement et multilatéralement. L'augmentation de 1986 à 1990 n'a fait que compenser l'accroissement de la population jusqu'en 1988; en 1989–1990, l'aide extérieure a légèrement dépassé la croissance de la population. L'orientation future dépendra de l'équilibre entre les dépenses multilatérales croissantes et la diminution potentielle des flux bilatéraux, étant donné l'évolution politique récente aux Etats-Unis d'Amérique et en Scandinavie.

4) Pendant les années 1980, les institutions multilatérales, particulièrement l'UNICEF et la Banque mondiale, ont joué un rôle plus important dans le financement de l'aide au secteur de santé que précédemment. Cette tendance à la croissance devrait s'accélérer dans les années 1990, dans la mesure où la Banque mondiale apparaît comme l'institution la plus importante dans le secteur de santé, et qui probablement surpassera bientôt l'US/AID en matière d'assistance bilatérale.

5) Si en valeur absolue, les Etats-Unis d'Amérique, la France et le Japon sont les plus gros pays donateurs, les pays nordiques et les Pays-Bas sont ceux qui, en proportion du PIB, contribuent le plus à l'aide extérieure au secteur de santé.

6) Près de la moitié de l'aide à la santé est dépensée pour le développement des infrastructures, par le biais de subventions aux services de santé et aux hôpitaux. L'autre moitié est affectée à des programmes de santé spécifiques. Si l'on compare les investissements au poids de la mor-

bidité, on observe des différences considérables de financement en fonction de la pathologie. Les pathologies qui bénéficient le plus du financement sont la lèpre, l'onchocercose, diverses autres maladies tropicales, les MST, l'infection à VIH et les affections cécitantes; toutes reçoivent plus de US$4 par DALY (*disability adjusted life years*: années de vie ajustées sur l'incapacité). Le PEV, le paludisme et le trachome reçoivent plus d'un dollar par DALY. Un certain nombre d'affections importantes sont comparativement sous-financées: les infections respiratoires aiguës, la presque totalité des maladies non transmissibles et l'ensemble des traumatismes reçoivent moins de US$0,10 par DALY.

7) Les pays les plus petits et les plus pauvres reçoivent une aide au secteur de santé plus importante que les pays ou grands ou riches, évaluée par habitant ou en proportion du PIB. Contrairement à une impression répandue, l'Afrique subsaharienne n'est pas bénéficiaire d'une aide plus importante que les autres régions, si l'on tient compte du revenu et de la taille de la population.

References

1. **Murray CJL, Govindaraj R, Musgrove P.** National health expenditures: a global analysis. *Bulletin of the World Health Organization*, 1994, **72**(4): 623–637.
2. **Drager N et al.** What determines aid for health: an empirical analysis of bilateral aid flows. *International Conference on Macroeconomics and Health in Countries in Greatest Need*. Document WHO/ICO/ME.CONF, 1992: 149–178.
3. **Howard L.** The evolution of bilateral and multilateral cooperation for health in developing countries. In: Reich M, Marui E, eds. *International cooperation for health: problems, prospects and priorities*. Dover, MA, Auburn House, 1989: 332–357.
4. **Jesperson E.** Social spending: how bilateral donors could do more. *Development journal*, 1991, **3**: 26–36.
5. **Parker D.** *The effectiveness of health aid: a literature review and research framework*. Princeton, NJ, Woodrow Wilson School of Public and International Affairs, Princeton University, 1990.
6. **United Nations. Administrative Committee on Coordination — Subcommittee on Nutrition**. Estimation of flows of external resources in relation to nutrition. *SCN news*, 1990, **5**: 22–36.
7. **United Nations Development Programme.** *The widening gap in global opportunities: human development report 1992*. Oxford, Oxford University Press, 1992.
8. **Murray CJL et al.** A study of financial resources devoted to research on health problems of developing countries. *Journal of tropical medicine and hygiene*, 1990, **93**: 229–255.
9. **United Nations Population Fund.** *Global population assistance report 1982–90*. New York, 1992.
10. **United Nations. Advisory Committee for Co-ordination of Information Systems.** *Register of development activities of the United Nations system 1990*. Geneva, United Nations, 1991.
11. **Organization for Economic Cooperation and Development.** *Creditor Reporting System database of bilateral ODA commitments*. Paris, 1992.
12. **Organization for Economic Cooperation and Development.** *Development cooperation report*. Paris, 1992.
13. **Organization for Economic Cooperation and Development.** *Consolidated version of the DAC sectoral breakdown of bilateral ODA commitments 1971–1990*. Paris, OECD (unpublished database).
14. **International Monetary Fund.** *International financial statistics yearbook, 1992*. Washington DC, 1993.
15. **Murray CJL.** Quantifying the burden of disease: the technical basis for disability-adjusted life years. *Bulletin of the World Health Organization*, 1994, **72**(3): 429–445.
16. **Murray CJL, Lopez AD, Jamison DT.** The global burden of disease in 1990: summary results, sensitivity analysis and future directions. *Bulletin of the World Health Organization*, 1994, **72**(3): 495–509.

Annex

Total flows from external assistance

Demographic region and country	To the health sector (in millions US$)	External assistance Per capita (US$)	As % of GDP	As % of total health expenditures
Sub-Saharan Africa	1251	2.5	0.45	10.4
Benin	33	7.0	1.61	37.3
Bostwana	29	22.9	1.02	16.5
Burkina Faso	42	4.7	6.12	72.3
Burundi	15	2.8	0.30	9.3
Cameroon	38	3.3	0.31	11.9

(Annex: continued)

Demographic region and country	To the health sector (in millions US$)	External assistance Per capita (US$)	As % of GDP	As % of total health expenditures
Cape Verde	13	34.3	3.40	53.7
Central African Republic	20	6.5	1.51	36.0
Chad	33	5.8	2.97	47.7
Comoros	3	6.9	1.32	24.5
Congo	14	6.1	0.48	12.1
Côte d'Ivoire	11	0.9	0.11	3.4
Equatorial Guinea	5	11.8	3.25	42.7
Ethiopia	43	0.8	0.71	18.8
Gabon	12	10.5	0.26	6.4
Gambia	10	11.4	3.84	51.0
Ghana	29	2.0	0.46	13.2
Guinea	20	3.5	0.78	20.0
Guinea-Bissau	8	8.1	4.06	49.8
Kenya	84	3.5	0.96	22.1
Lesotho	16	9.1	2.93	35.2
Liberia	6	2.4	5.63	68.3
Madagascar	17	1.5	0.55	21.4
Malawi	22	2.5	1.16	23.3
Mali	36	4.3	1.47	28.4
Mauritania	11	5.5	1.14	30.0
Mauritius	14	13.3	0.58	13.3
Mozambique	45	2.9	3.12	53.3
Namibia	9	4.9	0.43	10.9
Niger	43	5.6	1.70	34.1
Nigeria	58	0.6	0.17	6.1
Rwanda	29	4.1	1.37	39.8
São Tome and Principe	2	20.6	4.99	54.2
Senegal	36	4.9	0.62	16.9
Seychelles	4	63.2	1.32	21.9
Sierra Leone	7	1.7	1.20	49.5
Somalia	31	4.0	0.78	51.6
South Africa	2	0.0	0.00	0.0
Sudan	39	1.5	0.15	4.5
Swaziland	17	21.8	2.47	34.2
Tanzania (United Rep. of)	53	2.1	2.55	54.0
Togo	14	3.9	0.87	7.0
Uganda	46	2.8	1.15	33.7
Zaire	48	1.3	0.63	26.7
Zambia	6	0.7	0.13	4.1
Zimbabwe	42	4.2	0.69	11.0
India	286	0.3	0.10	1.6
China	77	0.1	0.02	0.6
Other Asia and islands	594	0.9	0.07	1.4
Bangladesh	128	1.2	0.59	18.5
Bhutan	4	2.9	1.44	28.5
Fiji	4	4.8	0.26	6.9
Indonesia	159	0.9	0.15	7.7
Lao People's Dem. Rep.	5	1.2	0.56	21.9
Malaysia	3	0.1	0.01	0.2
Mongolia	2	1.1	0.13	1.9
Nepal	33	1.8	1.15	25.4
Papua New Guinea	7	1.8	0.21	4.8
Philippines	69	1.1	0.15	7.4
Rep. of Korea	32	0.7	0.01	0.2
Samoa	1	8.0	1.17	39.7

(Annex: continued)

Demographic region and country	External assistance			
	To the health sector (in millions US$)	Per capita (US$)	As % of GDP	As % of total health expenditures
Singapore	1	0.2	0.00	0.1
Solomon Islands	2	7.3	0.14	6.3
Sri Lanka	26	1.5	0.32	8.6
Thailand	36	0.7	0.05	0.9
Tonga	1	9.3	0.95	14.8
Vanuatu	2	15.3	1.29	22.8
Viet Nam	25	0.4	0.28	13.3
Latin America and the Caribbean	591	1.3	0.05	1.3
Antigua and Barbuda	1	8.7	0.16	3.6
Argentina	11	0.3	0.01	0.2
Barbados	2	6.1	0.10	1.9
Belize	2	12.8	0.63	10.7
Bolivia	37	5.1	0.82	20.5
Brazil	84	0.6	0.02	0.4
Chile	10	0.7	0.03	0.7
Colombia	26	0.8	0.06	1.6
Costa Rica	4	1.6	0.08	1.2
Dominica	2	27.9	1.17	14.5
Dominican Republic	11	1.5	0.15	4.0
Ecuador	31	3.0	0.28	6.8
El Salvador	44	8.5	0.86	14.7
Guatemala	32	3.4	0.46	12.6
Guyana	15	18.4	4.58	44.2
Haiti	33	5.1	1.33	19.0
Honduras	20	4.0	0.35	7.7
Jamaica	19	7.8	0.48	9.5
Mexico	65	0.8	0.03	0.9
Nicaragua	27	6.9	1.77	20.6
Panama	15	6.1	0.31	4.3
Paraguay	10	2.4	0.19	6.7
Peru	29	1.4	0.07	2.2
St Kitts and Nevis	1	29.9	0.85	14.1
Suriname	2	3.8	0.12	4.1
Trindad and Tobago	1	1.1	0.03	0.6
Uruguay	5	1.7	0.06	1.4
Venezuela	2	0.1	0.01	0.1
Middle Eastern crescent	453	0.9	0.04	1.2
Algeria	2	0.1	0.00	0.1
Cyprus	5	6.6	0.41	10.3
Egypt	111	2.1	0.20	7.7
Islamic Republic of Iran	2	0.0	0.00	0.0
Israel	3	0.6	0.01	0.1
Jordan (E. Bank)	18	5.9	0.41	10.8
Kuwait	2	0.8	0.01	0.1
Morocco	20	0.8	0.08	3.1
Oman	1	0.9	0.02	0.5
Pakistan	76	0.7	0.19	5.5
Qatar	0	0.1	0.00	0.0
Saudi Arabia	1	0.1	0.00	0.0
Syrian Arab Republic	20	1.6	0.08	4.0
Tunisia	18	2.3	0.15	3.0
Turkey	23	0.4	0.02	0.5
Turkmenistan	2	0.5	0.02	0.4
United Arab Emirates	0	0.3	0.00	0.1
Yemen	25	2.2	0.36	11.3

Design, content and financing of an essential national package of health services[*]

J.-L. Bobadilla,[1] P. Cowley,[2] P. Musgrove,[3] & H. Saxenian[4]

A minimum package of public health and clinical interventions, which are highly cost-effective and deal with major sources of disease burden, could be provided in low-income countries for about US$ 12 per person per year, and in middle-income countries for about $22. Properly delivered, this package could eliminate 21% to 38% of the burden of premature mortality and disability in children under 15 years and 10–18% of the burden in adults. The cost would exceed what governments now spend on health in the poorest countries but would be easily affordable in middle-income countries. Governments should ensure that, at the least, poor populations have access to these services. Additional public expenditure should then go either to extending coverage to the non-poor or to expansion beyond the minimum collection of services to an essential national package of health care, including somewhat less cost-effective interventions against a larger number of diseases and conditions.

Introduction

No country in the world can provide health services to meet all the possible needs of the population, so it is advisable to establish criteria for which services to provide. Two basic criteria are the size of the burden caused by a particular disease, injury or risk factor and the cost-effectiveness of interventions to deal with it. The World Bank's *World development report 1993: investing in health* (*1*) applies these criteria to the design of an *essential* national package of health services. Because epidemiological profiles differ among countries, even at the same income level, the national package must be tailored to a country's circumstances. However, it should always include a *minimum* package of both public health measures and individual clinical services which are highly cost-effective and help resolve major health problems. Governments should ensure universal access to its national package by financing it directly or, when public resources are inadequate, by promoting private expenditure on the clinical interventions in the package. This article makes a case to justify such a package. It explains what the minimum package contains and how the component services were chosen, and estimates what it could cost, how

much it could improve health, and what it implies for investment in facilities, equipment and personnel. Defining a package also clarifies the trade-off between coverage of the population and the cost-effectiveness of health care interventions that are provided, especially in poor countries.

Creating a package

Justification

Why is it advisable to collect various health services into a "package", and what does that mean? Governments could and often do proceed in other ways. They can simply agree to pay for, or guarantee to provide, any of a list of services, without considering possible relations between one intervention and another. Or they could choose not to specify outputs at all, and agree to pay for, or provide, a particular collection of inputs: medical professionals would then decide which services were actually provided, whether by delivering services they thought were justified or by responding to patients' demand. The second approach is incompatible with maximizing value for money, or getting the maximum health gain per dollar spent, because people often demand services offering little health improvement and do not always seek those that cost less or provide a greater health gain. Medical professionals also commonly seek to provide, and to generate demand for, services of questionable value. In any case, it is impossible to decide which inputs to finance without some idea of what services they are meant to provide. The first approach—choosing interventions but not packaging them—takes no account of joint costs or co-morbidi-

[*] From the Population, Health and Nutrition Department, the World Bank, Washington, DC 20433, USA.
[1] Senior Health Specialist. Requests for reprints should be sent to this author.
[2] Consultant.
[3] Principal Economist.
[4] Senior Economist.

Reprinted from *Bulletin of the World Health Organization*, 1994, **72** (4): 653-662.

171

ty; so the interventions chosen in this way will cost more than they should, or will reach fewer people.

The principal argument for a collection of services to be provided jointly is to minimize the total cost of the package by exploiting the shared use of inputs and by reducing the cost to patients of obtaining services. Clustering of interventions improves cost-effectiveness through at least three mechanisms: synergism between treatment and prevention activities; joint production costs; and improved use of specialized resources through the screening of patients at the first level of care, to ensure that a small share of high-risk cases can be recognized and referred to hospital. Sometimes a cluster of diseases can be treated together, because they share diagnostic procedures or treatment protocols, or even the same drugs. And sometimes services can be organized to reach related individuals, e.g., integration of maternal and child care. Thus the package becomes more than simply a list of interventions: properly understood, it is also a vehicle for orienting demand and improving referral.

These are primarily medical reasons why services should be packaged in order to increase the health gain from a given collection of inputs. Other justifications for a package of care have to do more with the limited capabilities of governments to set priorities and to plan investment. The national package is a starting point, a way of assuring that the highest priority services are not slighted; governments that adopt it will have a better basis for setting other priorities and deciding what else to pay for in health care. It also simplifies the task of planning investment in buildings and equipment, in training people, and in purchasing drugs and supplies. The minimum output of services defines a minimum need for inputs. And in very poor countries, concentration on a package rather than on individual inputs or outputs makes it easier to estimate the need for external assistance and to use donor resources well. Finally, the definition of an explicit package of services for government to finance helps establish the boundary between the public and private sectors and may focus the attention of governments on their own capacities and responsibilities. When this boundary is not clear, governments easily waste resources by trying to do too much instead of doing what matters most.

Criteria for which services to be included

A health package could be designed purely to deal with a country's principal health *problems*; services would then be included to treat problems in descending order of importance, as measured by the loss in disability-adjusted life years (DALYs) (2). Unfortu-

nately, the only solutions for some such problems may yield very small health gains or very high costs, or both. An alternative is to design the package on the basis of *interventions*, according to their cost-effectiveness. This is the ratio of the cost of providing the intervention once (where that is appropriate) — or during a year (where treatment must be repeated) — to the health gain (in DALYs). The lower the cost per DALY obtained, the more cost-effective the intervention is.

Estimates of the cost-effectiveness of interventions, which were used to design the package come, with some modifications, from Jamison et al. (3). Fig. 1 shows dollar costs and health gains from 47 interventions: higher points represent most effective interventions and points farther to the right represent cheaper ones. The diagonal lines are contours of equal cost per DALY, decreasing away from the origin. Individual interventions can differ in cost from less than one dollar to more than $ 10 000. They can differ just as widely in health gains: an intervention which saves one person's life and prevents infection of others can gain between 10 and 100 years of healthy life, whereas the improvement from some other interventions may amount to only a few hours or days of complete health. There is little correlation between what an intervention costs and how much additional health it provides: neither cost nor results alone is a guide to cost-effectiveness. The cost per DALY gained also varies greatly, by much more than the likely errors of estimation or the variation in cost-effectiveness from one country or epidemiological situation to another. It matters which services are included in a package; this would not be the case if the cost per healthy life-year gained were about the same for all services.

However, some cost-effective interventions deal with problems making only small contributions to ill health, because the condition is rare or the individual health loss from it is negligible. Including all such

Fig. 1. US dollar costs and health gains in DALYs from 47 interventions.

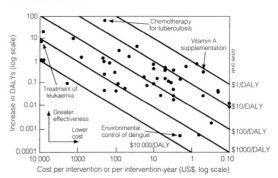

interventions would make the package very complicated to administer and might multiply the requirements for specialized, seldom used inputs, which
could raise costs and overtax health system capacities. The World Bank's report therefore proposes a
minimum package based on both problems and
interventions: the services included are highly cost-
effective and deal with major threats to health (1).
(Cost-effective interventions against health problems, which cause large losses to individuals but are
so rare as to produce little overall health loss, may
belong in a larger, essential national package).

Content of the package

In communities with moderate or high mortality, a
few causes typically account for a large share of
deaths. The interventions included in the minimum
package address such causes and some of the risk
factors that produce them. In 1990 an estimated 55%
of the burden of disease was concentrated in children
under 15 years old, with 660 million DALYs lost.
Just ten disease conditions or clusters cause 71% of
this loss, as shown in Table 1. Except for congenital
malformations,[a] all these causes correspond to very
cost-effective interventions, at less than $100 per
DALY. Protein-energy malnutrition and vitamin-A
deficiency can produce death or disability directly or
through other diseases; Table 1 counts only the
direct loss. The total loss attributable to these conditions is five to six times larger when their indirect
effect is included.

The burden of disease in the adult population is
less concentrated than that of children under 15 years
old: the ten main classes of disease and injuries
account for only about 50% of the adult burden.
Although most interventions to control these diseases
are quite cost-effective, the impact is moderate
because they prevent or treat only a small fraction of
the problem. Overall, it is estimated that only 10–18%
of the adult disease burden could be eliminated with
the interventions in the minimum package, whereas
the interventions for children could reduce their burden by 21–28%. Of course, separating the interventions for different age groups is artificial, because
many services such as immunization with hepatitis
vaccine are given to children but the benefits accrue
throughout life. A similar but more indirect case can

be made for the effect of reducing infection in childhood on improved well-being in adult life (e.g., treatment of helminthic diseases improves cognitive abilities which in turn increases educational attainment).
Mosley & Gray (4) and Elo & Preston (5) have identified many diseases in children that affect health in
adulthood. Interventions applied to adults can also
produce substantial benefits in children, as is the
case with prenatal and delivery care and AIDS prevention programmes.

Another way of analysing the burden of disease
is by way of risk factors. Current understanding of
the attributable risk for most of the important risk
factors is quite limited. There is no agreed classification of risk factors, nor is there a standard methodology to avoid double counting of deaths and disabilities when comparing disease burdens due to
different risk factors. The *World development report
1993* estimated the DALYs lost to nine risk factors
or clusters of risk factors, based on the evidence published in the scientific literature on the attributable
risks. Indoor air pollution, the most important risk
factor accounting for about 13% of the burden, cannot be matched with a cost-effective intervention,
making it a high research priority. The second, inadequate water and sanitation, explaining about 10% of
the burden, is matched with a well known intervention, but the cost-effectiveness is unfavourable, at
more than $1000 per DALY. The reason for this
somewhat counter-intuitive result is that cost-effectiveness is able to capture only the health benefits of
interventions; water and sanitation produce substantial non-health improvements in the welfare of
households, and their provision or facilitation could
be justified on those grounds (6). Protein-energy
malnutrition and vitamin-A deficiency together
explain about 10% of the DALYs in developing
countries, unsafe sex 4%, alcohol abuse 3%, excess
fertility 2.4%, and tobacco consumption only 1%.
The interventions available to deal with these risk
factors, with the exception of food supplementation,
are included in the minimum package because of
their favourable cost-effectiveness.

When diseases or risk factors change rapidly,
the present burden of disease is not a good indicator
of the priority for their control. Tobacco consumption and AIDS transmission through unsafe sex are
increasing very rapidly in many developing countries; the priority for controlling these risk factors is
high because in the next few decades the diseases
caused by tobacco and AIDS will be among the main
causes of death and disability. It is estimated that
deaths due to tobacco consumption will increase
from three million in 1990 to ten million in about 30
years, with most of the increase occurring in developing countries. Similarly AIDS is the first cause of

---

[a] Potentially cost-effective interventions exist to prevent some of
the congenital malformations of the nervous system and treat
the most common congenital errors of metabolism, but they
address only a very small fraction of the total burden due to this
cluster of causes. Middle-income countries with low infant mortality should consider these interventions for inclusion in the
national essential package.

Table 1: **Main cause of disease burden in children and adults in demographically developing countries in 1990 and the cost-effectiveness of the interventions available for their control**

Disease and injuries	No. of DALYs lost[a] (million)	Main intervention	Cost-effectiveness ($ per DALY)
Children			
Respiratory infections	98 (14.8)[b]	Integrated management of the sick child (IMSC)	30–100
Perinatal morbidity and mortality	96 (14.6)	(a) Prenatal and delivery care	30–100
		(b) Family planning	20–150
Diarrhoeal disease	92 (14.0)	IMSC	30–100
Childhood cluster (diseases preventable through immunization)	65 (10.0)	Expanded programme of immunization EPI-plus[c]	12–30
Congenital malformation	35 (5.4)	Surgical operations	High (unknown)
Malaria	31 (4.7)	IMSC	30–100
Intestinal helminths	17 (2.5)	School health programme	20–34
Protein-energy malnutrition	12 (1.8)	IMSC	30–100
Vitamin-A deficiency	12 (1.8)	EPI-plus[c]	12–30
Iodine deficiency	9 (1.4)	Iodine supplementation	19–37
Subtotal	467 (71.0)	—	—
Total DALYs lost	660 (100)	—	—
Adults			
Sexually transmitted diseases (STD) and HIV infection	49.2 (8.9)	Condom subsidy plus IEC[d]	3–18
Tuberculosis	36.6 (6.7)	Short-course chemotherapy	3–7
Cerebrovascular disease	31.7 (5.8)	Case management	High (unknown)
Maternal morbidity and mortality	28.1 (5.1)	Prenatal and delivery care	30–110
Ischaemic heart disease	24.9 (4.5)	Tobacco control programme	35–55
Chronic obstructive pulmonary disease	23.4 (4.3)	Tobacco control programme	35–55
Motor vehicle accidents	18.4 (3.3)	Alcohol control programme	35–55
Depressive disorders	15.7 (2.9)	Case management	500–800
Peri- endo- and myocarditis and cardiomyopathy	12.4 (2.2)	Case management	High (unknown)
Homicide and violence	12.2 (2.2)	Alcohol control programme	35–55
Subtotal	252.6 (48.6)	—	—
Total DALYs lost	550.0 (100)	—	—

[a] DALYs lost (for specific diseases and the total) are taken from the 1993 World Development Report (1). The total for children and adults include DALYs lost in 1990 due to all diseases and injuries.
[b] Figures in parentheses are percentages.
[c] EPI-plus includes the six vaccines of the Expanded Programme on Immunization (EPI), plus the vaccine against hepatitis B and vitamin A supplementation.
[d] IEC: activities dedicated to information, education and communication.

death in many African cities and is likely to become a major cause of death in Sub-Saharan Africa, India and other Asian countries unless action is taken soon to prevent HIV transmission.

Table 2 presents the health interventions included in the minimum package, and some basic information on their cost and potential effect in low- and middle-income countries. These scenarios were modelled with data from Sub-Saharan Africa and from Latin America and the Caribbean, respectively. The cost of labour and other health inputs, the epidemiological profile and magnitude of the burden of disease, and population age structure vary between the two cases. Low-income countries are characterized by younger populations and higher mortality and fertility rates; higher incidence of certain diseases; and lower labour costs. Two major contributors to the potential DALY gain in low-income countries are the prenatal and delivery care cluster and the treatment of tuberculosis, both of which are

Table 2: **Cost-effectiveness of the health interventions (and clusters of intervention) included in the minimum package of health services in low- and middle-income countries**

Interventions	Cost per beneficiary	Cost per capita	DALYs potentially gained[a] (per 1000 population)	Effectiveness[b]	Cost per DALY($)
Low-income countries					
I. *Public health*					
Expanded programme of immunization plus[c]	14.6	0.5	45	0.77	12–17
School health programme	3.6	0.3	4	0.58	20–25
Tobacco and alcohol control programme	0.3	0.3	12	0.14	35–55
AIDS prevention programme[d]	112.2	1.7	35	0.58	3–5
Other public health interventions[e]	2.4	1.4	—	—	—
Subtotal	—	4.2	—	—	14
II. *Clinical services*					
Chemotherapy against tuberculosis	500.0	0.6	34	0.51	3–5
Integrated management of the sick child	9.0	1.6	184	0.25	30–50
Family planning	12.0	0.9	7	0.70	20–30
STD treatment	11.0	0.2	26	0.42	1–3
Prenatal and delivery care	90.0	3.8	57	0.42	30–50
Limited care[f]	6.0	0.7	—	0.03	200–300
Subtotal	—	7.8	—	—	—
Total	—	12.0	—	—	—
Middle-income countries					
I. *Public health*					
Expanded programme of immunization plus[c]	28.6	0.8	4	0.77	25–30
School health programme	6.5	0.6	5	0.58	38–43
Tobacco and alcohol control programme	0.3	0.3	9	0.14	45–55
AIDS prevention programme[d]	132.3	2.0	15	0.58	13–18
Other public health interventions[e]	5.2	3.1	—	—	—
Subtotal	—	6.9	—	—	—
II. *Clinical services*					
Chemotherapy against tuberculosis	275.0	0.2	6	0.51	5–7
Integrated management of the sick child	8.0	1.1	21	0.25	50–100
Family planning	20.0	2.2	6	0.70	100–150
STD treatment	18.0	0.3	3.7	0.42	10–15
Prenatal and delivery care	255.0	8.8	25	0.42	60–110
Limited care[f]	13.0	2.1	—	0.03	400–600
Subtotal	—	14.7	—	—	133
Total	—	21.5	—	—	—

[a] Sum of losses to premature mortality and to disability, including losses to others because of secondary transmission of disease.
[b] Calculated by multiplying efficacy, diagnostic accuracy (when applicable) and compliance.
[c] Plus refers to vaccine against hepatitis B and vitamin A supplementation.
[d] DALYs lost from AIDS include dynamic effects (probability of transmission to others) only in the first year, which understates the value of preventing cases and thus the cost-effectiveness of preventive interventions.
[e] Includes information, communication, and education on selected risk factors and health behaviours, plus vector control and disease surveillance.
[f] Includes treatment of infection and minor trauma; for more complicated conditions, includes diagnosis, advice and pain relief, and treatment as resources permit.

largely neglected. Practically all the preventive and some of the therapeutic activities of the package involve behavioural changes. Since supplying services does not necessarily induce acceptance by the potential beneficiaries, much of the cost of these activities is dedicated to information, education and communication (IEC). These are sometimes needed not only for the consumers but also for the providers of health services.

Cost and payment

For low-income countries, the minimum package is estimated to cost about $12 per person per year. This rises to an estimated $22 per person per year in middle-income countries. About one-third of the total would go for public health activities and the remaining two-thirds for the essential clinical services. To verify the robustness of the estimates, the costs of the package were calculated in two ways. One approach was based on the cost of specific activities, estimated from existing studies in many countries of service delivery costs by type of intervention. In the other approach, costs were estimated for a prototype district health system able to deliver the minimum package, consisting of a district hospital, health clinics, and outreach activities. (The minimum package presented in Table 2 requires about one district hospital bed per 1000 population, 0.1 physicians per 1000 population, and between two and four nurses per physician). The two estimates were then compared to identify and correct errors or inconsistencies. Detailed cost estimates for specific countries must take into account prevailing demographic and epidemiological conditions and input costs. And it is important to recognize that the estimates should reflect what it would cost to carry out the intervention effectively, not what the intervention costs at present. For example, a country's tuberculosis programme may be treating only a small fraction of those with tuberculosis. The package should be designed not with these current programme costs, but with the estimated costs of effectively reaching a much larger population. The content of the package is chosen to provide the greatest possible health gain for a limited expenditure, independently of who is to pay for it.

Countries may choose to finance the whole package, for the whole population, from public resources. If they do not, there are still two criteria for what governments should finance. One is that certain services are so nearly public goods, or provide such substantial external benefits, that private markets will provide too little of them. For such interventions to be available, they must be financed by governments. The other criterion is that governments have a special responsibility for the health of the poor, who can pay for very little health care. User fees to recover part of the cost from poor people would have to be very low; they could only be justified by assuring greater technical efficiency in service provision, as for example if the revenues were retained and used locally to guarantee supplies of drugs. The contribution to total operating costs would be insignificant. The poor also tend to suffer worse health than the non-poor, but that would not matter if they could pay for the corresponding care. It happens that the services included in the package deal with problems which particularly affect the poor, but no intervention is included simply because

the corresponding problem is associated with poverty: it must also be cost-effective. Poverty, like public goods, is relevant to who pays for the package but not to what goes into it.

Beyond assuring the provision of cost-effective public health interventions to everyone, and the access of the poor to the entire minimum package of services, governments face two issues about what health services to finance. One is what to include in an *essential national package*, which would start with the minimum package but could be much larger, including a variety of other services. Everything beyond the essential set of services is considered *discretionary*, and should be financed entirely from private sources (out-of-pocket or through insurance) or by way of mandated social insurance. Such services should not be subsidized from general public revenues. The other issue is how far to pay for services, even those in the essential national package, for the nonpoor part of the population. This involves the choice of where to draw the poverty line between the two groups, and how in practice to distinguish the poor from the nonpoor. For a given level of public spending, the more the package is targeted to the poor, the more comprehensive it can be.

Most low-income countries currently need to use all their public expenditure on health, simply to pay for the minimum package for the poor. They cannot afford an essential package which includes much more than the minimum. And they may be unable to finance even the minimum package completely for the nonpoor: in low-income countries governments spend, on average, just $6 per person for health and the total health spending (both public and private) is about $14 per person. Funding the minimum package in these settings would require a combination of an increase in public spending for health, a reorientation of current government health outlays away from discretionary services, and targeting public spending on clinical services to the poor.

This situation is shown on the left side of Fig. 2: choices on the essential package and on priority for the poor define four combinations of a population group with a set of health services. The vertical axis indicates the degree of public subsidy, which should be equal or close to 100% for the minimum package for the poor. The subsidy should fall, perhaps quite sharply, as public expenditure is extended either to the nonpoor or to interventions outside the minimum package. This condition can be stated in the form of two rules for public expenditure: it should not pay for any services for the nonpoor which it does not also assure for the poor, and it should not pay for a less cost-effective service unless and until it has paid for all services which are more cost-effective. Anything else would be inequitable, favouring those who

Fig. 2. **Health care choices in a low-income and middle-income country.** The vertical axis indicates the level of public subsidy, the right-side horizontal axis refers to the population volume classified as poor and non-poor, and the left-side horizontal axis represents clinical health services divided into the minimum and the essential packages. Public subsidies should be close to 100% for the minimum package for the poor. In low-income countries the subsidy should fall, perhaps quite sharply, as resources extend to the non-poor or to interventions outside the minimum package. In middle-income countries the subsidy could extend to the non-poor and can finance part of the essential package only if the minimum package is assured for the poor and all cost-effective services are covered for the entire population.

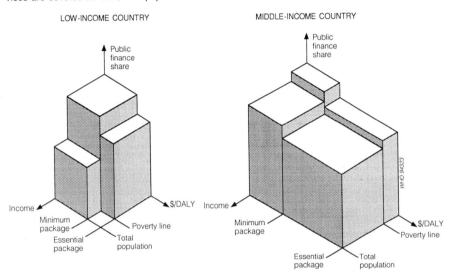

can afford to pay over those who cannot, or inefficient, favouring interventions which yield less value for money over those which are more justified.

The right side of Fig. 2 shows the situation of a middle-income country, where current public spending on health averages about $62 per capita. Such countries can afford an essential package which goes well beyond the minimum, to cover less cost-effective interventions that address a wider spectrum of diseases and injuries. The poor are a smaller share of the population, and resources are adequate even to subsidize less cost-effective services for the nonpoor. There may still be differences in the degree of public subsidy, but they can be smaller, or involve less targeting to the poor, than in low-income countries.

Implications for public policy

A government wishing to adopt an essential national health care package faces a number of requirements and choices: these involve needs for information, choices about how to deliver and pay for services, and questions as to how to influence decisions in the private sector or in subnational levels of government.

Data needs for the design of the package. The analytical requirements for a rigorously designed nation-

al package are substantial. But countries can design provisional packages quickly while the analytical database is built up. They can develop a national essential package by using proxies for the data, or alternatively, by adopting the minimum package described above (perhaps with some adjustments) as the preliminary national package. Over the longer term, the package is best designed from results of a national burden of disease estimation and the local level analysis of the cost-effectiveness of interventions. The national burden of disease can be calculated over a period of months if data on morbidity and mortality are available. If these data are missing, indirect estimation can be used, or, as an interim proxy, regional disease burden estimates (*1*) can be adjusted for a particular country. Local estimates of intervention costs (and assumed effectiveness) should also be developed, at least for the most important health interventions. This can also take months, depending on the cost data available.

Implementation of the package. Once a national package is designed, the challenge is how to implement it. Government budgets are not organized by disease intervention: allocations are made across organizations (ministries of health, affiliated foundations, governmental research institutions, third-party insurers), across facilities (hospitals and health clinics), and across input categories (personnel, supplies, drugs, maintenance, training, transport, and the like).

Where governments finance and provide health services, they can use input availability, norm setting, training, and consumer education to affect which services are utilized. It would be neither possible nor desirable for governments to supervise the providers' day-to-day clinical decisions. But governments can facilitate the delivery of the package by financing the inputs needed (drugs, personnel, supplies, equipment). Similarly, not financing specialist physicians, sophisticated equipment, and drugs for discretionary services diminishes the likelihood that services outside the national package will be provided at public facilities. "Essential equipment lists" can be developed to identify equipment needs for the essential package. Norm-setting also influences what is delivered. Governments usually establish norms about what types of services should be provided in different levels of public facilities. Again, including essential services and excluding discretionary services are important. Governments can also ensure that medical and nursing curricula give adequate attention to the national essential package. In many countries, the curriculum is not up-to-date regarding diagnosis and treatment of sexually transmitted diseases, tuberculosis treatment, and even family planning methods. And in-service staff training should support the essential package, to facilitate its delivery. Finally, governments can, through education campaigns, inform the public about the package—about the services guaranteed to be offered in different types of facilities, and when to seek such services.

Public finance and private provision of the package. Governments can also choose to finance all or part of the package through private providers. Reimbursement mechanisms can be designed in a variety of ways, including payment according to diagnosis or on a per capita basis. Governments can also contract with nongovernmental organizations or other private groups to provide care to subgroups of the population. In any event, monitoring mechanisms will be needed to ensure that the intended services are provided to the target population.

Mandating the package. In countries where states or municipalities are responsible for service delivery but funding is largely federal, the national government can require that lower levels of government provide at least those services in the national essential package, to qualify for federal transfers. And the cost of the package can guide per capita intergovernmental resource flows. The government can influence private as well as public finance of the national package, by requiring that all private insurers provide, at a minimum, the elements of the national package. This would in no way prevent insurers from providing additional, discretionary services, but it would ensure that the national package's highly cost-effective services are included in any insurance package.

Making the transition. In many developing countries the existing stock of health facilities, equipment, and health personnel is poorly matched to the requirements for delivery of a national essential package. Many countries have too many tertiary public hospital beds and physicians in urban areas, while rural areas still lack health clinics and primary care providers. Because it may be difficult politically to redress this imbalance in infrastructure by closing large public facilities, it is critical that new physical and human resource investments be directed at the inputs needed to deliver the national package in order to correct this imbalance over time. And to the extent feasible, governments can improve resource allocation by redirecting *recurrent* spending toward lower-level facilities, which provide most of the cost-effective interventions.

Achieving the potential health gains from the package. Designing a cost-effective package that addresses major disease burdens, and reallocating funds for that package, does not guarantee success. Programmes must also operate efficiently. The minimum package outlined in Table 3 assumes that a well-functioning referral system connects health outreach, health clinics and district hospitals. It assumes that vehicles are available to transport obstetric emergencies to district hospitals; that staff can be attracted to work in remote areas; that drugs are available when needed in the health system; and that operating rooms are available for obstetric emergencies, and are not closed because of a shortage of key supplies. Careful attention to technical efficiency is just as important as allocative efficiency to the successful implementation of the national essential package.

Discussion and conclusions

The notion of an essential national package of health services presented here derives from a series of efforts over the past decade and a half to determine health sector priorities. The earliest attempts usually refer to interventions characterized by low cost and a low level of complexity but not to well-defined packages. These efforts to define priority health interventions in order to make more efficient use of resources include the WHO primary health care approach (7); the somewhat narrower selective primary health care proposal of Walsh & Warren (8), directed to children's health and selected tropical diseases; the UNICEF concentration on a small number of interventions directed at mothers and children (9); and a World Bank Policy Paper on health (10). A more complex exercise is the PAHO health sector planning approach (11), which starts with disease priorities and derives needs for such inputs as staff and facilities.

All these recommendations or partial packages were designed from very incomplete information on the burden of disease, particularly noncommunicable diseases among adults and other health problems that cause disability as well as, or instead of, mortality. Partly in consequence, and partly because of the emphasis on children, for whom most of the disease burden is due to premature mortality, health gains were measured chiefly or exclusively by reduction in deaths. Data on cost-effectiveness were also limited to a few childhood problems and some parasitic diseases. The minimum package proposed here represents an advance over earlier efforts because it draws on information about all the major health problems of low- and middle-income countries and all age groups, deals with disability as well as mortality, and is based on both disease burden and cost-effectiveness rather than on such partial criteria as cost alone or complexity of interventions. It also provides guidance for expanding from a minimum collection of services to a larger essential package, and relates this choice to decisions about public finance of health care.

One limitation on cost-effectiveness for allocating health resources is that many interventions significantly improve not only health but also income and welfare. Sometimes the health benefits alone justify the interventions (e.g., the education of girls). In other cases such as water and sanitation, the cost per DALY gained is high; but the consumers' willingness to pay for the associated non-health benefits may allow for part of the cost to be recovered, lowering the *public expenditure* per unit of health gain. More generally, cost-effectiveness alone is not a justification for public expenditure. Public finance needs to be justified by the additional health gains, compared to what would result from private finance; or by a reduction in costs; or because the intervention is at least partly a public good; or because the beneficiaries are too poor to pay for the intervention, even through insurance in some circumstances, cost-effectiveness may conflict with another objective of public spending on health care, which is to reduce inequities. Universal coverage with an intervention may raise marginal costs substantially above average costs, because part of the population lives in remote areas. Since such people are more likely to be poor,

concentrating public resources on the poor is a partial solution to this problem; but it still may be true that much more health gain could be achieved, even for the poor, if some otherwise cost-effective interventions were not extended to areas of very high cost. The relative importance of cost-effectiveness versus equity will then determine whether to modify the package by leaving out some interventions, providing mobile services rather than fixed facilities, concentrating on public health rather than clinical interventions for the high-cost population, or sacrificing some efficiency in order to preserve equity.

In exceptional cases paying a high marginal cost to cover the whole population may be justified on efficiency grounds, because the disease—like smallpox and perhaps poliomyelitis—can be eradicated. Such dynamic arguments, which are not based only on the present burden of disease and the cost-effectiveness of interventions, also underlie the package's emphasis on reducing tobacco use and controlling the spread of AIDS. Finally, since public budgets for health reflect the inertia of past investments, adoption of an appropriate package and the corresponding allocation of spending is also a dynamic problem: how quickly and effectively an essential national package can be introduced depends on how much new investment and training may be needed and on the technical, administrative and political capacity of the existing health system to analyse health problems and respond to them.

Acknowledgements

We thank our co-authors of the *World development report 1993*, Dean Jamison, Robert Hecht, Kenneth Hill, Jee-Peng Tan, and (part-time) Seth Berkley and Christopher Murray, as well as all the epidemiologists, clinicians and social scientists who participated in the several background consultations to this report.

Résumé

Structure, contenu et financement d'un module national de services de santé essentiels

Au cours des 15 dernières années, plusieurs propositions ont été faites pour identifier les interventions de santé qui devraient bénéficier de la priorité, parmi lesquelles les services pédiatriques, la prévention de la mortalité prématurée, les mesures de prévention et de santé publique, les interventions à faible coût, les soins médicaux de faible complexité et les gestes et interventions que le personnel des centres de niveau primaire ayant relativement peu de formation peut réaliser. La présente étude utilise beaucoup de données nouvelles sur l'incidence de la maladie et de l'incapacité, et sur les coûts et les résultats des interventions, pour définir un module *minimal* de soins de santé. Ce module repose sur deux critères destinés à maximiser les bénéfices pour la santé et à maîtriser les coûts dans les systèmes de santé dont les capacités sont limitées: d'une part les problèmes de santé qui représentent une fraction importante du poids de la morbidité — y compris les conséquences de l'incapacité chronique et de la mortalité précoce — et, d'autre part, les interventions à bon rapport coût-efficacité destinées à traiter ces problèmes et qui apportent, à faible coût, une année supplémentaire de vie en bonne santé ou sans incapacité. La mise en œuvre de ce module minimal exigerait une dotation en personnel comprenant environ un médecin, deux à quatre infirmières et dix lits par hôpital de premier niveau pour 10 000 habitants. Quand les ressources le permettent, ce module minimal pourrait être élargi et devenir un module national *essentiel* de soins de santé, où les interventions pourraient être de rapport coût-efficacité légèrement plus faible et viser un plus grand nombre de pathologies.

Que de plus les autorités publiques soient ou non le prestateur de services, il leur est possible de financer la totalité du module national pour la population entière, et de laisser au financement privé tous les soins non essentiels ou relevant d'une libre décision. Lorsque les ressources publiques ne couvrent pas toutes les interventions à bon rapport coût-efficacité pour tous, il est souhaitable de concentrer les actions sur les plus défavorisés — lesquels ne peuvent payer qu'une très faible partie des soins de santé, soit directement, soit par un système d'assurance — et sur les interventions qui concernent le domaine public ou qui apportent des bénéfices extérieurs si importants que les marchés privés ne les assureront pas convenablement. Parmi ces interventions, plusieurs ont pour but l'information du public sur les risques pour la santé ou les changements de comportement. Les pouvoirs publics peuvent également exiger la couverture du module essentiel par les assurances privées ou un système d'assurance sociale obligatoire.

Le coût estimé du module minimal est de US$12 par personne et par an dans les pays à faible revenu, qui tous actuellement dépensent moins que ça pour la santé. Le coût s'élèverait à environ US$22 par personne dans les pays à revenu intermédiaire, ce qui permettrait de mettre sur pied un module essentiel plus généreux. Le module minimal permettrait à lui seul d'éliminer, en fonction de la situation épidémiologique existante, de 10 à 18% du poids actuel de la morbidité chez l'adulte de plus de 15 ans. Les bénéfices seraient encore plus élevés pour l'enfant: 21 à 38% du poids de la morbidité pourrait être éliminé.

References

1. **World Bank.** *World development report 1993: investing in health.* New York, Oxford University Press, 1993.
2. **Murray C.** Quantifying the burden of disease: the technical basis for disability-adjusted life years. *Bulletin of the World Health Organization*, 1994, **72**(3): 429–445.
3. **Jamison D et al.** eds. *Disease control priorities in developing countries.* New York, Oxford University Press (for the World Bank), 1993.
4. **Mosley WH, Gray R.** Childhood precursors of adult morbidity and mortality in developing countries: implications for health programs. In: Gribble J, Preston SH, eds. *The epidemiological transition. Policy and planning implications for developing countries.* Washington DC, National Research Council, National Academy Press, 1993.
5. **Elo IT, Preston SH.** Effects of early life conditions on adult mortality: a review. *Population Index*, 1992, **58**(2): 186–212.
6. **World Bank.** *World development report 1992.* New York, Oxford University Press, 1992.
7. *Primary health care. Report of the International Conference on Primary Health Care, Alma Ata, September 1978.* Geneva, World Health Organization, 1978.
8. **Walsh JA, Warren K.** Selective primary health care—an interim strategy for disease control in developing countries. *New England journal of medicine*, 1979, **301**: 967–974.
9. **Cash R et al.** *Child health and survival: the UNICEF-GOBI-FFF Program.* Wolfeboro, NH, Croom Helm, 1987.
10. **Golladay FL.** *Health: sector policy paper.* Washington DC, World Bank, 1980.
11. **Ahumada J et al.** *Health planning: problems of concept and method*, 2nd edition. Washington DC Pan American Health Organization, 1967 (PAHO Scientific Publication No. 111).

Cost-effectiveness analysis and policy choices: investing in health systems

C.J.L. Murray,[1] J. Kreuser,[2] & W. Whang[3]

The role of health systems infrastructure in studies of cost-effectiveness analysis and health resource allocation is discussed, and previous health sector cost-effectiveness analyses are cited. Two substantial difficulties concerning the nature of health system costs and the policy choices are presented. First, the issue of health system infrastructure can be addressed by use of computer models such as the Health Resource Allocation Model (HRAM) developed at Harvard, which integrates cost-effectiveness and burden of disease data. It was found that a model which allows for expansion in health infrastructure yields nearly 40% more total DALYs for a hypothetical sub-Saharan African country than a model which neglects infrastructure expansion. Widespread use of cost-effectiveness databases for resource allocations in the health sector will require that cost-effectiveness analyses shift from reporting costs to reporting production functions. Second, three distinct policy questions can be treated using these tools, each necessitating its own inputs and constraints: allocations when given a fixed budget and health infrastructure, or when given resources for marginal expansion, or when given a politically constrained situation of expanding resources. Confusion concerning which question is being addressed must be avoided through development of a consistent and rigorous approach to using cost-effectiveness data for informing resource allocations.

Introduction

Cost-effectiveness analysis of health sector interventions was first applied in the 1960s based on methods developed to analyse military investments (*1*). Since 1970, the number of published studies using cost-effectiveness analysis has been steadily rising, reflecting a growing concern for the appropriate use of scarce health sector resources (*2*). Initially, most cost-effectiveness studies reported results using indicators such as the cost per case diagnosed and treated of a particular disease or the cost per fully immunized child. These studies using outcome or benefit measures that are very disease or context specific have been gradually replaced by studies using more general measures of health outcome. With more widespread reporting of results in terms of costs per quality-adjusted life year (QALY) or other general health measure, comparisons of the cost-effectiveness of interventions targeting different health problems have become possible. League tables of the cost-effectiveness of different interventions are a natural consequence (*3–8*).

Two landmark policy analyses have provided an impetus to using cost-effectiveness to compare a wide range of health interventions. These exercises provide enough information so that cost-effectiveness analysis for the first time can be used to inform resource allocations across the entire health sector. First, the Oregon Health Services Commission (*9–18*) examined 714 condition-treatment pairs (called interventions in the rest of the following discussion) and calculated the cost per QALY. The valuation of outcomes from medical intervention and the rankings from cost-effectiveness analysis were then subject to extensive public review through a series of town meetings. The rank list of interventions from this process can then be used for selecting the interventions that Medicaid will finance in the State, which plans to fund (in order of the rank list) each intervention maximally until the budget runs out. This sectoral application of cost-effectiveness is now being implemented (*18*). The second major policy review was the Health Sector Priorities Review undertaken by the World Bank from 1987 to 1993 (*7*). Twenty-six major health problems of developing countries were reviewed by teams of economists, public health specialists and epidemiologists. The cost-effectiveness of more than 50 specific health interventions were evaluated using a standard methodology for costs

[1] Associate Professor of International Health Economics, Harvard Center for Population and Development Studies, 9 Bow Street, Cambridge, MA 02138, USA. Requests for reprints should be sent to this author.

[2] Information Officer, Information Engineering Unit, Organization and Business Practices Department, The World Bank, Washington DC, USA.

[3] Columbia University College of Physicians and Surgeons, New York NY, USA.

Reprinted from *Bulletin of the World Health Organization*, 1994, **72** (4): 663–674.

181

and benefits.[a] These databases provide useful information on cost-effectiveness which will help determine resource allocations across the entire health sector.

Building largely on the Health Sector Priorities Review, the World Bank has promoted in the *World development report 1993: investing in health* (WDR) the concept of using cost-effectiveness of health sector interventions and the burden of disease of health problems to develop essential packages of clinical and preventive care (*23*). The WDR also proposes that cost-effectiveness analysis be used to determine the package of services covered by insurance schemes and to inform health research priorities. In this issue of the *Bulletin*, Bobadilla et al. (*24*) provide details on the method and rationale for selection and of interventions and their quantities in the proposed package. In brief, estimates of the current burden of disease are combined with a cost-effectiveness rank list of interventions, to derive packages of services that, for a given budget, will purchase the largest improvement in health as measured by DALYs (disability-adjusted life years). Given the considerable attention garnered by the WDR, it is important to examine carefully the implications of this new and more extensive application of cost-effectiveness analysis.

Limitations of sectoral cost-effectiveness

In recent years, the theoretical basis for using cost-effectiveness analysis to guide health sector resource allocations has been discussed: the validity of DALY or QALY maximization as a goal for the health sector (*25–30*), the nature of individual preferences for health states and how these preferences are incorporated into QALYs (*31–35*), the importance of marginal costs that change as a function of output (*36, 37*), the effect of intervention-specific fixed costs (*36, 38*), and the sensitivity of conclusions to abstract concepts such as discounting (*39–51*). These technical issues are important and likely to be vigorously debated for many years but probably do not have a profound effect on the sectoral application of cost-effectiveness to policy choice, although further research may indicate important modifications and refinements are needed in the methods.

Two more general and potentially important criticisms are concerned with the focus of cost-effectiveness analysis. First, cost-effectiveness analysis of health interventions, which are more often than not

disease specific, tends to neglect the role of the health system in delivering these interventions. There are no explicit analyses of the cost-effectiveness of improving the physical or human infrastructure of the health system, which provide for direct comparisons between investing in the delivery system and purchasing more specific interventions delivered by the health system. Some may be concerned that the intervention focus of cost-effectiveness analysis may shift the focus of policy debate from who delivers health services to satisfying specific targets or goals for particular activities. In the extreme, some accuse cost-effectiveness analysis of fostering a vertical approach to disease control as opposed to the horizontal approach embodied in the primary health care movement. Second, there is a potential for considerable confusion, including in the WDR, on the policy choice that should be informed by cost-effectiveness analysis. For example, should cost-effectiveness analysis be used to suggest the reallocation of resources between programmes that will lead to the greatest improvement in health or should it only be used to suggest how marginal increases in health sector resources could best be allocated to improve health?

In this paper, we present in brief a proposed method by which the cost-effectiveness of investing in the physical and human infrastructure of the health system can be evaluated. A resource allocation model, the technical details of which are described elsewhere (*36*), is illustrated with an application to sub-Saharan Africa. The model is then used to address the second issue of the range of policy questions that can be addressed with cost-effectiveness analysis. Finally, some implications for future cost-effectiveness studies are highlighted.

Cost-effectiveness of investing in the health system

The accepted standard for reporting the results of cost-effectiveness studies in the literature and unpublished reports is to provide information on the average cost per unit of health output (such as a DALY) at one level of production. Average cost equals the sum of general or infrastructure fixed costs, programme-specific fixed costs, and variable costs divided by total output. Arbitrary rules are promulgated to allocate the general infrastructure fixed costs, such as the costs of hospitals and health centres to specific interventions undertaken in those facilities. These arbitrary divisions of joint production costs are usually based on some proxy measure of activity, such as staff hours, bed-days, or square-feet occupied. The treatment of the costs of maintain-

---

[a] To make the results of the Health Sector Priorities Review consistent with the Global Burden of Disease, benefits were measured using disability-adjusted life years. See Murray et al. (*19–22*) for details of the method of calculating benefits.

ing the physical and human infrastructure of the health system in this arbitrary manner leads to two major problems with the cost-effectiveness approach when applied to sectoral decisions.

First, the average cost-list approach used in the WDR (23) ignores existing infrastructure and implicitly assumes that hospitals and health centres can be built in infinitely divisible quantities.[b] The average cost of an intervention includes a component due to the general fixed costs divided by the volume of output at the time of the assessment. Allocating resources according to average unit costs implies that fractions of facilities, e.g., 2% of a health centre, can be built as required. Concomitantly, existing facilities can be used in shares less than one while the costs for the rest of the facility are not incurred. A resource allocation based on an average cost list may include only the costs of running 45% of district hospitals, ignoring the fact that hospitals and health centres come in indivisible units. For example, the package of essential clinical services proposed by the World Bank for low-income countries does not include all the costs of maintaining and operating the existing referral and district hospitals. Even the fractional costs of facilities depend on operating each new fraction at the same level of output as was included in the analysis. Otherwise the general fixed costs divided by output, which figures in average cost, would be different.

Second, even if shares of facilities could be built or closed at will, the joint costing rules artifactually penalize interventions that are more technically efficient. Fig. 1 shows a production function for a health centre that undertakes only two activities: the expanded programme of immunization (EPI) and prenatal care. The area within the curve shows all possible combinations of the two activities, given the current staffing levels and operating budget for the health centre. The production possibilities frontier which is the curved line shows what could be achieved with maximal technical efficiency for both activities.

Many health centres operate far from the production possibilities frontier. Consider a health centre at point A in Fig. 1; joint costing rules would allocate equal shares of the health centre's overhead costs to EPI and prenatal care. Imagine a new regional manager who works to increase the efficiency of EPI such that at no extra cost to the health centre it now operates at point B. Joint costing rules would now attribute a much higher share of the over-

[b] While the cost-effectiveness analysis methods used in developing the packages of care for the WDR do not explicitly address the health system, the WDR devotes the whole of Chapter 6 to the need for developing health systems.

Fig. 1. **Production function for hypothetical health centre undertaking only two activities—prenatal care and expanded programme on immunization; misallocation of overhead costs through use of joint-costing rules.** Point A represents a typical level of output and point B the increased level achieved through improved management.

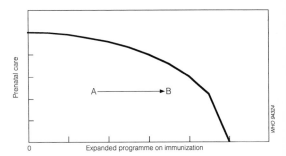

head costs to EPI than before. Clearly, fixed costs have not increased; only productivity has increased. The joint costing approach to calculating average costs entails a very real risk of penalizing with higher estimated unit costs those programmes that are more efficient.

To examine investments in human and physical health infrastructure in a cost-effectiveness framework, a more sophisticated approach to resource allocation questions is required. Correa (52) and Torrance et al. (38) developed hypothetical planning models to choose health maximizing mixes of interventions under various constraints. Torrance et al. (38) discussed the possibility of designing a resource allocation model that would directly incorporate the limits on service delivery imposed by the current health system infrastructure and the possibility of improving the health system. At least four optimization models for the health sector applied to specific interventions that maximize a measure of health status given a budget constraint and a variety of possible interventions have been developed (37, 53–55). None of these applications, however, attempted to incorporate the health system into the modelling exercise.

Health Resources Allocation Model (HRAM)

In order to deal with these problems, we have developed at Harvard an optimization model for the health sector based on the burden of disease, the cost-effectiveness of available health interventions, and the available health system infrastructure. Our model has been developed in the General Algebraic Modeling System (GAMS), a computer system which facilitates the development of algebraic models in days, which previously took months (56). GAMS has been extensively used in other fields such as agriculture, education and industry to deal with complex non-linear optimization problems. Our model, HRAM, has also been designed to address technical problems related to intervention fixed costs, rising marginal costs, and regional heterogeneity. The details on the latter and the technical specifications of the model are provided elsewhere (36) and are not discussed in this paper in detail. The following discussion describes the general strategy used to incorporate the health system into a cost-effectiveness framework.

In order to put the appraisal of infrastructure in cost-effectiveness terms, we have defined several budget constraints that include interchangeable dollars and a series of constraints reflecting the current capacity of the health system to deliver various types of services. While there is flexibility in the design of the model to specify various types of budget constraints, we have so far included constraints for services delivered at referral hospitals, district hospitals and health centres. Given current facilities and staffing levels, the Ministry of Health begins with a constraint on the volume of services it can provide through referral hospitals, district hospitals and health centres. For referral and district hospitals, we have used bed-days as the unit of service delivery, and for health centres we have used patient-contact equivalents.

Each intervention or activity may consume referral hospital bed-days, district hospital bed-days or health centre contacts in addition to interchangeable dollars. In other words, the use of the general health system infrastructure is captured in terms of units of service rather than using arbitrary joint costing rules. Table 1 provides examples of production functions for several health interventions. In choosing an optimal allocation of health resources across activities, when the available budget of district hospital bed-days is exhausted, no further interventions using district hospitals can be bought. The same limitation would apply to referral hospital bed-days and health centre contacts. However, the government may choose to build new referral hospitals, district hospitals or health centres in order to relax the service constraint. In addition to the set of interventions included in the model, three more are added: construction and staffing of a referral hospital, district hospital or health centre. For health centres, we have also included a geographical access constraint. It is not sufficient to have an adequate total number of health centre contacts for the population; health centres must be positioned close enough to the community so that they can use them. In the simulations for sub-Saharan Africa, expanding geographical access

to health centres, particularly in remote areas, is a major force driving the expansion of infrastructure in an optimal resource allocation. While not included so far, geographical access constraints could also be added for district hospitals.

At each budget level, the resource allocation model searches to see if the total output of the system in terms of DALYs avoided could be increased by using some resources to expand the health system rather than spending it on particular activities delivered with the current health infrastructure. In other words, the ability of computers to undertake repetitive calculations at high speed is used to test if the total output of the health sector in terms of DALYs would be higher or lower by improving the health system. Improvements in the health system can be undertaken in this model by building, staffing and operating new referral hospitals, district hospitals or clinics.[c] In this framework, infrastructure investments can be evaluated in terms of the increase in the number of DALYs or equivalent measure of health status.

As one purchases an intervention such as measles immunization at the point where all children are immunized, the marginal cost per DALY reaches infinity because no more health benefits are gained by expanding coverage beyond 100%. While technically correct in micro-economic jargon, it is a cumbersome approach to capturing the practical limits of each intervention. More intuitive is to constrain the purchase of each intervention by the total amount of DALYs that can be addressed with a particular intervention in a particular community. The link between the burden of disease or the total number of DALYs lost due to a particular health problem and cost-effectiveness is thus established. The example of the model, which is described below, makes use of the Global Burden of Disease study results (19) for sub-Saharan Africa. The estimates of the current burden of disease had to be modified to remove the impact of currently financed health interventions on the measured burden of disease.

To explore the use of such an optimization model, we have used the World Bank's Health Sector Priorities Review database on the cost-effectiveness of some 50 interventions (7), the same database utilized by Bobadilla et al. (24). Each estimate of

---

[c] In this version of the model, we are able to build new infrastructure and use it in the same time period. The costs of opening and operating new units of infrastructure are the annual operating fixed costs plus the equivalent annual capital cost. As the model is not a multi-period model, we do not take into account the necessary time lag between the decision to improve the physical or human infrastructure of the health system and its implementation.

Table 1: **Data for the Health Resource Allocation Model for five interventions**

Intervention	Segment[a]	Programme-specific fixed costs (US $)	Marginal cost function (US $)	Per DALY Referral hospital (bed-days)	Per DALY District hospital (bed-days)	Per DALY Health centre (contacts)
ARI screening	0	40 000	24.23	0	0.20	4.00
	1		27.26			
	2		30.29			
	3		33.32			
	4		36.35			
Poliomyelitis immunization	0	60 000	9.17	0	0	5.52
	1		14.66			
	2		18.33			
	3		36.66			
	4		183.30			
School-based anti-helminthic chemoprophylaxis	0	100 000	4.79	0	0	0
	1		4.79			
	2		5.99			
	3		7.19			
	4		7.19			
Short-course chemotherapy for sputum smear-positive tuberculosis	0	53 000	1.71	0	3.85	0
	1		2.74			
	2		3.42			
	3		6.84			
	4		34.20			
Tetanus referral	0	200 000	24.08	2.29	0	0
	1		32.10			
	2		40.13			
	3		48.16			
	4		56.18			

[a] To approximate the increasing marginal cost, the nonlinear marginal cost curve for each intervention within a region is broken up into five linear segments numbered from 0 to 4.

cost-effectiveness was reviewed and modified to increase the comparability across interventions. Despite our attempts to unearth details, frequently only average cost results are reported in the literature or reports on cost-effectiveness. Where necessary, expert judgement was used to develop the intervention production functions and form of the marginal cost curve, examples of which are provided in Table 1.[d]

The model was run for a hypothetical sub-Saharan African country with a population of 10 million and a GDP per capita of $340, using the regional GBD results adjusted to the total population to determine the DALY limits for each disease. A digression on the burden of disease is necessary. The results of the Global Burden of Disease study provide an estimate of the current burden of disease. Current or

measured burden incorporates the impact of currently financed health interventions; for example, if measles immunization coverage is 70%, then a significant share of the burden of measles has already been avoided. There are three levels of the burden of disease relevant to this discussion of resource allocation: first, the current burden of disease; second, the burden of disease that would be present if currently financed health interventions were stopped; and third, the lowest achievable burden given a technical and allocative efficiency within a budget constraint. The resource allocation model used as an input estimated the burden in the absence of currently financed health interventions in order to calculate the lowest achievable burden of disease for a given budget.

Fig. 2 shows the expansion path for the optimal allocation of health resources to maximize DALYs averted at each budget level. For reference, current expenditure in sub-Saharan Africa excluding South Africa is US$ 14 per capita. The equivalent annual capital cost of the existing health infrastructure and the fixed operating costs of the health system are

[d] Table 1 provides a stepped marginal cost function for five interventions. For convenience, we divided non-linear marginal cost functions into five linear steps or segments which are summarized in the Table.

Fig. 2. **DALY retrieval expansion path for sub-Saharan Africa.**

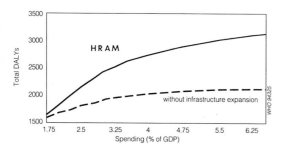

nization, and hygiene promotion. With increases over current budget levels, the major gainers are chemotherapy for sputum smear-negative tuberculosis cases, oral rehydration therapy, malaria control and hygiene promotion.

Fig. 2 shows two expansion paths. The top line is the expansion path for the complete model. The second line is the expansion path when the options of adding infrastructure are removed from the model. Simple inspection shows that expanding the infrastructure is a tremendously important component of health improvement. At current expenditure levels in sub-Saharan Africa, expanding the health system produces nearly 40% more total DALYs.

US$ 3.27 per capita. This health sector production function indicates that with increasing expenditure the marginal cost of each DALY purchased increases rapidly. For all budget ranges included, the marginal cost per DALY is higher than average cost. Table 2 shows the number of new referral hospitals, district hospitals and health centres bought at three budget levels. Even at current levels of health expenditure, nearly 25% of the budget should be spent on expanding the health system. The remainder should be spent on the set of interventions listed. The Table also provides the utilization rates of the three types of facilities modelled at each budget level. Referral hospital bed-occupancy is less than 1%. The implication is that there is excess referral hospital capacity but a shortage of district hospital capacity. If closure or down-sizing of referral hospitals were politically feasible, this desirable option could be added as an additional intervention in the model.

Table 3 shows the allocation to specific interventions at three budget levels. Some highlights are worth discussing. Comparison with the WDR's $12 per capita package for low-income countries is difficult, as their package is based on a marginal increase of $12 per capita, given current expenditures. At current budget levels, the most important interventions by expenditure are screening and treatment of acute respiratory infections (ARI), malaria control, tuberculosis chemotherapy, measles immunization, oral rehydration therapy, breast-feeding, tetanus immu-

Policy choice and sectoral cost-effectiveness

Having illustrated a model that incorporates health system investment choice into a cost-effectiveness framework, we can return to the nature of policy questions that can be treated with these analytical tools. Three distinct policy questions using burden of disease and cost-effectiveness results can be framed.

(1) *Ground-zero.* Given a fixed budget and health infrastructure, how can non-fixed resources be spent so as to maximally reduce the burden of disease?

(2) *Marginal expansion.* Given an existing health infrastructure and a set of currently financed activities, none of which can be changed, how best can marginal increases in the health sector resources be spent so as to maximally reduce the burden of disease?

(3) *Politically constrained ground-zero.* Given an existing health infrastructure, for political or other reasons there may be a set of services or activities that are deemed to be 'protected' from changes in budget and a set of other services or activities that could be expanded or contracted. For a fixed health sector budget, how can health resources be reallocated to maximally reduce the burden of disease without reducing the resources allocated to 'protected' activities?

Table 2: **Infrastructure expansion and rising budget levels**

Facility type	At 3% of GDP		At 4% of GDP		At 5% of GDP	
	Additional facilities	Utilization rate (%)	Additional facilities	Utilization rate (%)	Additional facilities	Utilization rate (%)
Referral hospital	0	0	0	0	0	0.61
District hospital	41	99	47	100	53	98
Clinic	411	56	53	64	578	74

Table 3: **Allocations to specific interventions at varying health budget levels for a hypothetical sub-Saharan African country**[a]

Intervention	At 3.0% of GDP		At 4.0% of GDP		At 5.0% of GDP	
	Spending ('000 $)	DALYS ('000 $)	Spending ('000 $)	DALYS ('000 $)	Spending ('000 $)	DALYS ('000 $)
Fixed infrastructure [b]	32 697		32 699		32 698	
ARI screening and referral	6 879	233	11 107	277	11 107	277
Oral rehydration therapy	789	12	4 831	53	15 661	123
BCG added to DPT	920	71	1 783	80	2 291	84
Hepatitis B immunization	391	8	505	9	505	9
Iodination of salt or water	249	32	249	32	249	32
Measles immunization	4 986	272	7 686	298	12 545	324
Poliomyelitis immunization	907	30	1 232	33	1 503	34
Semiannual vitamin-A dose for children 0–5 years	577	38	881	41	881	41
Tetanus immunization	1 651	213	2 042	222	2 042	222
Breast-feeding promotion w/education or hospital routine for diarrhoeal diseases	2 564	74	2 755	77	2 755	77
Improved weaning practices from education	1 526	46	1 526	46	1 526	46
Oral iron supplementation during pregnancy	70	1	70	1	70	1
Chlamydia treatment w/antibiotics	107	6	107	6	107	6
Gonorrhoea treatment w/antibiotics	111	9	111	9	111	9
Syphilis treatment w/antibiotics	147	156	147	156	147	156
HIV blood screening	911	39	962	40	962	40
Annual breast examinations	0	0	0	0	312	1
Antibiotics for rheumatic heart disease	0	0	388	3	722	5
Cataract surgery	860	9	935	10	935	10
CVD preventive programme	0	0	0	0	287	2
Improved domestic and personal hygiene	0	0	5 306	47	9 658	72
Injected insulin and health education for IDDM[c]	0	0	0	0	231	0
Leprosy multidrug clinic	537	6	541	7	541	7
Low-cost management of acute MI[c]	0	0	0	0	780	3
Pap smear at 5-year intervals	246	1	227	2	422	2
Pneumococcal vaccine	884	16	2 543	32	3206	36
Schizophrenia	248	3	331	3	331	3
School-based anti-helminthic chemoprophylaxis	597	12	597	12	597	12
Short-course chemotherapy for sputum-negative patients	6 688	372	10 208	415	14 120	443
Short-course chemotherapy for sputum-positive patients	3 498	453	5 018	484	5 218	487
Sugar or salt fortified with iron	124	19	124	19	124	19
Tetanus referral case management	0	0	0	0	1 176	3
Vector control for malaria	12 123	304	16 587	348	18 942	364
Added infrastructure	20 713		24 502		27 238	
Total costs ('000 $)	102 000	2 435	136 000	2 762	170 000	2 950
Total cost per capita ($)	10.20		13.60		17.00	

[a] Population is assumed to be 10 million and GDP per capita $340.
[b] Fixed infrastructure reports the costs of construction, maintenance and staffing of the clinics, district hospitals and referral hospitals, which are assumed to have been constructed previously. Assumptions are based on infrastructure data for sub-Saharan African countries.
[c] IDDM: insulin-dependent diabetes mellitus. MI: myocardial infarction.

All three and combinations of (2) and (3) can be addressed using the burden of disease and cost-effectiveness information, as described above for sub-Saharan Africa. The inputs to the process, however, to answer each of these questions will be different. Table 4 shows that the budget constraint on the purchase of interventions is fixed at the current level to answer questions (1) and (3), while for the second question there is a marginal increase in the budget available to buy further interventions.

Table 4: **Setting health sector priorities: different inputs to answer different policy questions**

	Inputs to optimization or packaging		
	Budget	Burden	Health system
1. Ground-zero	Current budget minus fixed cost of operating current health infrastructure	Burden in absence of currently financed health interventions	Total available capacity
2. Marginal expansion	Marginal increase in budget	Current burden	Unused capacity
3. Politically constrained ground-zero	Current budget minus fixed cost of operating health infrastructure and cost of protected activity	For protected, current burden For remainder, burden in absence of currently financed health interventions	Total capacity, less capacity used for protected services

The burden of disease estimates that should be used either in HRAM or in the World Bank packaging exercise will be different for the three questions. The first question, which can be labelled the ground-zero exercise, was the one addressed by the HRAM applied to sub-Saharan Africa. The burden of disease in the absence of currently financed interventions is the required input. To allocate marginal increases in resources, maintaining currently financed activities, the currently observed burden of disease is the appropriate input. Finally, to answer the third question, we would want to use the current burden of disease for those conditions affected by currently financed and protected activities and the burden of disease in the absence of currently financed activities for those activities that are not protected.

Finally, the approach to the infrastructure constraints would also be different for the three questions. The ground-zero exercise would use total available capacity at each level of the health system as the constraint on service delivery with the option for building new infrastructure. The input to the marginal budget exercise would be the unused capacity at each level with the option of building new infrastructure. The politically constrained exercise would use total capacity at each level minus the capacity used to deliver 'protected' services.

In the WDR, the World Bank proposes a package of essential public health and clinical services that would cost $12 in a low-income country. This package is meant to be a marginal package of expenditure and health gain on top of currently financed activities. Some confusion is generated when the World Bank states, "In fact, in the poorest countries total current public spending of $6 per person is about $6 short of the cost of the package. Total per capita spending, including private spending, is about $14, about the same as the proposed package." (23, page 67). The package, however, has been described at several junctures as addressing the marginal burden of disease and has been calculated using the current burden, not the burden in the absence of current-

ly financed activities.[e] In other words, by the nature of its calculation, the World Bank package is a marginal package on top of current expenditure. Paying for the package in a low-income country is not a question of resource reallocation but a question of increasing health expenditure by $12 per capita or a doubling of total health sector expenditure in a low-income country; if the increase was to come entirely from the public sector it would entail a tripling of publicly financed health expenditure. Potential confusion around the policy question that is being asked and the appropriate method of calculation by the World Bank highlights the importance of developing a consistent and internally rigorous approach to using cost-effectiveness for informing sectoral resource allocation questions.

Implications

The cost-effectiveness of interventions, the burden of disease, and information on the human and physical infrastructure in a health system can be combined to answer a host of resource allocation questions including variations of protected expenditures and marginal budget increases. Using a computer program like the one illustrated here, investments in the health system can be directly compared with expanding resources for particular interventions for a given level of the health system. The preliminary work presented on such models can easily be developed to incorporate other investments in health system quality or coverage. Investments in health information systems or training can be included as long

---

[e] The method used to calculate the package is different for different interventions. Some of the package is based on a cost per person receiving a service and an estimate of the desired coverage of the service so that this is closer to the ground-zero analysis. For others, including most of the clinical services, the package is estimated, based on the current burden of disease and the cost per DALY averted.

as the chain of causation between these investments and improvement in health through the delivery of specific health interventions can be traced. More sophisticated versions of such a computer program could take into account the delay between the decision to improve the health system and the completion of new construction or training. A multi-period model would also allow for incorporating expected changes in the burden of disease due to demographic and epidemiological changes (57, 58).

If more widespread use of cost-effectiveness databases to inform health sector resource allocation is intended, then it will be important to alter the standards of reporting cost-effectiveness studies in the literature. Frequently studies report only an average cost per unit of service delivered or health benefit such as a DALY. Details on the component costs are often not provided. In order to examine the cost-effectiveness of investing in the health system, we must shift to reporting the different resources used in providing a health intervention rather than costs. Table 1 illustrates crude forms of such resource use profiles where the component inputs such as bed-days, clinic contacts, or outreach workers are denominated. More detailed resource use profiles could be provided outlining specific inputs and the necessary quality of the inputs such as nursing or surgeons' time, etc. There is an urgent need to develop a simple but useful categorization of the inputs to health service production that provides sufficient detail for sectoral analysis.

Another major benefit from a shift to reporting production functions would be to increase the transferability of cost-effectiveness results from one environment to another. In the WDR, studies on the cost-effectiveness of a programme in the United Republic of Tanzania are directly compared with results of studies in Brazil where the same input such as nursing time can be ten times more expensive in dollar terms; nevertheless, the World Bank is well aware of these limitations and the urgent need to refine methods to transfer cost-effectiveness results from one context to another. Such comparisons obscure the real use of resources for health programmes which would be transparent if resource use is reported directly. We hope that the World Bank and the World Health Organization will take the lead in developing a standard approach to reporting health intervention resource use profiles and ultimately production functions.

In this paper, we have argued that cost-effectiveness results, information on the burden of disease, and details on the available health system resources can be combined to provide useful insights into a wide range of questions on allocation of health sector resources. All these questions, however, are com-

plicated and require at present the assistance of sophisticated computer algorithms to define preferable patterns of resource allocation. Given the early stage of development of this sectoral application of cost-effectiveness, it appears that computer programs, such as HRAM, will remain an essential adjunct to policy analysis. Ultimately, as these methods are tested in a range of countries, simpler decision rules may be developed that will allow for more rapid application of the cost-effectiveness and disease burden results to questions of resource allocation.

Despite the challenges raised in this paper, the method proposed by the WDR and others remains a much better alternative to current practice. We should not let the perfect be the enemy of the good. The World Bank's Health Sector Priorities Review and the 1993 WDR have advanced technical analysis of health policy choices in developing countries by years if not decades. On the other hand, we must always remain cognizant of the fact that technical analysis of health sector priorities using the burden of disease, the cost-effectiveness of interventions, and the available resources is only one input to the policy process and is not intended to be a rigid prescription for all health system ailments.

Acknowledgements

We gratefully acknowledge the extensive efforts of John Kim and Robert Ashley. Comments and suggestions from Julio Frenk, Dean Jamison, Jose-Luis Bobadilla, Philip Musgrove, and Peter Berman have been very helpful.

Résumé

Investigation du secteur de santé: analyse coût-efficacité et choix politiques

Les études actuelles sur l'affectation des ressources en fonction du rapport coût-efficacité — notamment l'*Oregon State plan* et le *Rapport sur le développement dans le monde 1993* de la Banque mondiale — prêtent le flanc à deux critiques importantes. Tout d'abord, les analyses coût-efficacité tendent à négliger le rôle des infrastructures de santé. Ensuite, se pose le problème des choix politiques qui devraient être documentés par une analyse coût-efficacité de l'affectation des ressources.

En premier lieu, les études qui négligent le rôle de l'infrastructure dans l'affectation des ressources d'après leur coût-efficacité supposent implicitement que l'infrastructure physique est infiniment divisible. La méthode utilisant la liste des coûts moyens (comme celle utilisée dans le rapport de la Banque mondiale) suppose que des fractions des installations, 2% d'un hôpital de district par exemple, peuvent être construites conformément aux normes. Une nouvelle difficulté intervient avec les effets indésirables de l'établissement conjoint des coûts.

Cet effet infrastructure peut être corrigé en utilisant un modèle informatisé tel que le *Harvard Health Resources Allocation Model* (HHRAM) qui, comme dans le rapport de la Banque mondiale, intègre le rapport coût-efficacité et le poids de la morbidité. Le HHRAM a été appliqué à un pays d'Afrique subsaharienne fictif, ayant une population de 10 millions d'habitants et un PIB par habitant de US$ 340; ce modèle, qui tient compte de l'expansion des infrastructures de santé dans l'affectation des ressources, donne un nombre total de DALY supérieur de 40% à ce que donne un modèle négligeant l'infrastructure. Au niveau des budgets actuels — qui pour l'Afrique subsaharienne, à l'exclusion de l'Afrique du Sud, est de US$ 14 par habitant — les interventions les plus importantes compte tenu des dépenses sont le dépistage et le traitement des infections respiratoires aiguës, la lutte antipaludique, la chimiothérapie antituberculeuse, la vaccination antirougeoleuse, la réhydratation orale, l'allaitement au sein, la vaccination antitétanique et l'amélioration de l'hygiène.

Le second point est que l'analyse coût-efficacité de l'affectation des ressources permet de traiter trois questions de politique distinctes, chacune avec ses propres contraintes budgétaires et infrastructurelles et ses propres estimations du poids de la morbidité. 1) Affectation à partir du niveau zéro: étant donnés un budget fixe et une infrastructure de santé, comment des ressources non fixées peuvent-elles être dépensées de façon à diminuer au maximum le poids de la morbidité? 2) Affectation de ressources à l'expansion marginale: étant donnés une infrastructure de santé et un ensemble d'activités actuellement financées, dont aucune ne peut être modifiée, comment les augmentations marginales des ressources du secteur de santé peuvent-elles être dépensées de façon à diminuer au maximum le poids de la morbidité ? 3) Affectation au niveau zéro politiquement limitée: le budget du secteur de santé étant fixé, comment les ressources pour la santé peuvent-elles être réaffectées pour diminuer au maximum le poids de la morbidité sans diminuer les ressources affectées aux activités «protégées». Le problème de savoir quelle est la question traitée par une étude doit être évité en élaborant une méthode cohérente et rigoureuse d'utilisation du rapport coût-efficacité pour documenter l'affectation de ressources.

Une conséquence de l'analyse ci-dessus est que pour examiner le rapport coût-efficacité de l'investigation des systèmes de santé, il faut rendre compte des fonctions de production des interventions de santé plutôt que des coûts. Nous souhaitons que la Banque mondiale et l'Organisation mondiale de la Santé donnent l'exemple en mettant au point une méthode codifiée pour l'évaluation des fonctions de production des interventions de santé.

Malgré les problèmes soulevés dans cet article, la méthode proposée par le rapport de la Banque mondiale et divers auteurs reste la meilleure alternative à la pratique actuelle. Toutefois, ne pas oublier que l'analyse technique des priorités du secteur de santé ne prétend pas être une prescription rigide destinée à traiter tous les maux des systèmes de santé.

References

1. **Klarman HE, Francis JOS, Rosenthal G.** Cost-effectiveness analysis applied to the treatment of chronic renal disease. *Medical care*, 1968, **6**: 48–54.
2. **Elixhauser A et al.** Health care CBA/CEA: an update on the growth and composition of the literature. *Medical care*, 1993, **31**: js1–js11.
3. **Williams AH.** Economics of coronary artery bypass grafting. *British medical journal*, 1985, **291**: 326–329.
4. **Torrance GW, Zipursky A.** Cost-effectiveness of antepartum prevention of Rh immunization. *Clinics in perinatology*, 1984, **11**: 267–281.
5. **Schulman KA et al.** Cost-effectiveness of low-dose zidovudine therapy for asymptomatic patients with human immunodeficiency virus (HIV) infection. *Annals of internal medicine*, 1991, **114**: 798–802.
6. **Drummond M, Torrance G, Mason J.** Cost-effectiveness league tables: more harm than good? *Social science and medicine*, 1993, **37**: 33–40.
7. **Jamison DT et al.**, eds. *Disease control priorities in developing countries*. New York, Oxford University Press, 1993.
8. **Allen D, Lee RH, Lowson K.** The use of QALYs in health service planning. *International journal of health planning and management*, 1989, **4**: 261–273.
9. **Oregon Health Services Commission.** *Oregon Medicaid priority setting project*. Portland, 1991.
10. **Brown LD.** The national politics of Oregon's rationing plan. *Health affairs*, 1991, **10**(2): 28–51.
11. **Dixon J, Welch HG.** Priority setting: lessons from Oregon. *Lancet*, 1991, **337**: 891–894.
12. **Fox DM, Leichter HM.** Rationing care in Oregon: the new accountability. *Health affairs*, 1991, **10**(2): 7–27.
13. **Garland MJ, Hasnain R.** Health care in common: setting priorities in Oregon. *Hastings Center report*, September-October 1990: 16–18.
14. **Hadorn DC.** Setting health care priorities in Oregon—cost-effectiveness meets the rule of rescue. *Journal of the American Medical Association*, 1991, **265**: 2218–2225.

15. **Klevit HD et al.** Prioritization of health care services—a progress report by the Oregon Health Services Commission. *Archives of internal medicine*, 1991, **151**: 912–916.

16. **Østbye T, Speechley M.** The Oregon formula: a better method of allocating health care resources. *Nordisk medicin*, 1992, **107**(3): 92–95.

17. **Eddy DM.** Oregon's methods—did cost-effectiveness analysis fail? *Journal of the American Medical Association*, 1991, **266**: 2135–2141.

18. **Kitzhaber JA.** Prioritising health services in an era of limits: the Oregon experience. *British medical journal*, 1993, **307**: 373–377.

19. **Murray CJL, Lopez AD, Jamison DT.** The global burden of disease in 1990: summary results, sensitivity analysis and future directions. *Bulletin of the World Health Organization*, 1994, **72**: 495–509.

20. **Murray CJL.** Quantifying the burden of disease: the technical basis for disability-adjusted life years. *Bulletin of the World Health Organization*, 1994, **72**: 429–445.

21. **Murray CJL, Lopez AD.** Quantifying disability: data, methods, and results. *Bulletin of the World Health Organization*, 1994, **72**: 481–494.

22. **Murray CJL, Lopez AD.** Global and regional cause-of-death patterns in 1990. *Bulletin of the World Health Organization*, 1994, **72**: 447–480.

23. **World Bank.** *World development report 1993: investing in health*. New York, Oxford University Press, 1993.

24. **Bobadilla J-L et al.** Design, content and financing of an essential national package of health services. *Bulletin of the World Health Organization*, 1994, **72**: 653–662.

25. **Garber AM, Phelps CE.** *Economic foundations of cost-effectiveness analysis*. Cambridge MA, National Board of Economic Research, 1992 (NEBR working paper 4164).

26. **Phelps CE, Mushlin AI.** On the (near) equivalence of cost-effectiveness and cost-benefit analyses. *International journal of technology assessment in health care*, 1991, **7**(1): 12–21.

27. **Loomes G, McKenzie L.** The use of QALYs in health care decision-making. *Social science and medicine*, 1989, **28**(4): 299–308.

28. **Birch S, Gafni A.** Cost-effectiveness/utility analyses—do current decision rules lead us where we want to be? *Journal of health economics*, 1992, **11**: 279–296.

29. **Johannesson M, Jönsson B.** Economic evaluation in health care: is there a role for cost-benefit analysis? *Health policy*, 1991, **17**: 1–23.

30. **Hammer JS.** *Prices and protocols in public health care*. Washington, World Bank, 1993 (Population Health and Nutrition Working Paper Series).

31. **Mehrez A, Gafni A.** Quality-adjusted life years, utility theory, and healthy-years equivalents. *Medical decision-making*, 1989, **9**: 142–149.

32. **Miyamoto JM, Eraker SA.** Parameter estimates for a QALY utility model. *Medical decision-making*, 1985, **5**(2): 191–213.

33. **Sackett DL, Torrance GW.** The utility of different health states as perceived by the general public. *Journal of chronic disease*, 1978, **31**: 697–704.

34. **Pliskin JS, Shepard DS, Weinstein MC.** Utility functions for life years and health status. *Operations research*, 1980, **28**(1): 206–224.

35. **Torrance GW.** Measurement of health state utilities for economic appraisal: a review. *Journal of health economics*, 1986, **5**: 1–30.

36. **Murray CJL, Kreuser J, Whang W.** *A cost-effectiveness model for allocating health sector resources*. Cambridge MA, Harvard Center for Population and Development Studies 1994 (Health Transition Working Paper).

37. **Forgy L.** Cost-effectiveness in child health: a minimum information approach to planning and forecasting. In: Hill K, ed., *Child health priorities for the 1990s*. Baltimore, Johns Hopkins University Institute for International Programs, 1992: 309–335.

38. **Torrance GW, Thomas WH, Sackett DL.** A utility maximization model for evaluation of health care programs. *Health services research*, Summer 1972: 118–133.

39. **Daniels N.** *Just health care*. New York, Cambridge University Press, 1985.

40. **Lind R.** Discounting for time and risk in energy policy. Baltimore, Johns Hopkins University Press, 1982.

41. **Little I, Mirrlees S.** *Project appraisal and planning for developing countries*, London, Heinemann, 1974.

42. **Hartman RW.** One thousand points of light seeking a number: a case study of CBO's search for a discount rate policy. *Journal of environmental economics and management*, 1990, **18**(suppl.):s3–s7.

43. **Martens LLM, van Doorslaer EKA.** Dealing with discounting. *International journal of technology assessment in health care*, 1990, **6**: 139–145.

44. **Hammit J.** Discounting health increments. *Journal of health economics*, 1993, **12**: 117–120.

45. **Krahn M, Gafni A.** Discounting in the economic evaluation of health care interventions. *Medical care*, 1993, **31**: 403–418.

46. **Olsen J.** On what basis should health be discounted? *Journal of health economics*, 1993, **12**: 39–53.

47. **Viscusi K, Moore M.** Rates of time preference and valuations of the durations of life. *Journal of public economics*, 1989, **38**: 297–317.

48. **Johanneson M.** On the discounting of gained life-years in cost-effectiveness analysis. *International journal of technology assessment in health care*, 1992, **8**(2): 359–364.

49. **Parsonage M, Neuberger H.** Discounting and health benefits. *Health economics*, 1992, **1**: 71–76.

50. **Messing SD.** Discounting health: the issue of subsistence and care in an underdeveloped country. *Social science and medicine*, 1973, **7**: 911–916.

51. **Keeler E, Cretin S.** Discounting of life-saving and other nonmonetary effects. *Management science*, 1983, **29**: 300–306.

52. **Correa H.** Health planning. *Kyklos international review for social science*, 1967, **20**(4): 909–923.

53. **Feldstein MS, Piot MA, Sundaresan TK.** Resource allocation model for public health planning: a case study of tuberculosis control. Geneva, 1973 (supplement to vol. 48 of the *Bulletin of the World Health Organization*).

54. **Chen MM, Bush JW.** Maximizing health system output with political and administrative constraints using math-

ematical programming. *Inquiry*, 1976, **13**: 215–227.

55. **Barnum H.** *A resource allocation model for child survival.* Cambridge MA, Oelgeschlager, Gunn and Hain, 1980.

56. **Brooke A, Kendrick D, Meeraus A.** *GAMS — a user's guide release 2.25.* South San Francisco, The Scientific Press, 1992.

57. **Omran AR.** The epidemiologic transition theory: a preliminary update. *Journal of tropical pediatrics,* 1983, **29**: 305–316.

58. **Bobadilla JL et al.** The epidemiologic transition and health priorities. In: Jamison DT et al., eds. *Disease control priorities in developing countries.* New York, Oxford University Press, 1993: 673–702.

Index

Index

Index